Immune Response and the Eye

Chemical Immunology and Allergy

Vol. 92

Immune Response and the Eye

2nd, revised edition

In Memoriam J. Wayne Streilein

Volume Editors

Jerry Y. Niederkorn, *Dallas, Tex.*
Henry J. Kaplan, *Louisville, Ky.*

25 figures, 7 in color, and 12 tables, 2007

KARGER

Basel · Freiburg · Paris · London · New York ·
Bangalore · Bangkok · Singapore · Tokyo · Sydney

Chemical Immunology and Allergy
Formerly published as 'Progress in Allergy' (Founded 1939)
continued 1990–2002 as 'Chemical Immunology'
Edited by Paul Kalos 1939–1988, Byron H. Waksman 1962–2000

Jerry Y. Niederkorn
Departments of Ophthalmology
and Microbiology
U.T. Southwestern Medical Center
Dallas, Tex., USA

Henry J. Kaplan
Department of Ophthalmology &
Visual Science
University of Louisville
Louisville, Ky., USA

Vol. 73 (1st edition)
Immune Response and The Eye
Editor: J. Wayne Streilein, Boston, Mass., USA
XII+226 p., 20 figures, 7 in color, and 14 tables, 1999. ISBN 978–3–8055–6893–7

Bibliographic Indices. This publication is listed in bibliographic services, including Current Contents® and Index Medicus.

www.karger.com
Printed in Switzerland on acid-free paper by Reinhardt Druck, Basel
ISSN 1660–2242
ISBN 978–3–8055–8187–5

Contents

Treatment of Immune-Mediated Ocular Diseases

Abbreviations used in this book

AC	anterior chamber
ACAID	anterior chamber-associated immune deviation
ADT-HIPIF	adoptively transferred-hapten immune pulmonary interstitial fibrosis
agr	accessory gene regulator
AH	aqueous humor
AIRE	autoimmune regulator
AKC	atopic keratoconjunctvitis
AMD	age-related macular degeneration
ARN	acute retinal necrosis
AU	anterior uveitis
BCR	B cell receptor
BM	bone marrow
BMZ	basement membrane zone
BRB	blood-retinal barrier
C3	complement 3
CB	ciliary body
CCC	chronic cicatrizing conjunctivitis
CFA	complete Freund's adjuvant
CGRP	calcitonin gene-related peptide
CNV	choroidal neovascularization
CRP	complement-regulatory proteins
CTL	cytotoxic T lymphocytes
CTLA-4	cytotoxic T lymphocyte antigen-4

DC	dendritic cell
DES	dry eye syndrome
DTH	delayed-type hypersensitivity
EAAU	experimental autoimmune anterior uveitis
EAU	experimental autoimmune uveoretinitis
EE	endogenous endophthalmitis
EIU	endotoxin-induced uveitis
EMIU	experimental melanin protein-induced uveitis
FasL	Fas ligand
GFP	green fluorescent protein
GI	gastrointestinal
GPC	giant papillary conjunctivitis
HEL	hen egg lysozyme
HSK	herpes stromal keratitis
HSV-1	herpes simplex virus type 1
I/CB	iris and ciliary body
ICAM-1	intercellular adhesion molecule-1
ICE	interleukin-1β-converting enzyme
IEL	intraepithelial lymphocytes
IFN	interferon
IL	interleukin
iNKT	invariant natural killer T (cell)
IRBP	interphotoreceptor retinoid binding protein
iT_{reg}	induced CD4+ CD25+ regulatory T cell
KC	the murine homologue of Gro-α
KCS	keratoconjunctivitis sicca
KO	knockout
LC	Langerhans cell
LFA-1	lymphocyte function-associated antigen-1
LPS	lipopolysaccharide
MAC	membrane attack complex
MCA	methylcholanthrene
MCSF	macrophage colony-stimulating factor
MHC	major histocompatibility complex
MICA/B	MHC class I chain-related proteins A and B
MIP	macrophage inflammatory protein
MMP	matrix metalloproteinase
MPO	myeloperoxidase
MSH	melanocyte stimulating hormone
MTU	*Mycobacterium tuberculosa* adjuvant-induced uveitis
MyD889	myeloid differentiation factor 88

MZ	marginal zone
NK	natural killer
NKT	natural killer T (cells)
NNR	neonatal neuronal retina
nT_{reg}	naturally occurring CD4+ CD25+ regulatory T cell
OCP	ocular cicatricial pemphigoid
OPG	osteoprotegerin
OVA	ovalbumin
PAC	perennial allergic conjunctivitis
PAMP	pathogen-associated molecular pattern
PDS	pigment dispersion syndrome
PE	pigmented epithelial
PEC	peritoneal exudate cells
PMN	polymorphonuclear neutrophils
POE	postoperative endophthalmitis
POMC	pro-opiomelanocortin
PTE	posttraumatic endophthalmitis
PUK	peripheral ulcerative keratitis
RA	rheumatoid arthritis
RGCs	retinal ganglion cells
RPE	retinal pigment epithelial
SAC	seasonal allergic conjunctivitis
sar	staphylococcal accessory regulator
SC	secretory component
SCF	stem cell factor
SOM	somatostatin
SRS	subretinal space
TCR	T cell receptor
TGF	transforming growth factor
Th	T helper (cells)
TLR	Toll-like receptor
TNF	tumor necrosis factor
TNFRII	TNF receptor II
T_{reg}	regulatory T cells
TSP	thrombospondin
VEGF	vascular endothelial growth factor
VIP	vasoactive intestinal polypeptide
VKC	vernal keratoconjunctivitis
VKH	Vogt-Koyanagi-Harada disease
VZV	varicella-zoster virus

Niederkorn JY, Kaplan HJ (eds): Immune Response and the Eye.
Chem Immunol Allergy. Basel, Karger, 2007, vol 92, pp 1–3

Rationale for Immune Response and the Eye

Jerry Y. Niederkorn[a], *Henry J. Kaplan*[b]

[a]Department of Ophthalmology, University of Texas Southwestern Medical Center, Dallas, Tex., [b]Department of Ophthalmology and Visual Science, University of Louisville, Louisville, Ky., USA

The second edition of *Immune Response and the Eye* was originally conceived to be an update to the first edition, which was published in 1999 and was edited by the late J. Wayne Streilein. At the time of his death, Wayne had set into motion plans to update the first edition and to introduce exciting new developments in the field of ocular immunology to the readers of this book. He recognized the enormous number of advances that had occurred since the publication of the previous edition and it was with great enthusiasm that he enlisted the authors of this edition to prepare their respective chapters. His untimely death in 2004 not only put this project on hold but robbed the world of a remarkable mentor, scientist, and role model. It has been a bittersweet experience for us to resume what Wayne started and to try to mold this edition of *Immune Response and the Eye* into a fitting tribute to his vision. We have attempted to retain the original roster of authors. It is noteworthy that, with only a few exceptions, each of the authors is a former trainee of J. Wayne Streilein, and thus his influence is felt throughout this edition of *Immune Response and the Eye.*

The purpose of this volume, like its predecessor, is to illuminate the remarkable nature of immune responses in the eye. Unlike many organs, the eye makes unique demands on the immune system and cannot tolerate the full array of immune responses that are available to the rest of the body. In the final analysis, the eye has only one known function – the unfettered transmission of light from the external environment to the photoreceptors of the retina and, from there, onto the visual cortex. Although the eye is only a few centimeters in diameter, it is composed of almost every type of tissue found in the rest of the body, as well as additional cellular and noncellular elements found nowhere else. This remarkable organ is an extension of the brain and, like the brain, conducts enormously complex neurological functions. The million ganglion cells of the retina transmit 500 electrical signals along the optic nerve each second, which in computer terms is roughly equivalent to 1.5×10^9 bits of information per second. This remarkable neurological system is paralyzed if the single cell layer that forms the corneal endothelium is damaged by inflammation or if immune-mediated injury is inflicted upon any of the cellular elements of the retina. Yet, a robust immune response and inflammation are necessary to control life-threatening infections. Wayne Streilein recognized this almost 30 years ago and characterized the immune response in the eye as a 'dangerous compromise' in which certain immune functions were downregulated to protect tissues of the eye from immune-mediated injury, while preserving a unique spectrum of immune responses that inflicted minimal damage to innocent bystander cells, yet simultaneously provided a degree of protection against pathogens that confronted the eye. This, accordingly to Wayne, was 'the way of immune privilege'. This concept has been widely adopted by vision and ophthalmology researchers and has found its way into mainstream immunology circles that have ignored the eye in the past, but now recognize that there are many immunological lessons to be learned from this remarkable organ.

This volume is not just about immune privilege in the eye, but also embraces the broad spectrum of immune functions that are uniquely expressed in the eye. The eye is continuously exposed to the external environment and as a result, it must adopt a specialized pattern of immune responses to protect against an array of pathogens that assault the ocular surface, as well as the interior of the eye. The immunological provisions that are made for such infectious diseases are discussed in this volume of *Immune Response and the Eye*. Other chapters highlight the occasional failures of immune regulation in the eye and the types of blinding, immune-mediated diseases that can ensue. The field of ocular immunology has made enormous advances, some of which offer glimmers of hope and potential therapeutic application ranging from corneal and retinal transplantation to the management of immune-mediated inflammation by re-imposing immune privilege onto an inflamed eye.

Many of the contributors to this volume of *Immune Response and the Eye* were profoundly influenced by J. Wayne Streilein, either as a trainee or collaborator. Wayne began his career as a research fellow with the eminent transplantation immunologist, Rupert Billingham. On the occasion of Billingham's death, Wayne sent his current and former fellows the following note to express his philosophy of science and mentoring: 'Throughout our lives, we experience losses through the deaths of individuals whom we know well and love. In my advancing maturity, I have come to realize that these are not merely irreplaceable losses. They can also be bittersweet opportunities to ponder the connectivities among individual lives, and the growth and evolution of shared ideas. I am cognizant of the flow of ideas that have passed to and through me, and I am fortunate to have found trainees willing to receive these ideas and able to fashion them into discoveries that bring truth closer and closer….'

This volume of *Immune Response and the Eye* is a manifestation of this philosophy that is now transmitted through each of the authors who must now carry on this tradition as scientist, mentor, and role model for the next generation of scientists.

Dr. Jerry Y. Niederkorn
Department of Ophthalmology, University of Texas Southwestern Medical Center
5323 Harry Hines Blvd.
Dallas, TX 75390–9057 (USA)
Tel. +1 214 648 3829, Fax +1 214 648 9061, E-Mail jerry.niederkorn@utsouthwestern.edu

Niederkorn JY, Kaplan HJ (eds): Immune Response and the Eye.
Chem Immunol Allergy. Basel, Karger, 2007, vol 92, pp 4–10

Anatomy and Function of the Eye

Henry J. Kaplan

Department of Ophthalmology and Visual Science, University of Louisville, Louisville, Ky., USA

Abstract

This text is not a generic book on the immunology of the eye, but instead is based on the theme of ocular immune privilege. In subsequent chapters it is apparent that the immunologic privilege within the eye is dependent upon novel anatomic and physiologic properties of the organ. The focus of this chapter is to provide a concise description of both the function and anatomy of the normal eye.

Vision

The greatest fear expressed by all patients is the loss of vision and the fear of blindness. The majority of patients have less of a concern about death from cancer, stroke or heart attack. The clarity of vision is recorded as visual acuity, which is a measurement of the smallest object a person can identify at a given distance. A patient with normal vision will have visual acuity of 20/20 – i.e. at 20 feet the patient can see a letter that subtends an angle of 20°. One definition of legal blindness is a visual acuity ≤20/400 – i.e. the smallest object the patient can identify at 20 feet is a letter that subtends an angle of 400° [1].

Light rays entering the eye are focused on the neurosensory retina, specifically the fovea, by the two major refractive surfaces of the eye – the cornea and the lens (fig. 1). Approximately two thirds of the refractive power of the eye are provided by the cornea with the remaining one third provided by the lens. If the axial lens of the eye is too short, the light rays entering the eye will be focused at a point (focal point) behind the fovea – i.e. far sighted or hyperopia. In contrast, if the axial lens of the eye is too long, the focal point or the incident light rays will be focused in front of the fovea – i.e. near sighted or myopia.

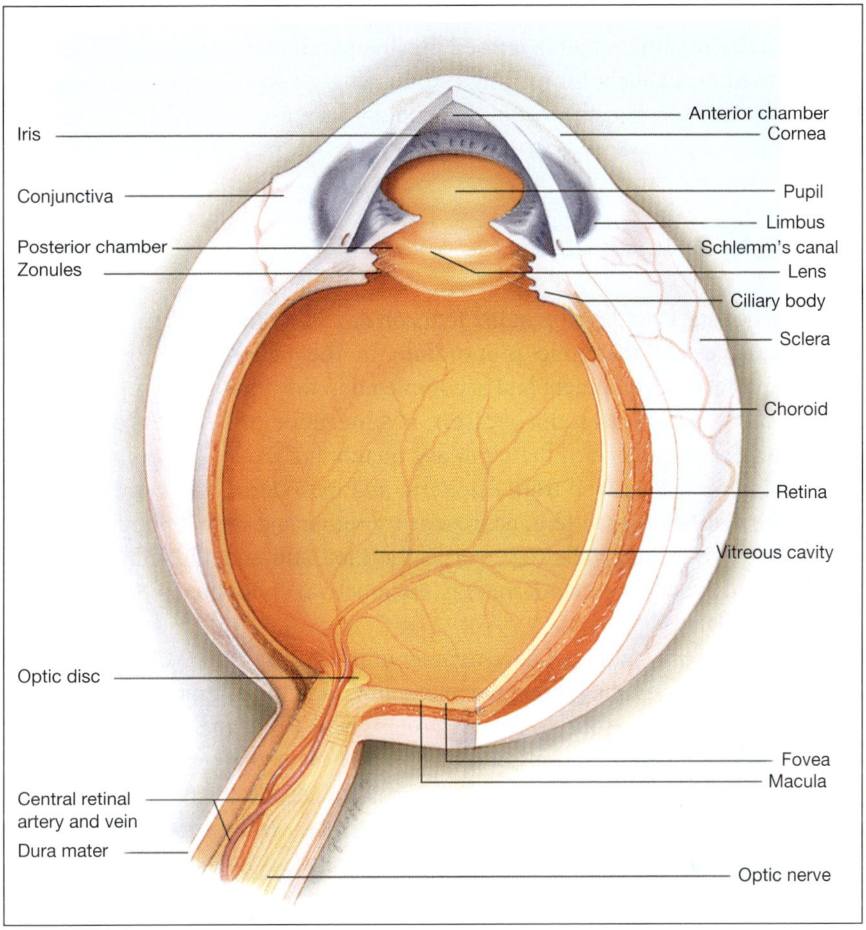

Fig. 1. A schematic cross-section of the eye demonstrating its major anatomical features (reproduced with permission of the American Academy of Ophthalmology [1]).

Spectacles, contact lenses, and refractive surgery can correct these optical errors and achieve normal distance vision.

Light rays from an object at a distance (i.e. >20 feet) are considered parallel to the visual axis of the eye. An object that is closer than 20 feet requires increased refractive power from the eye to maintain the focal point on the fovea of the retina. This increase in refractive power for the eye is accomplished by the ability of the ciliary muscle to contract and the lens to become more convex, a process called accommodation. The lens of every eye undergoes progressive hardening with age with the loss of the ability to change its shape. This loss of accommodation is experienced as a decreased ability to focus on near objects – i.e. difficulty reading – and is termed presbyopia. It can be corrected by either glasses used exclusively for reading (i.e. reading glasses) or the lower segment of glasses used for distance vision that contain increased power (i.e. the bifocal segment).

Development of the Eye

The eye starts to develop in the fetus on day 22 following fertilization with the appearance of the optic primordium in the neural folds. It continues throughout fetal development and is completed in the 9th month with the development of the peripheral retinal vessels, myelinization of the fibers of the optic nerve and disappearance of the pupillary membrane [2, 3]. The embryonic tissues of the eye are derived from ectoderm and mesoderm. The ectoderm gives rise to the neuroectoderm (e.g. neurosensory retina and retinal pigment epithelium), the neural crest cells (e.g. corneal stroma and endothelium, as well as choroid) and the surface ectoderm (e.g. conjunctival epithelium, corneal epithelium, and lens).

The embryonic and fetal development of the human eye involves a series of sequential steps, including inductive interactions and the migration of cells from distinct regions of the embryo. Three elements have been identified as important in this process: growth factors, homeobox genes, and neural crest cells.

Growth factors are soluble molecules that provide the chemical signals in the earliest stages of embryonic development. There are certain substances that participate and control the normal development of the eye influencing the migration, proliferation, and differentiation of cells. Fibroblast growth factor, transforming growth factor-β and insulin-like growth factor-I are essential for the normal development of the eye [4]. They not only provide signals for the differentiation of cells in the region of the eye, but they also regulate the level of expression of homeobox genes. These latter genes function as the mechanism for controlling the overall arrangement of the eye as an organ. Visual acuity is dependent upon the precise spatial arrangement of the cells of the eye. Therefore, the expression of homeobox genes at the appropriate level and time are critical.

Homeobox genes contain a distinctive segment of DNA, 180 base pairs in length, that encodes an almost identical sequence of 60 amino acids. Since these genes control the activity of other subordinate genes, homeobox genes are considered 'master' genes. These genes act as transcription factors and bond to specific DNA sequences of subordinate genes, resulting in activation or repression of their expression. Thus, the spatial and temporal expression of homeobox genes is critical to the normal embryonic development of the eye [5, 6].

The neuroectoderm located at the crest of the neural folds gives rise to the neural crest cells. They migrate to different regions of the embryo where differentiation occurs; therefore, they are a transient population of cells. The signals these cells encounter during migration guide the cells along the correct pathway to their appropriate destination. The secretion of extracellular matrix molecules such as collagen, fibronectin, and proteoglycans is influenced by growth factors, which, thus, also have a role in regulating the migration of neural crest cells. Early in development the neural crest cells are multipotent, but their final differentiation is considerably influenced by local factors.

The Anatomy of the Eye

Immune privilege of the eye involves the globe and its contents. Thus, only a passing reference will be made to the orbit and eyelids. The orbit is the bony, concave cavity in the skull that houses the globe, extraocular muscles, blood vessels and nerves of the eye. There is a very thin orbital floor (consisting of the maxillary, palatine, and zygomatic bones), a medial wall (consisting of the frontal process of the maxilla, lacrimal bone, orbital plate of the frontal bone, and lesser wing of the sphenoid), an orbital roof (consisting of the frontal bone), and a lateral wall (consisting of the zygomatic and greater wing of the sphenoid) (fig. 2) [8].

The globe is protected by the eyelids and lubrication of the ocular surface. The upper and lower eyelids are comprised of skin, subcutaneous connective tissue, and muscle. In addition, the tarsal plates in each lid consist of dense connective tissue and cartilage. They contain the meibomian glands – modified holocrine sebaceous glands – that are oriented vertically in two parallel rows through the tarsus. Movement of the eyelids assists lubrication of the surface of the globe, as well as protection from inadvertent trauma [9].

The surface of the cornea is protected by the tear film. It is a trilaminar layer consisting of an anterior lipid layer, a middle aqueous phase, and a posterior mucin layer [10]. The anterior layer of the tear film contains polar and non-polar lipids secreted primarily by the meibomian (tarsal) glands. The sebaceous glands in the lid margin are in close relation to the eyelashes and also secret lipids (fig. 3). The middle aqueous layer is secreted by the main and accessory lacrimal glands. The main lacrimal gland is located in a shallow depression within the orbital plate of the frontal bone. The accessory lacrimal glands of Krause and Wolfring are located in the conjunctival fornices. The mucin layer of the tear film coats the superficial corneal epithelial cells and conjunctival surface. Tear mucins are secreted normally by the conjunctival goblet cells.

The thick outer coat of the eye, the sclera, is white and opaque. The transparent front window of the eye, which serves as the major refractive surface, is

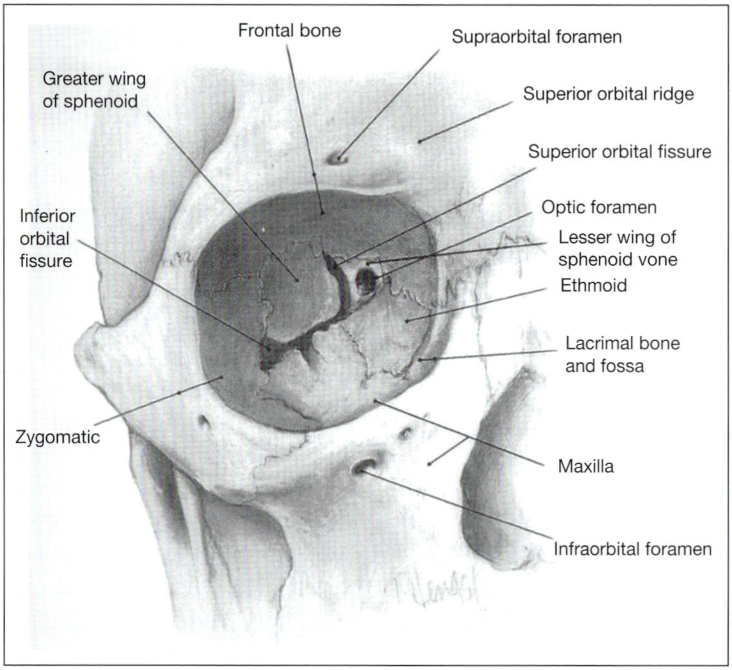

Fig. 2. Frontal view of the bony right orbit (reproduced with permission of Lippincott Williams & Wilkins [7]).

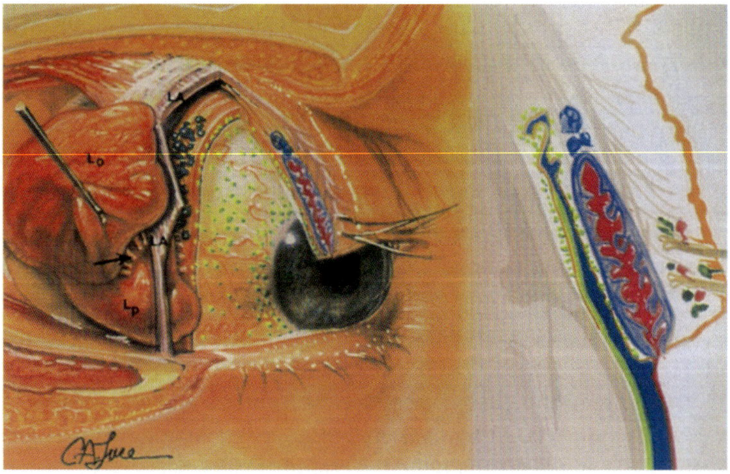

Fig. 3. Cross-section of the upper eyelid (reproduced with permission of Lippincott Williams & Wilkins [3]).

the cornea (fig. 1). Light rays pass through the cornea into the anterior chamber which is filled with aqueous humor. The rays then continue as they pass through the lens, the major internal refractive structure of the eye. The rays then enter the clear vitreous cavity and impinge upon the neurosensory (neural) retina. The pigmented epithelium of the retina (retinal pigment epithelium) provides nourishment and support to the outer layers of the neurosensory retina – the photoreceptors (rods and cones). Nourishment for the photoreceptors is derived from the vessels within the choroid. The choroid extends anteriorly and with the ciliary body and iris comprises the uveal tract of the eye.

As light passes through the inner retina it is absorbed by the photoreceptors in the neuorsensory retina. Light is either absorbed by rhodopsin, which is concentrated in the outer segment membrane of rods, or by opsin, which is located in cones. Phototransduction is the process by which light is captured by the photoreceptors and the small amount of energy is converted into a neural response. Through a series of biochemical reactions in the neural retina, the ganglion cells are depolarized and transmit a visual signal to the lateral geniculate nucleus of the central nervous system [11].

Anatomy of Immune Privilege

Immune privilege within the eye is dependent upon many molecular biochemical interactions, as well as novel anatomic features – e.g. the alymphatic status of the internal structures of the eye and the blood ocular barrier. The conjunctiva is a mucous membrane consisting of non-keratinized squamous epithelium with numerous goblet cells and a rich vascularized substantia propria. The latter contains lymphatic vessels as well as bone-marrow-derived inflammatory cells. Specialized aggregations of conjunctiva-associated lymphoid tissue (CALT) are present and thought to be analogous to mucosa-associated lymphoid tissue (MALT), which is present in the intestine. These aggregations are comprised of T and B lymphocytes, as well as antigen-presenting cells and epithelium [12].

The fluid compartments of the eye (aqueous humor and vitreous) are separated from blood by various tight junctions (zonulae occludens) between endothelial or epithelial cells. The capillaries of the retinal vascular circulation (i.e. endothelium), as well as the interdigitating surfaces of the retinal pigment epithelium and non-pigmented epithelium of the ciliary processes, contain zonulae occludens [13]. They constitute an effective barrier to soluble molecules and contribute to the novel constitution of the aqueous humor and vitreous. Both the alymphatic status of the inner globe and the blood ocular barrier have been postulated to be important anatomical contributions to the existence of immune privilege. In various diseases the blood ocular barrier is disrupted and associated with the loss of immune privilege within the eye. The presence of collateral lymphatic channels within the normal eye, as well as during disease, has been postulated but remains an unresolved issue to date [14, 15].

References

1 Bradford CA: Basic Ophthalmology, ed 8, revised. San Francisco, American Academy of Ophthalmology, 2004.
2 Ocular Development; in Basic and Clinical Science Course; Section 2: Fundamentals and Principles of Ophthalmology. San Francisco, American Academy of Ophthalmology, 2003–2004, pp 132–163.
3 Tripathi BJ, Tripathi RC: Development of the human eye; in Bron AJ, Tripathi RC, Tripathi BJ (eds): Wolff's Anatomy of the Eye and Orbit, ed 8. London, Chapman & Hall, 1997.
4 Tripathi BJ, Tripathi RC, Livingston AM, et al: The role of growth factors in the embryogenesis and differentiation of the eye. Am J Anat 1991;192:442–471.
5 Matsuo T: The genes involved in the morphogenesis of the eye. Jpn J Ophthalmol 1993;37: 215–251.
6 Monaghan AP, Davidson DR, Sime C, et al: The Msh-like homeobox genes define domains in the developing vertebrate eye. Development 1991;112:1053–1061.
7 Doxanas MT, Anderson RL: Clinical Orbital Anatomy. Baltimore, Lippincott Williams & Wilkins; 1984.
8 Orbit and Ocular Adnexa; in Basic and Clinical Science Course; Section 2: Fundamentals and Principles of Ophthalmology. San Francisco, American Academy of Ophthalmology, 2003–2004, pp 5–13.
9 Eyelids; in Basic and Clinical Science Course; Section 2: Fundamentals and Principles of Ophthalmology. San Francisco, American Academy of Ophthalmology, 2003–2004, pp 24–32.
10 Tear Film; in Basic and Clinical Science Course; Section 2: Fundamentals and Principles of Ophthalmology. San Francisco, American Academy of Ophthalmology, 2003–2004, pp 303–311.
11 Retina; in Basic and Clinical Science Course; Section 2: Fundamentals and Principles of Ophthalmology. San Francisco, American Academy of Ophthalmology, 2003–2004, pp 355–360.
12 Knop N, Knop E: Conjunctiva-associated lymphoid tissue in the human eye. Invest Ophthalmol Vis Sci 2000;41:1270–1279.
13 Kaufman PL, Alm A: Adler's Physiology of the Eye, ed 10, revised. St. Louis, Mosby, 2003.
14 Junghans BM, Wadley RB, Crewther SG, Crewther DP: X-ray elemental analysis differentiates blood vessels and lymphatic vessels in the chick choroids. Aust NZ J Ophthalmol 1999;27:244–246.
15 Liang H, Crewther SG, Crewther DP, Junghans BM: Structural and elemental evidence for edema in the retina, retinal pigment epithelium, and choroids during recovery from experimentally induced myopia. Invest Ophthalmol Vis Sci 2004;45:2463–2474.

Dr. Henry J. Kaplan
Department of Ophthalmology and Visual Science, University of Louisville
301 East Muhammad Ali Boulevard
Louisville, KY 40202 (USA)
Tel. +1 502 852 5466, Fax +1 502 852 4595, E-Mail hank.kaplan@louisville.edu

Niederkorn JY, Kaplan HJ (eds): Immune Response and the Eye.
Chem Immunol Allergy. Basel, Karger, 2007, vol 92, pp 11–26

Regional Immunity and Immune Privilege

Henry J. Kaplan[a], *Jerry Y. Niederkorn*[b]

[a]Department of Ophthalmology and Visual Science, University of Louisville, Louisville, Ky., [b]Department of Ophthalmology, University of Texas Southwestern Medical Center, Dallas, Tex., USA

Abstract

The immune system is confronted with an endless array of potential pathogens and immunogens and it must make a decision regarding the nature of the response that is invoked. Robust immune-mediated inflammation is necessary to purge some life-threatening infections. In other conditions, immune responses must be tempered to reduce the risk of irreparable damage to tissues that possess a limited capacity for regeneration. The diversity of pathogens is remarkable and includes microorganisms that range in size from the microscopic picornaviruses to tapeworms that measure up to 35 feet in length. The immune system must adjust its response to take into consideration the nature of the pathogen and the organs that are affected. In some conditions, this amounts to a compromise in which immune-mediated inflammation is restrained or diverted in a manner that inflicts minimal injury to host cells. In still other cases, the immune response is all but silenced. These immunological adjustments are the basis for regional immunity and immune-privileged sites.

The renowned Irish writer and satirist Jonathan Swift is credited with the quotation (roughly paraphrased) '… big fleas have little fleas upon their back to bite them, and lesser fleas have even lesser fleas, and so on ad infinitum'. Parasitologists sometimes use this quote to illustrate the universal threat that infectious diseases pose to the existence of virtually all organisms – even parasites themselves have parasites! The immune system has evolved as a sophisticated and highly successful adaptation for reducing the risk of infection and for eliminating pathogenic microorganisms.

The immune system is composed of two functionally distinct components: the innate immune system and the adaptive immune system. The innate immune system is characterized by its nimble response to pathogens that express pathogen-associated molecular patterns. Cellular elements of the innate immune system express receptors that recognize pathogen-associated molecular patterns and, thus, identify pathogens for elimination by phagocytosis or cytolysis. Macrophages and neutrophils are rapidly activated by molecules elaborated by microorganisms and are the first responders to infections. They are professional phagocytes and are efficient in controlling bacterial and fungal infections. Although cytotoxic T lymphocytes (CTLs) effectively kill virus-infected cells, they must first engage antigen-presenting cells (APCs) expressing the relevant viral peptides expressed on major histocompatibility complex (MHC) class I molecules, and then undergo clonal expansion before they can acquire cytolytic activity. By contrast, antigen presentation and clonal expansion are not needed for natural killer (NK) cells of the innate immune system to lyse virus-infected cells.

The complement system is a complex array of serum-borne molecules with enzyme activity that is generated in a cascade-like fashion. The complement cascade can be activated by one of three pathways. One of these, the alternative pathway, is triggered directly by many bacteria. Once activated, complement components serve as opsonins and facilitate phagocytosis by cells of the innate immune apparatus. Other complement components produce osmotic lysis through the formation of cell membrane pores. Since the complement cascade can be directly activated by either bacterial products or by antigen-antibody interactions, it straddles the innate and adaptive immune systems.

The innate immune response plays a critical role in initiating an adaptive immune response. Macrophages and dendritic cells present antigens to T and B cells, which is facilitated by components of the complement system [1]. Moreover, elements of the innate immune apparatus serve to activate APCs and enhance antigen presentation and the clonal expansion of T and B cells. Recent evidence suggests that the third component of complement acts as a co-stimulatory molecule for activating T-cell responses [1]. T and B cells have the capacity to generate an endless array of receptors that facilitate the formation of antibodies and T-cell receptors, which provide exquisitely specific recognition of potential pathogens. Once the receptor-bearing T and B cells have matured, they are poised to recognize and respond to pathogens. The second encounter with antigens results in a swifter and more robust expansion of the antigen-specific T and B cells. B cells undergo further maturation, culminating in the production of copious amounts of antibody, which can opsonize pathogens, activate complement, or serve as a ligand for engaging Fc-bearing effector cells such as NK cells and macrophages. Engagement of the T-cell receptor triggers CTLs, which are highly effective in killing virus-infected cells. Signaling through the T-cell receptor also activates cells that mediate inflammatory responses such as delayed-type hypersensitivity.

Coordination of the innate and adaptive immune responses is crucial for protecting hosts from a wide array of pathogens. However, the immune rcsponsc does not adhere to the notion that 'one size fits all'. Some pathogens, such as helminths, trigger the preferential production of a unique pattern of cytokines by cells of the innate immune apparatus. In particular, the production of interleukin (IL)-4 tilts the adaptive immune response toward a Th2 pathway, which favors the production of antibodies, especially those of the IgE isotype. Th2 cytokines also stimulate eosinophilia and the activation of mast cells. The Th2 pattern of immunity involves a constellation of humoral and cellular components that are uniquely adapted to eliminate parasitic infections. By contrast, other pathogens, such as intracellular parasites, frequently infect macrophages and stimulate the production of IL-12. IL-12 in turn induces the secretion of interferon-γ, which favors the development of Th1 immunity. Elements of the Th1 immune response preferentially activate macrophages, rendering them highly effective in eliminating intracellular pathogens such as *Toxoplasma gondii* and *Mycobacterium tuberculosis*. Th1 immunity also culminates in the expansion of antigen-specific CTL, which are crucial for eliminating virus-infected cells. Thus, the adaptive immune response to antigens is shaped by the nature of the innate immune system's interpretation of the pathogens and antigenic peptides that it processes.

The Th1 and Th2 immunological dimorphism is an adaptation for preferentially activating the most effective immune effector elements for eliminating pathogens. However, the immune response is also influenced by the microenvironment in which antigens or pathogens are encountered. In some organs, immune responses, whether innate or adaptive, can be deleterious if they inflict nonspecific collateral injury to tissues that have limited regenerative capacities. This immunological dilemma creates the need for immune-privileged sites and sites which express unique regional immunity.

Mucosal Immune System

Mucosal surfaces, especially the gastrointestinal (GI) tract, are examples of sites displaying highly specialized regional immunity. The most common portal of entry for microorganisms is through the mucosal surfaces of the body, which, in humans, is over 400 ft^2 and far exceeds the surface area of the skin [2]. The mucus blanket of the GI and respiratory tracts forms a protective barrier that restricts the adherence of potential pathogens to epithelial cells of these organs. Antigens that gain entry via mucosal surfaces, such as the GI tract, are processed by gut-associated lymphoid tissues, which typically leads to the generation of secretory IgA antibody and, in many cases, regulatory T (T_{reg}) cells [3].

The tear film that coats the ocular surface and the mucus layer of the GI and respiratory tracts are richly endowed with secretory IgA antibodies, which are secreted by B cells of the common mucosal immune system [4, 5]. The importance of IgA antibody is reflected by the commitment of the immune system to its production. IgA accounts for 70% of all the immunoglobulin secreted by the mammalian immune system and more IgA is produced each day than all of the other immunoglobulin isotypes combined [2, 6]. Secretory IgA antibody seems to be ideally suited for the protection of mucosal surfaces, as it is highly effective in blocking adhesion of pathogens to epithelial surfaces [2, 4, 7]. Moreover, IgA is a poor activator of the complement system and does not provoke inflammation. This in turn reduces the risk of chronic inflammation in organs such as the GI tract that are repeatedly exposed to foreign molecules present in foods.

Each day our GI and respiratory tracts are exposed to a bewildering array of foreign molecules that are present in the air we breathe and the food we ingest. When encountering these foreign substances, the immune system must make a decision to either attack or tolerate the alien molecules. Many of the foreign molecules and microorganisms are tolerated as demonstrated by the enormous population of commensal intestinal bacteria that not only thrive in our GI tracts, but are necessary for maintaining homeostasis. Indeed, the intestinal bacterial flora account for over 90% of the cells in the human body!

The immunological decision to tolerate antigens expressed on foodstuffs is based in part on the unique immune regulatory mechanism termed oral tolerance. Oral tolerance, or more accurately, mucosal tolerance, is induced when antigens are introduced via mucosal surfaces and are subsequently processed by APCs within the common mucosal immune system. There are varying reports as to whether mucosal tolerance is due to clonal anergy, clonal deletion, or active suppression by T_{reg} cells [3, 8–11]. The nature of oral tolerance is also affected by the dose of antigen and the presence or absence of mucosal adjuvants such as cholera toxin [3, 8–11]. Although it was recognized almost 100 years ago, mucosal tolerance remains an enigma, but is crucial for maintaining the homeostasis of mucosal surfaces [10, 12].

Immune Privilege of the Brain

Multiple sites in the body express varying degrees of immune privilege including the anterior chamber of the eye, brain, hamster cheek pouch, hair follicle, and pregnant uterus. The earliest explanation for the immune privilege of the brain suggested that the absence of conventional lymphatic vessels prevented antigens from leaving the brain and reaching regional lymph nodes, and the tight junctions between vascular endothelial cells in the brain created a blood-brain barrier that retarded extravasation of immune elements into the brain. However, subsequent studies demonstrated that thc movcmcnt of macromolecules and cells into and out of the brain was not restricted [13]. Antigens introduced into the brain were able to leave the brain by both the venous and lymphatic routes, although the lymphatic pathway was less efficient [14, 15].

Not only do antigens introduced into the CNS escape and accumulate in cervical lymph nodes, once there, they also induce a form of immune deviation termed brain-associated immune deviation in which delayed-type hypersensitivity is actively suppressed in an antigen-specific manner [14, 16, 17]. Brain-associated immune deviation is believed to contribute to the immune privilege of the brain and to coincidentally reduce the risk for immune-mediated inflammation in the CNS.

In addition to the brain-associated immune deviation, the immune privilege of the brain is enhanced by the expression of cell membrane molecules that delete inflammatory cells. It is well recognized that ocular immune privilege relies on the widespread expression of Fas ligand (FasL; CD95L) on cells within the eye [18]. Multiple cells in the CNS also express FasL; these include: astrocytes, oligodendrocytes, microglia, and the vascular endothelium [19]. Interestingly, the microvascular endothelial cells in the CNS are believed to reduce the risk for inflammation by expressing FasL, which limits the extravasation of viable inflammatory cells [20, 21].

Immune Privilege at the Maternal/Fetal Interface

The allogeneic fetus confronts the maternal immune system with paternal alloantigens and, thus, is a potential target for immune rejection. However, the reproductive success of placental mammals is a testament to the efficacy of immune privilege of the maternal/fetal unit. The villous trophoblast, which is in direct contact with maternal blood vessels, lacks MHC class I and II molecules [22]. The absence of conventional MHC class I molecules on the villous trophoblast renders the allogeneic fetus less likely to be recognized and attacked by allospecific CTLs. However, the immune privilege of the allogeneic fetus is due to more than the simple absence of MHC class I and II molecules on the villous trophoblast. Like the brain and the anterior chamber of the eye, multiple anatomical, physiological, and immunoregulatory processes conspire to prevent the induction and expression of immune-mediated inflammation of the allogeneic fetus.

The absence of MHC class Ia molecules in the eye, brain, and trophoblast creates an immunological dilemma, as it arouses the attention of NK cells, which are programmed to lyse MHC class I-negative cells [23]. This is especially important for the allogeneic fetus, as NK cells account for 70% of the lymphocytes found in the pregnant uterus [22]. To compensate for the paucity or frank absence of MHC class Ia molecules, the trophoblast expresses nonclassical MHC class Ib molecules such as HLA-G and HLA-E [24–28]. HLA-G and HLA-E have the capacity to engage the NK-inhibitory receptor CD94/NKG2 and shut off NK cell-mediated lysis [25, 26, 29].

Immune-mediated inflammation at the maternal/fetal interface is also inhibited by multiple molecules and mechanisms that either buffer against the pro-inflammatory properties of the complement cascade or induce apoptosis of inflammatory cells [30]. These include: (a) complement-regulatory proteins; (b) indoleamine dioxygenase, which starves T cells due to tryptophan deprivation; (c) FasL, and (d) tumor necrosis factor-related apoptosis-inducing ligand, which induces apoptosis of macrophages and neutrophils [30].

Immune deviation may also contribute to the immune privilege of the allogeneic fetus. Transforming growth factor (TGF)-β is the critical cytokine that promotes the development of tolerizing APCs in the eye and it appears to play a similar role at the maternal/fetal interface. The TGF-β content of seminal plasma is among the highest of any biological fluids [31]. Moreover, the TGF-β level in uterine luminal fluid rises over threefold immediately following insemination [32]. Exposure to semen promotes the generation of tolerance to the male-specific histocompatibility antigen, which can be demonstrated by prolonged survival of male skin grafts transplanted to pregnant female recipients [33, 34]. Moreover, immunization with paternal cells in the presence of semen induces tolerance to paternal MHC class I antigens [35]. Studies indicate that the tolerance to paternal MHC antigens in pregnant mice is transient and disappears shortly after parturition [36]. Anecdotal evidence suggests that a similar, if not identical form of tolerance to paternal alloantigens may occur in humans. Live birth rates following in vitro fertilization are significantly improved when women are exposed to semen at the initiation of pregnancy [37]. In both mice and humans, there is a steep increase in the numbers of CD4+ CD25+ T_{reg} cells during pregnancy [38, 39]. Depletion of CD4+ CD25+ T cells prevents the development of the allogeneic offspring [38]. Thus, the immune privilege of the allogeneic fetus is the result of multiple mechanisms that restrict the induction and expression of alloimmunity.

Ocular Immune Privilege

In 1948, Medawar [40] observed that genetically incompatible tumor cells could often grow when transplanted into the anterior chamber of the eye or brain, but not when implanted subcutaneously. He interpreted this unexpected growth potential as failure of the immune system to reject allogeneic grafts and coined the term, 'immune privileged'. Thus, immune-privileged sites are defined as sites in the body where foreign tissue grafts can survive for extended periods of time whereas similar grafts placed in conventional sites are acutely rejected by the host. It has subsequently been recognized that destruction by the host immune system could not only be abrogated in specific sites, but that certain tissues appeared to have protection as well. Billingham and Boswell [41] provided evidence that the cornea of the eye is an immunologically privileged tissue giving rise to this concept. However, controversy surrounded the immunologically privileged status of the anterior chamber of the eye until inbred strains of rats were used to definitively demonstrate its existence [42]. Skin grafts transplanted across both major and minor histocompatibility barriers enjoyed prolonged survival within the anterior chamber. However, several factors were found to restrict privilege exhibited by this site – the magnitude of immunogenetic disparity between donor and recipient, graft size, type of tissue grafted, and, at least in the case of thyroid grafts, the endocrine status of the host.

Medawar [40] initially proposed that the prolonged survival of allogeneic tissue grafts was a consequence of 'immunologic ignorance' – namely that alloantigens within the anterior chamber of the eye were sequestered from recognition by the host immune response. In 1970, Kaplan and Streilein [43, 44] made the surprising observation that allogeneic lymphoid cells injected into the anterior chamber of normal rat eyes induced a deviant form of systemic immunity. Rather than being ignored by the host immune system, the alloantigens on injected lymphoid cells induced a robust antigen-specific antibody response. Moreover, the recipient rats had an impaired ability to reject orthotopic skin allografts genetically identical to the injected cells. The term 'immune deviation' was used to describe this phenomenon. Subsequent studies by Niederkorn et al. [45], Niederkorn [46], and Streilein et al. [47] indicated that the immune deviation induced by the anterior chamber inoculation of antigen was not a function of the injected lymphoid cells, but was a characteristic of the anterior chamber. They coined the term 'anterior chamber-associated immune deviation (ACAID)' to characterize this phenomenon [48]. Subsequently, hundreds of publications have demonstrated the presence of ACAID using a wide range of antigens including soluble proteins, particulate antigens (e.g. viral proteins and hapten-derivatized cells), histocompatibility antigens, and tumor antigens. Recent studies on the existence of immune privilege in the eye have focused on allogeneic tumor cell implants and have demonstrated its existence not only in the anterior chamber, but also in the vitreous cavity and subretinal space [49, 50]. It is now recognized that immune privilege promotes survival of intraocular tumor growth by inhibition of both the adaptive and innate immune effector responses.

Biologic Importance of Ocular Immune Privilege

The host immune response has developed and evolved to protect the organism from invasion and damage by a wide range of infectious pathogens – ranging from viruses to bacteria to parasites. With time, the immune system has developed distinctive responses that are specific for pathogens as well as tissues. For example, an antigen-specific immune response, coupled with significant leukocyte inflammation, might effectively eliminate a pathogen in an organ such as the lung or liver without irreparable damage to that organ through the destruction of tissue by the nonspecific inflammation associated with the leukocyte response (i.e. the bystander effect). In contrast, such tissue injury might have a devastating effect on the function of an organ, such as the eye, or the host, if it occurred within the brain. For example, if the fovea of the retina (which measures <500 μm) or the respiratory center in the brain were inadvertently destroyed by bystander inflammation the result would be devastating. Blindness would result from destruction of the fovea; death would result from damage to the respiratory center.

The existence of ocular immune privilege is dependent upon multiple factors including the blood-ocular barrier, unconventional lymphatic drainage pathways within the eye, soluble immunomodulatory factors in the aqueous humor, immunomodulatory ligands on the surface of ocular parenchymal cells, regulation of the complement system within the eye, and tolerance-promoting APCs. The details of the blood-ocular barrier are described in a previous section by Kaplan [pp 4–10]. It results in the relative sequestration of the anterior chamber, vitreous cavity and neurosensory retina from the host immune system. To date, no patent lymphatic vessels have been demonstrated anatomically in the anterior chamber, vitreous cavity, or neural retina in mammals – although lymphatic vessels have been demonstrated in the subconjunctival space, as well as the outer avian choroid [51, 52]. In rodents, several studies have demonstrated that both soluble antigens and tumor cells injected into the anterior chamber can be detected in ipsilateral lymph nodes draining the head and neck region as early as 24 h after the intracameral injections suggesting the existence of lymphatic drainage channels serving the anterior segment of the eye [53–59]. Aqueous humor from the anterior chamber drains through the trabecular meshwork into the canal of Schlemm which empties directly into the venous circulation. A separate venous network, the posterior ciliary vein, drains the neurosensory retina.

Establishment of Ocular Immune Privilege

Three different strategies are used by the host immune system to modify the innate and adaptive immune responses within the eye: immunologic ignorance, peripheral tolerance to ocular-derived antigens and development of an intraocular immunosuppressive microenvironment.

Immunologic Ignorance

Although Medawar's original hypothesis that the absence of lymphatic drainage within the eye contributed to the inability of the host immune system to detect alloantigens is incorrect, recent studies have shown that specific ocular tissues have novel mechanisms that promote immunologic ignorance [60]. For example, the expression of MHC class I antigens is reduced, especially by corneal epithelial cells, and no corneal cells expressed MHC class II antigens [61, 62].

Alloreactive T cells of the 'direct' type have T-cell receptors that can recognize allogeneic MHC class I or II molecules directly. These cells are important mediators of allograft rejection. Since the normal cornea lacks MHC class II APCs, sensitization to foreign histocompatibility antigens and corneal graft rejection must await migration of recipient APCs into the graft bed, where they capture alloantigen from donor cells and result in sensitization of the indirect alloreactive effector T cells [63–66]. Since the normal cornea lacks patent lymphatic vessels, APCs carrying donor antigens show delayed trafficking to draining lymph nodes until lymphangiogenesis develops [67]. Thus, there is delayed corneal allograft rejection at least in part because of the lack of MHC class II APCs in the cornea.

A more detailed analysis of the immunologic ignorance and immune privilege of corneal tissue has been addressed in detail previously [68]. The minor role of alloreactive CD8+ cytotoxic T cells, as well as the importance of CD4+ T cells in corneal graft rejection has been reviewed elsewhere [60, 69–71]. The immunologic privilege of corneal cells also stems from their ability to prevent the generation of new blood and lymphatic vessels within the graft after corneal transplantation [72]. Angiostasis is achieved by neutralization of angiogenic factors that promote vessel formation into the graft and graft bed [67].

Peripheral Tolerance of Ocular Antigens

Despite the limited or unconventional lymphatic drainage from the inner structures of the eye, as well as the tight junctions presented by the pigment epithelium, antigens placed within the anterior chamber of the eye (as well as the vitreous cavity [73] and subretinal space [74]) elicit a deviant systemic immune response referred to as ACAID. The immunologic hallmarks of ACAID include the generation of primed cytotoxic (CD8+) T and B cells that produce non-complement-fixing antibodies, as well as the inhibition of delayed-type hypersensitivity (CD4+ Th1) and B cells that secrete complement-fixing antibodies [43, 44, 47, 75, 76]. An important feature in the development of ACAID is the camero-splenic access through which antigen, APCs, and soluble inhibitory molecules migrate directly into the bloodstream through the ocular trabecular meshwork and traffic preferentially to the spleen. The role of F4/80+ APCs in the induction of ACAID to soluble antigens is well established [77]. However, particulate antigens such as trinitrophenol-labeled T cells and HSV1 may induce a soluble ACAID-inducing signal [78–80].

The details of the cellular mechanism involved in the generation of ACAID are discussed in a subsequent chapter by Niederkorn [pp 27–35]. However, it should be emphasized that the antigen-specific T_{reg} cells that mediate ACAID consist of two populations – an afferent T_{reg} cell and an efferent T_{reg} cell. The afferent T_{reg} cell is CD4+ and suppresses the initial activation and differentiation of T cells into Th1 effector cells. The efferent T_{reg} cell population is CD8+ and inhibits the expression of Th1-mediated immunity such as delayed-type hypersensitivity. Thus, the afferent T_{reg} cells of ACAID are effective in secondary lymphoid organs, whereas the efferent T_{reg} cells of ACAID act in the periphery [81–83].

Intraocular Immunosuppressive Microenvironment

Although systemic mechanisms exist to prevent the development of an intraocular inflammatory response that will unnecessarily damage critical structures within the eye, there are also local factors within the eye that inhibit the components of the immune response to reinforce the protection provided by immune privilege. These local factors suppress both the molecules and the cells that mediate innate and adaptive immunity.

Although the soluble factors in aqueous humor may have multiple effects, there appear to be distinctive properties possessed by each. For example, the neuropeptides vasoactive intestinal peptide and somatostatin inhibit antigen- and mitogen-driven T cell proliferation [84], whereas α-melanocyte-stimulating hormone prevents T cells from secreting pro-inflammatory cytokines such as interferon-γ and can suppress the activation and effector function of bystander T cells [85, 86]. Thus, effector CD4+ T cells that enter the anterior chamber can be converted into T_{reg} cells that suppress intraocular inflammation and avoid damage to the inner structures of the eye.

Soluble factors in the aqueous humor are also directed at the regulation of innate immunity. For example, calcitonin gene-related peptide inhibits the production of nitric oxide by activated macrophages [87]; macrophage migration-inhibitory factor inhibits NK cells from lysing their targets [87, 88]; soluble CD95L interferes with CD95-induced activation of neutrophils [89], and α-melanocyte-stimulating hormone inhibits neutrophil effector functions [90].

An important component of innate immunity evolved in the protection of the eye from infectious pathogens is the complement system. At least two soluble inhibitors of complement activation exist in the aqueous humor – one that prevents antibody binding to C1q and another that prevents C3 conversion to C3b [91]. However, the aqueous humor has no inhibitory effect on non-complement-fixing, neutralizing antibodies. A soluble complement factor is also important in the development of ACAID. The ligation of the complement C3 activation product iC3b to complement receptor type 3 on APCs results in the sequential production of TGF-β_2 and IL-10, which are essential to the induction of ACAID [92].

In addition to soluble factors in the aqueous humor that modulate the intraocular immune response, ocular parenchymal cells express at least four different molecules that can modify the immune effector response within the eye. CD95L, which is expressed constitutively by cells of the eye, is at least partially responsible for the acceptance of orthotopic corneal allografts by the apoptosis of T cells that threaten corneal transplants. The membrane complement regulatory proteins (i.e. CD46, CD55, CD59 and complement receptor-related protein, Crry) are membrane-associated inhibitors of complement and are present on intraocular cells [93], as well as in soluble form in the aqueous humor [94, 95]. These molecules play an important role in controlling the low level of complement activation that is always present in the anterior chamber to protect the eye from infection, while simultaneously preventing widespread nonspecific inflammation which would be detrimental to the eye. The neutralization of Crry in rats provoked spontaneous inflammation in the anterior segment [96]. The immune co-stimulator B7-2 (CD86) is constitutively expressed on iris pigment epithelial cells. When this molecule binds to CTL antigen 4 (CTLA4) on T cells, these cells are inhibited from proliferation and interferon-γ production, and are converted into T_{reg} cells [97]. Another apoptosis-inducing molecule has been identified in the eye, tumor necrosis factor-related apoptosis-inducing ligand [98, 99]. The molecule is a member of the tumor necrosis factor super family and has been demonstrated to induce apoptosis in several tumors. Its mRNA and protein are constitutively expressed on the cornea and retina, and function in vitro and in vivo to kill tumor cells. Thus, the intraocular immune system has both soluble and insoluble molecules that can effectively regulate both the innate and adaptive immune response.

Effect of Inflammation on Ocular Immune Privilege

A more detailed explanation of the effect of inflammation on ocular immune privilege will appear in a subsequent chapter written by Mo et al. [pp 155–165]. Since inflammation and infection dramatically alter the blood-ocular barrier, as well as perhaps the normally dormant lymphatic vessels within the choroid, it is reasonable to inquire whether immune privilege and the immunosuppressive microenvironment are still contained under such an assault. It has been demonstrated that the aqueous humor maintains an immunosuppressive profile in eyes that are inflamed although the factors responsible for the inhibition are significantly altered [100–103]. With breach of the blood-ocular barrier, plasma proteins enter the eye and degrade the neuropeptides that are normally present in aqueous humor. Although the immunosuppressive properties of the aqueous humor are immediately neutralized by this occurrence, an immunosuppressive milieu is reestablished through the presence of active TGF-β_2. In normal aqueous humor, latent TGF-β_2 contributes very little to immunosuppression. However, ocular inflammation upregulates IL-6 production within the eye and it, in turn, activates local macrophages to convert latent TGF-β_2 to its active form. These findings have been confirmed in several different experimental models of intraocular inflammation [103].

Thus, the evolution of immune privilege as a protective mechanism for the function of vital organs such as the eye and the brain has resulted in a complex system with multiple regulatory safeguards for the control of both innate and adaptive immunity. The consequences of inadvertent bystander tissue destruction by antigen-nonspecific inflammation can be so catastrophic to the organ or host that a finely tuned and dynamic regulatory system is needed to ensure the integrity of these tissues. With the ability of infectious pathogens to constantly adapt to protective mechanisms, it is probably a continuous process with the emergence of new molecular and cellular protective mechanisms in response to pathogenic adaptations.

References

1 Heeger PS, Lalli PN, Lin F, et al: Decay-accelerating factor modulates induction of T cell immunity. J Exp Med 2005;201:1523–1530.

2 Staats HF, Jackson RJ, Marinaro M, et al: Mucosal immunity to infection with implications for vaccine development. Curr Opin Immunol 1994;6:572–583.

3 Garside P, Millington O, Smith KM: The anatomy of mucosal immune responses. Ann NY Acad Sci 2004;1029:9–15.

4 Mestecky J: The common mucosal immune system and current strategies for induction of immune responses in external secretions. J Clin Immunol 1987;7:265–276.

5 Sullivan DA: Immunology of the lacrimal gland and tear film. Dev Ophthalmol 1999;30:39–53.

6 Mazanec MB, Nedrud JG, Kaetzel CS, Lamm ME: A three-tiered view of the role of IgA in mucosal defense. Immunol Today 1993;14:430–435.

7 Niederkorn JY: The role of the innate and adaptive immune responses in *Acanthamoeba* keratitis. Arch Immunol Ther Exp (Warsz) 2002;50:53–59.

8 Dubois B, Goubier A, Joubert G, Kaiserlian D: Oral tolerance and regulation of mucosal immunity. Cell Mol Life Sci 2005;62:1322–1332.

9 Garside P, Mowat AM: Mechanisms of oral tolerance. Crit Rev Immunol 1997;17:119–137.

10 Mowat AM, Parker LA, Beacock-Sharp H, Millington OR, Chirdo F: Oral tolerance: overview and historical perspectives. Ann NY Acad Sci 2004;1029:1–8.

11 Wu HY, Weiner HL: Oral tolerance. Immunol Res 2003;28:265–284.

12 Wells HG: Studies on the chemistry of anaphylaxis. III. Experiments with isolated proteins, especially those of hen's egg. J Infect Dis 1911;9:147–171.

13 Barker CF, Billingham RE: Immunologically privileged sites. Adv Immunol 1977;25:1–54.

14 Harling-Berg C, Knopf PM, Merriam J, Cserr HF: Role of cervical lymph nodes in the systemic humoral immune response to human serum albumin microinfused into rat cerebrospinal fluid. J Neuroimmunol 1989;25:185–193.

15 Yamada S, DePasquale M, Patlak CS, Cserr HF: Albumin outflow into deep cervical lymph from different regions of rabbit brain. Am J Physiol 1991;261:H1197–H1204.
16 Harling-Berg CJ, Knopf PM, Cserr HF: Myelin basic protein infused into cerebrospinal fluid suppresses experimental autoimmune encephalomyelitis. J Neuroimmunol 1991;35:45–51.
17 Wenkel H, Streilein JW, Young MJ: Systemic immune deviation in the brain that does not depend on the integrity of the blood-brain barrier. J Immunol 2000;164:5125–5131.
18 Griffith TS, Brunner T, Fletcher SM, Green DR, Ferguson TA: Fas ligand-induced apoptosis as a mechanism of immune privilege. Science 1995;270:1189–1192.
19 Choi C, Benveniste EN: Fas ligand/Fas system in the brain: regulator of immune and apoptotic responses. Brain Res Brain Res Rev 2004;44:65–81.
20 Sata M, Suhara T, Walsh K: Vascular endothelial cells and smooth muscle cells differ in expression of Fas and Fas ligand and in sensitivity to Fas ligand-induced cell death: implications for vascular disease and therapy. Arterioscler Thromb Vasc Biol 2000;20:309–316.
21 Walsh K, Sata M: Is extravasation a Fas-regulated process? Mol Med Today 1999;5:61–67.
22 Moffett-King A: Natural killer cells and pregnancy. Nat Rev Immunol 2002;2:656–663.
23 Ljunggren HG, Ohlen C, Hoglund P, Franksson L, Karre K: The RMA-S lymphoma mutant: consequences of a peptide loading defect on immunological recognition and graft rejection. Int J Cancer Suppl 1991;6:38–44.
24 Ishitani A, Geraghty DE: Alternative splicing of HLA-G transcripts yields proteins with primary structures resembling both class I and class II antigens. Proc Natl Acad Sci USA 1992;89: 3947–3951.
25 Kovats S, Main EK, Librach C, et al: A class I antigen, HLA-G, expressed in human trophoblasts. Science 1990;248:220–223.
26 Rouas-Freiss N, Goncalves RM, Menier C, Dausset J, Carosella ED: Direct evidence to support the role of HLA-G in protecting the fetus from maternal uterine natural killer cytolysis. Proc Natl Acad Sci USA 1997;94:11520–11525.
27 Rouas-Freiss N, Khalil-Daher I, Marchal-Bras Goncalves R, et al: Role of HLA-G in maternal-fetal immune tolerance. Transplant Proc 1999;31:724–725.
28 Rouas-Freiss N, Khalil-Daher I, Riteau B, et al: The immunotolerance role of HLA-G. Semin Cancer Biol 1999;9:3–12.
29 Lee N, Llano M, Carretero M, et al: HLA-E is a major ligand for the natural killer inhibitory receptor CD94/NKG2A. Proc Natl Acad Sci USA 1998;95:5199–5204.
30 Niederkorn JY: Immune privilege of the eye and fetus: parallel universes? Transplantation 2005;80:1139–1144.
31 Robertson SA, Ingman WV, O'Leary S, Sharkey DJ, Tremellen KP: Transforming growth factor beta – a mediator of immune deviation in seminal plasma. J Reprod Immunol 2002;57: 109–128.
32 Tremellen KP, Seamark RF, Robertson SA: Seminal transforming growth factor β_1 stimulates granulocyte-macrophage colony-stimulating factor production and inflammatory cell recruitment in the murine uterus. Biol Reprod 1998;58:1217–1225.
33 James E, Chai JG, Dewchand H, et al: Multiparity induces priming to male-specific minor histocompatibility antigen, HY, in mice and humans. Blood 2003;102:388–393.
34 Lengerova A, Vojtiskova M: Prolonged survival of syngeneic male skin grafts in parous C57B1 mice. Folia Biol (Praha) 1963;9:72–74.
35 Robertson SA, Mau VJ, Hudson SN, Tremellen KP: Cytokine-leukocyte networks and the establishment of pregnancy. Am J Reprod Immunol 1997;37:438–442.
36 Tafuri A, Alferink J, Moller P, Hammerling GJ, Arnold B: T cell awareness of paternal alloantigens during pregnancy. Science 1995;270:630–633.
37 Tremellen KP, Valbuena D, Landeras J, et al: The effect of intercourse on pregnancy rates during assisted human reproduction. Hum Reprod 2000;15:2653–2658.
38 Aluvihare VR, Kallikourdis M, Betz AG: Regulatory T cells mediate maternal tolerance to the fetus. Nat Immunol 2004;5:266–271.
39 Somerset DA, Zheng Y, Kilby MD, Sansom DM, Drayson MT: Normal human pregnancy is associated with an elevation in the immune suppressive CD25+ CD4+ regulatory T-cell subset. Immunology 2004;112:38–43.

40 Medawar PB: Immunity to homologous grafted skin. III. The fate of skin homografts transplanted to the brain, to subcutaneous tissue, and to the anterior chamber of the eye. Br J Exp Pathol 1948;29:58–69.
41 Billingham RE, Boswell T: Studies on the problem of corneal homografts. Proc R Soc Lond B Biol Sci 1953;141:392–406.
42 Kaplan HJ, Stevens TR: A reconsideration of immunological privilege within the anterior chamber of the eye. Transplantation 1975;19:203–209.
43 Kaplan HJ, Streilein JW: Immune response to immunization via the anterior chamber of the eye. I. F1-lymphocyte-induced immune deviation. J Immunol 1977;118:809–814.
44 Kaplan HJ, Streilein JW: Immune response to immunization via the anterior chamber of the eye. II. An analysis of F1 lymphocyte-induced immune deviation. J Immunol 1978;120:689–693.
45 Niederkorn J, Streilein JW, Shadduck JA: Deviant immune responses to allogeneic tumors injected intracamerally and subcutaneously in mice. Invest Ophthalmol Vis Sci 1981;20:355–363.
46 Niederkorn JY: Immune privilege in the anterior chamber of the eye. Crit Rev Immunol 2002;22:13–46.
47 Streilein JW, Niederkorn JY, Shadduck JA: Systemic immune unresponsiveness induced in adult mice by anterior chamber presentation of minor histocompatibility antigens. J Exp Med 1980;152: 1121–1125.
48 Streilein JW, Niederkorn JY: Induction of anterior chamber-associated immune deviation requires an intact, functional spleen. J Exp Med 1981;153:1058–1067.
49 Jiang LQ, Jorquera M, Streilein JW: Subretinal space and vitreous cavity as immunologically privileged sites for retinal allografts. Invest Ophthalmol Vis Sci 1993;34:3347–3354.
50 Wenkel H, Chen PW, Ksander BR, Streilein JW: Immune privilege is extended, then withdrawn, from allogeneic tumor cell grafts placed in the subretinal space. Invest Ophthalmol Vis Sci 1999;40:3202–3208.
51 Junghans BM, Wadley RB, Crewther SG, Crewther DP: X-ray elemental analysis differentiates blood vessels and lymphatic vessels in the chick choroid. Aust NZ J Ophthalmol 1999;27: 244–246.
52 Liang H, Crewther SG, Crewther DP, Junghans BM: Structural and elemental evidence for edema in the retina, retinal pigment epithelium, and choroid during recovery from experimentally induced myopia. Invest Ophthalmol Vis Sci 2004;45:2463–2474.
53 Boonman ZF, van Mierlo GJ, Fransen MF, et al: Intraocular tumor antigen drains specifically to submandibular lymph nodes, resulting in an abortive cytotoxic T cell reaction. J Immunol 2004;172:1567–1574.
54 Camelo S, Kezic J, Shanley A, Rigby P, McMenamin PG: Antigen from the anterior chamber of the eye travels in a soluble form to secondary lymphoid organs via lymphatic and vascular routes. Invest Ophthalmol Vis Sci 2006;47:1039–1046.
55 Camelo S, Shanley A, Voon AS, McMenamin PG: The distribution of antigen in lymphoid tissues following its injection into the anterior chamber of the rat eye. J Immunol 2004;172:5388–5395.
56 Egan RM, Yorkey C, Black R, et al: Peptide-specific T cell clonal expansion in vivo following immunization in the eye, an immune-privileged site. J Immunol 1996;157:2262–2271.
57 Liu Y, Hamrah P, Zhang Q, Taylor AW, Dana MR: Draining lymph nodes of corneal transplant hosts exhibit evidence for donor major histocompatibility complex (MHC) class II-positive dendritic cells derived from MHC class II-negative grafts. J Exp Med 2002;195:259–268.
58 Niederkorn JY, Lynch MG: Reconsidering the immunologic privilege and lymphatic drainage of the anterior chamber of the eye. Transplant Proc 1989;21:259–260.
59 Niederkorn JY, Streilein JW: Alloantigens placed into the anterior chamber of the eye induce specific suppression of delayed-type hypersensitivity but normal cytotoxic T lymphocyte and helper T lymphocyte responses. J Immunol 1983;131:2670–2674.
60 Niederkorn JY: Immunology and immunomodulation of corneal transplantation. Int Rev Immunol 2002;21:173–196.
61 Abi-Hanna D, Wakefield D, Watkins S: HLA antigens in ocular tissues. I. In vivo expression in human eyes. Transplantation 1988;45:610–613.
62 Wang HM, Kaplan HJ, Chan WC, Johnson M: The distribution and ontogeny of MHC antigens in murine ocular tissue. Invest Ophthalmol Vis Sci 1987;28:1383–1389.

63 Hamrah P, Liu Y, Zhang Q, Dana MR: The corneal stroma is endowed with a significant number of resident dendritic cells. Invest Ophthalmol Vis Sci 2003;44:581–589.
64 Lee RS, Grusby MJ, Glimcher LH, Winn HJ, Auchincloss H Jr: Indirect recognition by helper cells can induce donor-specific cytotoxic T lymphocytes in vivo. J Exp Med 1994;179:865–872.
65 Shoskes DA, Wood KJ: Indirect presentation of MHC antigens in transplantation. Immunol Today 1994;15:32–38.
66 Streilein JW, Toews GB, Bergstresser PR: Corneal allografts fail to express Ia antigens. Nature 1979;282:326–327.
67 Cursiefen C, Chen L, Dana MR, Streilein JW: Corneal lymphangiogenesis: evidence, mechanisms, and implications for corneal transplant immunology. Cornea 2003;22:273–281.
68 Streilein JW: Ocular immune privilege: therapeutic opportunities from an experiment of nature. Nat Rev Immunol 2003;3:879–889.
69 Hegde S, Beauregard C, Mayhew E, Niederkorn JY: CD4+ T-cell-mediated mechanisms of corneal allograft rejection: role of Fas-induced apoptosis. Transplantation 2005;79:23–31.
70 Hegde S, Niederkorn JY: The role of cytotoxic T lymphocytes in corneal allograft rejection. Invest Ophthalmol Vis Sci 2000;41:3341–3347.
71 Niederkorn JY: The immunology of corneal transplantation. Dev Ophthalmol 1999;30:129–140.
72 Hori J, Streilein JW: Role of recipient epithelium in promoting survival of orthotopic corneal allografts in mice. Invest Ophthalmol Vis Sci 2001;42:720–726.
73 Jiang LQ, Streilein JW: Immune privilege extended to allogeneic tumor cells in the vitreous cavity. Invest Ophthalmol Vis Sci 1991;32:224–228.
74 Wenkel H, Streilein JW: Analysis of immune deviation elicited by antigens injected into the subretinal space. Invest Ophthalmol Vis Sci 1998;39:1823–1834.
75 Ksander BR, Geer DC, Chen PW, et al: Uveal melanomas contain antigenically specific and nonspecific infiltrating lymphocytes. Curr Eye Res 1998;17:165–173.
76 Wilbanks GA, Streilein JW: Distinctive humoral immune responses following anterior chamber and intravenous administration of soluble antigen. Evidence for active suppression of IgG2-secreting B lymphocytes. Immunology 1990;71:566–572.
77 Lin HH, Faunce DE, Stacey M, et al: The macrophage F4/80 receptor is required for the induction of antigen-specific efferent regulatory T cells in peripheral tolerance. J Exp Med 2005;201:1615–1625.
78 Ferguson TA, Herndon JM: The immune response and the eye: the ACAID inducing signal is dependent on the nature of the antigen. Invest Ophthalmol Vis Sci 1994;35:3085–3093.
79 Ferguson TA, Kaplan HJ: The immune response and the eye. I. The effects of monoclonal antibodies to T suppressor factors in anterior chamber-associated immune deviation (ACAID). J Immunol 1987;139:346–351.
80 Waldrep JC, Kaplan HJ: Anterior chamber-associated immune deviation induced by TNP-splenocytes (TNP-ACAID). II. Suppressor T-cell networks. Invest Ophthalmol Vis Sci 1983;24:1339–1345.
81 Skelsey ME, Mayhew E, Niederkorn JY: CD25+, interleukin-10-producing CD4+ T cells are required for suppressor cell production and immune privilege in the anterior chamber of the eye. Immunology 2003;110:18–29.
82 Stein-Streilein J, Streilein JW: Anterior chamber associated immune deviation (ACAID): regulation, biological relevance, and implications for therapy. Int Rev Immunol 2002;21: 123–152.
83 Streilein JW, Masli S, Takeuchi M, Kezuka T: The eye's view of antigen presentation. Hum Immunol 2002;63:435–443.
84 Taylor AW, Yee DG: Somatostatin is an immunosuppressive factor in aqueous humor. Invest Ophthalmol Vis Sci 2003;44:2644–2649.
85 Namba K, Kitaichi N, Nishida T, Taylor AW: Induction of regulatory T cells by the immunomodulating cytokines α-melanocyte-stimulating hormone and transforming growth factor-β_2. J Leukoc Biol 2002;72:946–952.
86 Taylor AW, Streilein JW, Cousins SW: Identification of α-melanocyte stimulating hormone as a potential immunosuppressive factor in aqueous humor. Curr Eye Res 1992;11:1199–1206.
87 Taylor AW, Yee DG, Streilein JW: Suppression of nitric oxide generated by inflammatory macrophages by calcitonin gene-related peptide in aqueous humor. Invest Ophthalmol Vis Sci 1998;39:1372–1378.

88 Apte RS, Sinha D, Mayhew E, Wistow GJ, Niederkorn JY: Cutting edge: role of macrophage migration inhibitory factor in inhibiting NK cell activity and preserving immune privilege. J Immunol 1998;160:5693–5696.
89 Gregory MS, Repp AC, Holhbaum AM, et al: Membrane Fas ligand activates innate immunity and terminates ocular immune privilege. J Immunol 2002;169:2727–2735.
90 Taylor AW: Ocular immunosuppressive microenvironment; in Streilein JW (ed): Immune Response and the Eye. Chem Immunol. Basel, Karger, 1999, vol 73, pp 72–89.
91 Goslings WR, Prodeus AP, Streilein JW, et al: A small molecular weight factor in aqueous humor acts on C1q to prevent antibody-dependent complement activation. Invest Ophthalmol Vis Sci 1998;39:989–995.
92 Sohn JH, Bora PS, Suk HJ, et al: Tolerance is dependent on complement C3 fragment iC3b binding to antigen-presenting cells. Nat Med 2003;9:206–212.
93 Bora NS, Gobleman CL, Atkinson JP, Pepose JS, Kaplan HJ: Differential expression of the complement regulatory proteins in the human eye. Invest Ophthalmol Vis Sci 1993;34:3579–3584.
94 Lass JH, Walter EI, Burris TE, et al: Expression of two molecular forms of the complement decay-accelerating factor in the eye and lacrimal gland. Invest Ophthalmol Vis Sci 1990;31:1136–1148.
95 Sohn JH, Kaplan HJ, Suk HJ, Bora PS, Bora NS: Complement regulatory activity of normal human intraocular fluid is mediated by MCP, DAF, and CD59. Invest Ophthalmol Vis Sci 2000;41:4195–4202.
96 Sohn JH, Kaplan HJ, Suk HJ, Bora PS, Bora NS: Chronic low level complement activation within the eye is controlled by intraocular complement regulatory proteins. Invest Ophthalmol Vis Sci 2000;41:3492–3502.
97 Yoshida M, Takeuchi M, Streilein JW: Participation of pigment epithelium of iris and ciliary body in ocular immune privilege. 1. Inhibition of T-cell activation in vitro by direct cell-to-cell contact. Invest Ophthalmol Vis Sci 2000;41:811–821.
98 Lee HO, Herndon JM, Barreiro R, Griffith TS, Ferguson TA: TRAIL: a mechanism of tumor surveillance in an immune privileged site. J Immunol 2002;169:4739–4744.
99 Wang S, Boonman ZF, Li HC, et al: Role of TRAIL and IFN-gamma in CD4+ T cell-dependent tumor rejection in the anterior chamber of the eye. J Immunol 2003;171:2789–2796.
100 Mo JS, Streilein JW: Immune privilege persists in eyes with extreme inflammation induced by intravitreal LPS. Eur J Immunol 2001;31:3806–3815.
101 Ohta K, Wiggert B, Yamagami S, Taylor AW, Streilein JW: Analysis of immunomodulatory activities of aqueous humor from eyes of mice with experimental autoimmune uveitis. J Immunol 2000;164:1185–1192.
102 Ohta K, Yamagami S, Taylor AW, Streilein JW: IL-6 antagonizes TGF-beta and abolishes immune privilege in eyes with endotoxin-induced uveitis. Invest Ophthalmol Vis Sci 2000;41:2591–2599.
103 Streilein JW, Ohta K, Mo JS, Taylor AW: Ocular immune privilege and the impact of intraocular inflammation. DNA Cell Biol 2002;21:453–459.

Dr. Henry J. Kaplan
Department of Ophthalmology and Visual Science, University of Louisville
301 East Muhammad Ali Bloulevard
Louisville, KY 40202 (USA)
Tel. +1 502 852 5466, Fax +1 502 852 4595, E-Mail hank.kaplan@louisville.edu

Niederkorn JY, Kaplan HJ (eds): Immune Response and the Eye.
Chem Immunol Allergy. Basel, Karger, 2007, vol 92, pp 27–35

The Induction of Anterior Chamber-Associated Immune Deviation

Jerry Y. Niederkorn

Department of Ophthalmology, University of Texas Southwestern Medical Center, Dallas, Tex., USA

Abstract

Evidence of ocular immune privilege was noted almost 130 years ago. The past 30 years have witnessed an explosion in research on ocular immune privilege. One of the primary mechanisms that contribute to ocular immune privilege is the unique form of immune deviation that is invoked when antigens are introduced into the anterior chamber (AC) of the eye – a phenomenon termed AC-associated immune deviation (ACAID). ACAID embodies a constellation of cellular interactions and at least four different organ systems: eye, thymus, spleen, and sympathetic nervous system. At least four different cell populations interact to generate CD8+ T regulatory cells that suppress both Th1- and Th2-mediated inflammation. The interactions that occur between F4/80+ antigen-presenting cells, CD4+ T regulatory cells, NK1.1+ T cells, $\gamma\delta$ T cells, B cells, and CD8+ T cells remain to be fully elucidated. Ocular immune privilege was originally perceived as a simple anatomic anomaly that has evolved to be one of the most sophisticated and intriguing forms of immune regulation.

The immune privilege of the eye is a widely recognized, but frequently oversimplified concept. The notion that the eye possessed unusual immunological characteristics was recognized in the 19th century by van Dooremaal [1] who observed prolonged survival of murine skin grafts transplanted into the anterior chamber (AC) of the dog eye. The term ocular 'immune privilege' was articulated by Medawar [2], who recognized that the extended survival of foreign grafts in the AC was a remarkable departure from the fate of similar grafts transplanted to sites outside of the eye. Medawar noted the conspicuous absence of major lymphatic drainage from the AC and proposed that the immune privilege of the eye was a consequence of antigen sequestration from the peripheral immune system. Thirty years would pass before the dynamic nature of ocular immune privilege would be recognized. The seminal studies of Kaplan et al. [3] demonstrated that alloantigenic cells introduced into the AC in fact did escape from the eye and induced a deviant immune response in which serum alloantibodies were generated, while systemic cell-mediated immune responses were suppressed in an antigen-specific manner. Subsequent studies in mice confirmed this AC-associated immune deviation (ACAID) and demonstrated that it is an important contributor to the immune privilege of the eye [4].

The Induction of Anterior Chamber-Associated Immune Deviation

As mentioned earlier, antigens introduced into the AC elicit a deviant immune response, which is characterized by the antigen-specific suppression of classical Th1 immune responses, such as delayed-type hypersensitivity (DTH) and complement-fixing antibodies, while preserving the generation of non-complement-fixing antibodies of the IgG1 isotype in the mouse [4, 5]. The suppression of Th1 immune responses and the impaired rejection of skin allografts from the same donors that were used for the alloantigenic cell injection in the AC, led some to suspect that ACAID was simply cross-regulation of the Th1 immunity produced by a robust Th2 response. This was supported by the observation that the benchmark Th1 cytokine, interferon-γ, was suppressed and the anti-inflammatory Th2 cytokine, interleukin (IL)-10, was upregulated following AC injection of antigens [6–8]. However, it was later noted that another Th2 cytokine, IL-4, was not required for the induction of ACAID [6] and that Th2-mediated allergic inflammatory lung diseases could be mitigated by inducing ACAID [9]. These observations indicate that ACAID is not simply a manifestation of a Th2-mediated cross-regulation of Th1 immune responses, but is a complex immunoregulatory phenomenon that involves multiple organ systems and cell populations.

Ocular Phase of Anterior Chamber-Associated Immune Deviation

The induction of ACAID begins with the introduction of antigen into the AC. The eye is an integral participant in the induction of ACAID, as enucleation within 3 days of AC injection prevents the induction of ACAID [10]. The absence of major lymphatic channels draining the AC led many to conclude that depositing antigens into the AC is tantamount to an intravenous injection. Moreover, the striking similarity between ACAID and the immune deviation

Table 1. ACAID and intravenously induced immune deviation are not the same immunoregulatory phenomenon

Requirement	ACAID	Intravenously induced immune deviation	References
IL-4	no	yes	[7]
IL-10	yes	no	[26]
B cells	yes	no	[31, 33, 47]
Efferent suppressor cells	yes	no	[48]
Blood-borne APC	yes	no	[20]
NKT cells	yes	no	[13]
β_2-Microglobulin	yes	no	[35]

that is induced by intravenous injection of antigen lent further support to the proposition that ACAID was simply a convoluted method for injecting antigens intravenously. However, a large body of data refutes this simplistic hypothesis. There is evidence that antigens introduced into the AC reach the submandibular lymph nodes of mice in 3 days [11]. In the primate eye, up to 25% of the contents of the AC can escape by the uveal/scleral pathway and reach lymphatic tissues [12]. Moreover, there are numerous fundamental differences in the cells and cytokine requirements involved in ACAID and intravenously induced immune deviation (table 1).

It is widely believed that within the eye, antigen is captured by F4/80+ macrophages, which under the influence of aqueous humor cytokines, such as transforming growth factor-β, are imprinted with a unique cytokine profile in which IL-12 synthesis is downregulated while IL-10 is upregulated. Ocular antigen presenting cells (APC) also acquire the capacity to secrete macrophage inflammatory protein-2, which is a potent chemokine that plays a critical role in the splenic phase of ACAID (discussed below) [13]. In addition to alterations in the cytokine and chemokine profile of ocular APC, apoptosis appears to be a crucial event that occurs during the processing of ocular antigens. Functional FasL must be expressed in the eye of the host and functional Fas receptor must be present on antigenic cells introduced into the AC [14, 15]. Fas-induced apoptosis of antigenic cells is required for the induction of ACAID, as hapten-derivatized cells from Fas-defective lpr/lpr mice cannot induce ACAID unless the haptenated cells are rendered apoptotic by alternative means such as γ-irradiation prior to AC injection [14]. Tumor necrosis factor-α (TNF-α) also contributes to the induction of apoptosis and the generation of ACAID [16]. TNF-α upregulates Fas receptor and promotes Fas-induced apoptosis and the subsequent induction of ACAID [16, 17]. Allogeneic cells and hapten-derivatized cells from TNFRII (TNF receptor II) knockout (KO) mice do not upregulate Fas receptor following exposure to TNF-α and do not induce ACAID [16, 17]. Interestingly, corneal allografts from C57BL/6 TNFRII KO mice fail to induce ACAID and experience a dramatic increase in the incidence of rejection compared to corneal grafts from C57BL/6 mice with intact TNFRII [17].

The induction of ACAID also requires ligation of the complement 3b (C3b) receptor on the surface of F4/80+ ocular APC [18]. This conclusion is based on findings indicating that neither C3 KO mice nor normal mice depleted of complement with cobra venom factor were able to develop ACAID [18]. Moreover, administration of OX-42 antibody, which blocks the C3 receptor on APC, prevents the induction of ACAID in wild-type mice. In vitro studies confirmed that ligation of the C3 receptor on F4/80+ ocular APC resulted in an increased secretion of IL-10, decreased production of IL-12, and an increased production of transforming growth factor-β, which is the classical phenotype of ACAID-inducing APC.

The processing of ocular antigen by F4/80+ ocular APC is swift. Removal of the eye within 1 day of AC injection of herpes simplex virus prevents the induction of ACAID and results in the development of positive DTH responses [14]. However, if the eye is left intact another 48 h, ACAID is induced. Within 48 h of AC injection, F4/80+ cells can be isolated from the blood and shown to induce ACAID if transferred to third-party recipients [19, 20]. The blood-borne F4/80+ APC produce an extraordinary amplification of the immune response; as few as 20 of these cells can induce ACAID if transferred to naïve recipients [20]. Expression of F4/80 and the major histocompatibility complex class I-like molecule, CD1d, on F4/80+ ocular APC is crucial for the subsequent cellular interactions that occur in the thymus and spleen, as ACAID cannot be induced in either F4/80 KO mice or CD1d KO mice, and macrophages from either of these KO mouse strains cannot adoptively transfer ACAID [21, 22].

Thymic Phase of Anterior Chamber-Associated Immune Deviation

There is evidence that the blood-borne F4/80+ APC follow two pathways after leaving the eye: one pathway leads to the thymus and the other ends in the spleen. The thymus is essential for the induction of ACAID [23]. Thymectomy prevents the generation of ACAID in either intact mice that are subsequently primed in the AC with antigen or in mice that receive intravenous injections of antigen-pulsed F4/80+ ocular macrophages that normally induce ACAID in euthymic animals [19]. Within 3 days of entering the thymus, F4/80+ APC induce the generation of CD4−, CD8− NK1.1+ thymocytes that are believed to enter the circulation as recent thymic emigrants and home to the spleen, where they contribute to the generation of splenic suppressor cells [24]. Other evidence indicates that F4/80+ ocular APC also migrate to the spleen, where they interact with natural killer T (NKT) cells and B cells, which in turn elicit the generation of CD4+ afferent and CD8+ efferent suppressor cells [13, 25, 26]. Both pathways of F4/80+ APC emigration from the eye ultimately culminate in the generation of CD8+ regulatory cells that are able to suppress the expression of DTH.

Splenic Phase of Anterior Chamber-Associated Immune Deviation

In all of the models of ACAID tested to date, an intact spleen is required for the induction and expression of ACAID [4, 27]. The splenic phase of ACAID requires 7 days for completion, as removal of this organ within 7 days of AC injection of antigen prevents the development of ACAID [28]. It is during this time that the F4/80+ APC that migrate from the eye interact with at least two different populations of spleen cells to culminate in the production of CD8+ suppressor cells. To achieve this, the F4/80+ ocular APC that enter the spleen must express CD1d, produce IL-10, IL-13, and macrophage inflammatory protein-2 and stimulate signal transducer and activator of transcription-6 [6, 13, 22, 26, 29, 30]. In the spleen, the F4/80+ cells interact with CD4+ NKT cells that secrete the chemokine, RANTES, which recruits other cells needed for the generation of end-stage regulatory cells of ACAID [29]. It is believed that the F4/80+ ocular APC secrete macrophage inflammatory protein-2, which attracts CD4+ NKT cells. The CD4+ NKT cells interact with CD1d on the F4/80+ ocular APC and secrete RANTES, which in turn recruits more F4/80+ ocular APC and T cells to the marginal zone of the spleen leading to the formation of clusters of F4/80+ ocular APC, CD4+ NKT, and T cells. The function and mechanisms evoked by this cellular triumvirate remain poorly understood, and must take into account at least four other cell populations that are required for the induction of ACAID: (a) B cells; (b) γδ T cells; (c) NK1.1− CD4+ T cells, and (d) CD8+ T cells.

There is compelling evidence that B cells participate in the induction of ACAID by acting as ancillary APC. ACAID cannot be induced in either B-cell KO mice or normal mice treated from birth with anti-immunoglobulin to deplete B-cell populations [31–33]. A combination of in vitro and in vivo studies have shown that F4/80+ ocular APC release antigen, which is captured and processed by splenic B cells [33, 34]. Following exposure to F4/80+ ocular

APC, splenic B cells can adoptively transfer antigen-specific ACAID to naïve mice [31, 33]. Studies utilizing transgenic mice carrying the hen egg lysozyme (HEL) B-cell receptor (BCR) confirmed that HEL BCR transgenic mice could develop ACAID using HEL, but not using other antigens such as ovalbumin [33]. These studies also demonstrated that antigen was regurgitated from F4/80+ ocular APC and captured via the BCR on the splenic B cells, internalized, and processed in acidified lysosomes before being presented to T cells [33]. A combination of in vitro and in vivo investigations analyzed the role of nonclassical class Ib molecules, namely Qa-1, in the presentation of antigens by ACAID B cells, and revealed that the induction of ACAID required the normal expression of β_2-microglobulin on both the B cells and the F4/80+ ocular APC, but not on the end-stage suppressor T cells [34]. The importance of β_2-microglobulin expression on F4/80+ ocular APC is consistent with previous results indicating that ACAID could not be induced in β_2-microglobulin-deficient mice [35]. The role of nonclassical class Ib molecule, Qa-1, in the presentation of antigenic peptides to regulatory T cells is reminiscent of studies by Noble et al. [36], who found that Qa-1+ B cells were needed for the generation of CD8+ T regulatory cells, which suppressed Th1 immune responses. It bears noting that F4/80+ APC, NK1.1+ T cells, and CD3+ T cells form clusters in the marginal zone of the spleen, which is an area rich in CD1+ B cells. We are attracted to the hypothesis that F4/80+ CD1d+ ocular APC interact with CD1d-dependent invariant CD4+ NK1.1+ T cells in the marginal zone of the spleen and release antigenic peptide fragments, which are captured and processed by CD1d+ B cells. The B cells in turn present the modified peptide fragments to CD8+ T cells, which differentiate into ACAID efferent suppressor cells.

In dissecting the splenic phase of ACAID, we must also take into account the observation that γδ T cells are necessary for the induction of ACAID [18]. γδ T cells represent a small population of lymphocytes that make up 2–10% of the total T-cell population and play critical, albeit poorly understood, roles in various forms of immune tolerance [37, 38]. Two independent studies have shown that γδ T cells are critical for the development of ACAID [39, 40]. It is not clear how γδ T cells contribute to the development of ACAID, but they are known to be potent producers of cytokines. It is noteworthy that γδ T cells produce significant quantities of two cytokines, IL-10 and transforming growth factor-β, which are essential for the induction and expression of ACAID. In addition, γδ T cells can inhibit the production of interferon-γ, and thus hamper the generation of Th1 immune responses. Recently, it has been demonstrated that γδ T cells can function as APC, raising the remote possibility that they might act as ancillary APC in the generation of ACAID suppressor cells [41].

Role of the Sympathetic Nervous System in Anterior Chamber-Associated Immune Deviation

The three organ systems involved in the induction of ACAID – eye, thymus, and spleen – have dense sympathetic innervations. The sympathetic nervous system influences systemic immunity, as chemical sympathectomy results in significant alterations in both DTH and antibody responses [42–45]. These observations prompted Li et al. [46] to examine the role of the sympathetic nervous system in ACAID. A series of in vitro and in vivo studies revealed that chemical sympathectomy did not affect the generation of F4/80+ ocular APC, yet it did prevent the induction of ACAID, most likely by impairing the generation of CD4+ NKT cells that are required for the generation of end-stage suppressor cells [46]. Thus, one more organ system (i.e. the sympathetic nervous system) appears to be crucial for the induction of ACAID.

Conclusions

The past 30 years have provided us with a wealth of information and insights into the mechanisms of ocular immune privilege. ACAID has emerged as a major component of immune privilege and what was initially thought of as a version of intravenously induced immune deviation, has evolved into a complicated immunoregulatory phenomenon that involves multiple organ systems including the eye, thymus, spleen, and sympathetic nervous system. The next 30 years will undoubtedly reveal even more complex cellular interactions that contribute to the generation of ACAID suppressor cells that extinguish the expression of both Th1- and Th2-based immune inflammation.

References

1 van Dooremaal JC: Die Entwicklung der in fremden Grund versetzten lebenden Gewebe. Albrecht von Graefes Arch Ophthalmol 1873;19:358–373.
2 Medawar PB: Immunity to homologous grafted skin. III. The fate of skin homografts transplanted to the brain, to subcutaneous tissue, and to the anterior chamber of the eye. Br J Exp Pathol 1948;29:58–69.
3 Kaplan HJ, Streilein JW, Stevens TR: Transplantation immunology of the anterior chamber of the eye. II. Immune response to allogeneic cells. J Immunol 1975;115:805–810.
4 Niederkorn JY: Immune privilege in the anterior chamber of the eye. Crit Rev Immunol 2002;22:13–46.
5 Streilein JW: Ocular immune privilege: therapeutic opportunities from an experiment of nature. Nat Rev Immunol 2003;3:879–889.
6 D'Orazio TJ, Niederkorn JY: A novel role for TGF-beta and IL-10 in the induction of immune privilege. J Immunol 1998;160:2089–2098.

7 Kosiewicz MM, Alard P, Streilein JW: Alterations in cytokine production following intraocular injection of soluble protein antigen: impairment in IFN-gamma and induction of TGF-beta and IL-4 production. J Immunol 1998;161:5382–5390.
8 Li XY, D'Orazio LT, Niederkorn JY: Role of Th1 and Th2 cells in anterior chamber-associated immune deviation. Immunology 1996;89:34–40.
9 Katagiri K, Zhang-Hoover J, Mo JS, Stein-Streilein J, Streilein JW: Using tolerance induced via the anterior chamber of the eye to inhibit Th2-dependent pulmonary pathology. J Immunol 2002;169:84–89.
10 Whittum JA, Niederkorn JY, McCulley JP, Streilein JW: Intracameral inoculation of herpes simplex virus type I induces anterior chamber associated immune deviation. Curr Eye Res 1982;2:691–697.
11 Egan RM, Yorkey C, Black R, et al: Peptide-specific T cell clonal expansion in vivo following immunization in the eye, an immune-privileged site. J Immunol 1996;157:2262–2271.
12 Sherman SH, Green K, Laties AM: The fate of anterior chamber fluorescein in the monkey eye. 1. The anterior chamber outflow pathways. Exp Eye Res 1978;27:159–173.
13 Faunce DE, Sonoda KH, Stein-Streilein J: MIP-2 recruits NKT cells to the spleen during tolerance induction. J Immunol 2001;166:313–321.
14 Griffith TS, Yu X, Herndon JM, Green DR, Ferguson TA: CD95-induced apoptosis of lymphocytes in an immune privileged site induces immunological tolerance. Immunity 1996;5:7–16.
15 Kawashima H, Yamagami S, Tsuru T, Gregerson DS: Anterior chamber inoculation of splenocytes without Fas/Fas-ligand interaction primes for a delayed-type hypersensitivity response rather than inducing anterior chamber-associated immune deviation. Eur J Immunol 1997;27:2490–2494.
16 Elzey BD, Griffith TS, Herndon JM, et al: Regulation of Fas ligand-induced apoptosis by TNF. J Immunol 2001;167:3049–3056.
17 Niederkorn JY, Mayhew E, Mellon J, Hegde S: Role of tumor necrosis factor receptor expression in anterior chamber-associated immune deviation (ACAID) and corneal allograft survival. Invest Ophthalmol Vis Sci 2004;45:2674–2681.
18 Sohn JH, Bora PS, Suk HJ, et al: Tolerance is dependent on complement C3 fragment iC3b binding to antigen-presenting cells. Nat Med 2003;9:206–212.
19 Wang Y, Goldschneider I, O'Rourke J, Cone RE: Blood mononuclear cells induce regulatory NK T thymocytes in anterior chamber-associated immune deviation. J Leukoc Biol 2001;69:741–746.
20 Wilbanks GA, Streilein JW: Studies on the induction of anterior chamber-associated immune deviation (ACAID). 1. Evidence that an antigen-specific, ACAID-inducing, cell-associated signal exists in the peripheral blood. J Immunol 1991;146:2610–2617.
21 Lin HH, Faunce DE, Stacey M, et al: The macrophage F4/80 receptor is required for the induction of antigen-specific efferent regulatory T cells in peripheral tolerance. J Exp Med 2005;201:1615–1625.
22 Sonoda KH, Stein-Streilein J: CD1d on antigen-transporting APC and splenic marginal zone B cells promotes NKT cell-dependent tolerance. Eur J Immunol 2002;32:848–857.
23 Wang Y, Goldschneider I, Foss D, et al: Direct thymic involvement in anterior chamber-associated immune deviation: evidence for a nondeletional mechanism of centrally induced tolerance to extrathymic antigens in adult mice. J Immunol 1997;158:2150–2155.
24 Goldschneider I, Cone RE: A central role for peripheral dendritic cells in the induction of acquired thymic tolerance. Trends Immunol 2003;24:77–81.
25 Sonoda KH, Exley M, Snapper S, Balk SP, Stein-Streilein J: CD1-reactive natural killer T cells are required for development of systemic tolerance through an immune-privileged site. J Exp Med 1999;190:1215–1226.
26 Sonoda KH, Faunce DE, Taniguchi M, et al: NK T cell-derived IL-10 is essential for the differentiation of antigen-specific T regulatory cells in systemic tolerance. J Immunol 2001;166:42–50.
27 Niederkorn J: Immune privilege of the eye; in Chan LS (ed): Animal Models of Human Inflammatory Skin Diseases. New York, CRC Press, 2004, p 564.
28 Streilein JW, Niederkorn JY: Induction of anterior chamber-associated immune deviation requires an intact, functional spleen. J Exp Med 1981;153:1058–1067.
29 Faunce DE, Stein-Streilein J: NKT cell-derived RANTES recruits APCs and CD8+ T cells to the spleen during the generation of regulatory T cells in tolerance. J Immunol 2002;169:31–38.

30 Nakamura T, Terajewicz A, Stein-Streilein J: Mechanisms of peripheral tolerance following intracameral inoculation are independent of IL-13 or STAT6. J Immunol 2005;175:2643–2646.
31 D'Orazio TJ, Niederkorn JY: Splenic B cells are required for tolerogenic antigen presentation in the induction of anterior chamber-associated immune deviation (ACAID). Immunology 1998;95:47–55.
32 Niederkorn JY, Mayhew E: Role of splenic B cells in the immune privilege of the anterior chamber of the eye. Eur J Immunol 1995;25:2783–2787.
33 Skelsey ME, Mayhew E, Niederkorn JY: Splenic B cells act as antigen presenting cells for the induction of anterior chamber-associated immune deviation. Invest Ophthalmol Vis Sci 2003;44: 5242–5251.
34 D'Orazio TJ, Mayhew E, Niederkorn JY: Ocular immune privilege promoted by the presentation of peptide on tolerogenic B cells in the spleen. II. Evidence for presentation by Qa-1. J Immunol 2001;166:26–32.
35 Hara Y, Okamoto S, Rouse B, Streilein JW: Evidence that peritoneal exudate cells cultured with eye-derived fluids are the proximate antigen-presenting cells in immune deviation of the ocular type. J Immunol 1993;151:5162–5171.
36 Noble A, Zhao ZS, Cantor H: Suppression of immune responses by CD8 cells. II. Qa-1 on activated B cells stimulates CD8 cell suppression of T helper 2 responses. J Immunol 1998;160: 566–571.
37 Cai JL, Tucker PW: Gamma-delta T cells: immunoregulatory functions and immunoprotection; in Bergstresser PR, Takashima A (eds): Gamma-Delta T Cells. Chem Immunol. Basel, Karger, 2001, vol 79, pp 99–138.
38 Holtmeier W, Kabelitz D: γδ T cells link innate and adaptive immune responses; in Kabelitz D, Schröder JM (eds): Mechanisms of Epithelial Defense. Chem Immunol Allergy. Basel, Karger, 2005, vol 86, pp 151–183.
39 Skelsey ME, Mellon J, Niederkorn JY: γδ T cells are needed for ocular immune privilege and corneal graft survival. J Immunol 2001;166:4327–4333.
40 Xu Y, Kapp JA: γδ T cells are critical for the induction of anterior chamber-associated immune deviation. Immunology 2001;104:142–148.
41 Brandes M, Willimann K, Moser B: Professional antigen-presentation function by human γδ T cells. Science 2005;309:264–268.
42 Bellinger DL, Lorton D, Romano TD, et al: Neuropeptide innervation of lymphoid organs. Ann NY Acad Sci 1990;594:17–33.
43 Madden KS, Felten SY, Felten DL, Sundaresan PR, Livnat S: Sympathetic neural modulation of the immune system. I. Depression of T cell immunity in vivo and vitro following chemical sympathectomy. Brain Behav Immun 1989;3:72–89.
44 Rice PA, Boehm GW, Moynihan JA, Bellinger DL, Stevens SY: Chemical sympathectomy increases the innate immune response and decreases the specific immune response in the spleen to infection with *Listeria monocytogenes*. J Neuroimmunol 2001;114:19–27.
45 Rook GA, Lightman SL, Heijnen CJ: Can nerve damage disrupt neuroendocrine immune homeostasis? Leprosy as a case in point. Trends Immunol 2002;23:18–22.
46 Li X, Taylor S, Zegarelli B, et al: The induction of splenic suppressor T cells through an immune-privileged site requires an intact sympathetic nervous system. J Neuroimmunol 2004;153:40–49.
47 Vella AT, Scherer MT, Schultz L, Kappler JW, Marrack P: B cells are not essential for peripheral T-cell tolerance. Proc Natl Acad Sci USA 1996;93:951–955.
48 Wilbanks GA, Streilein JW: Characterization of suppressor cells in anterior chamber-associated immune deviation (ACAID) induced by soluble antigen. Evidence of two functionally and phenotypically distinct T-suppressor cell populations. Immunology 1990;71:383–389.

Dr. Jerry Y. Niederkorn
Department of Ophthalmology, University of Texas Southwestern Medical Center
5323 Harry Hines Boulevard
Dallas, TX 75390–9057 (USA)
Tel. +1 214 648 3829, Fax +1 214 648 9061, E-Mail jerry.niederkorn@utsouthwestern.edu

Niederkorn JY, Kaplan HJ (eds): Immune Response and the Eye.
Chem Immunol Allergy. Basel, Karger, 2007, vol 92, pp 36–49

Anatomy and Immunology of the Ocular Surface

Erich Knop[a], *Nadja Knop*[b]

[a]Research Laboratory of the Eye Clinic CVK, Charité-University School of Medicine, Berlin, [b]Department for Cell Biology in Anatomy, Hannover Medical School, Hannover, Germany

Abstract

The ocular surface, in a strict sense, consists of the cornea and its major support tissue, the conjunctiva. In a wider anatomical, embryological, and also functional sense, the ocular mucosal adnexa (i.e. the lacrimal gland and the lacrimal drainage system) also belong to the ocular surface. This definition includes the source and the eventual drainage of the tears that are of utmost importance to ocular surface integrity. The ocular surface is directly exposed to the external environment, and therefore is endangered by a multitude of antigens and pathogenic microorganisms. As a mucosa, it is protected by the mucosal immune system that uses innate and adaptive effector mechanisms present in the tissue and tear film. Immune protection has two partly opposing tasks: the destruction of invading pathogens is counterbalanced by the limitation of inflammatory events that could be deleterious to the subtle structure of the eye. The immune system of the ocular surface forms an eye-associated lymphoid tissue (EALT) that is recognized as a new component of the mucosal immune system. The latter consists of the mucosa-associated lymphoid tissues in different organs of the body. Mucosa- and hence eye-associated lymphoid tissues have certain characteristics that discriminate them from the central immune system. The mechanisms applied are immunological ignorance, tolerance, or an immunosuppressive local microenvironment, all of which prefer non-reactivity and anti-inflammatory immunological responses. The interaction of these mechanisms results in immune privilege of the ocular surface. During eye closure, the ocular surface appears to have different requirements that make an innate pro-inflammatory environment more attractive for immune defense. The structural and functional components that contribute to this special immune regulation will be the focus of this chapter.

Anatomy of the Immune System at the Ocular Surface and Adnexa

Cornea

The cornea consists of a transparent connective tissue (stroma) covered by epithelia on both sides. The endothelium that lines the anterior chamber is a monolayer and the outer border of the cornea is a stratified non-keratinized squamous epithelium that is 5–7 cells thick [1]. It seals the stroma from the external environment by luminal junctions and forms a physical barrier against external antigens. This is supplemented by a physicochemical barrier of the epithelial-derived mucin layer that protects against the adhesion and entrance of antigens and by mechanical washing effects of the tear fluid and lid wiping combined with the action of protective proteins [2].

In the normal cornea, very few cells can assist in immune defense. Lymphoid cells do not occur under physiological conditions. The central cornea is avascular because blood and lymph vessels end in the limbal zone [3] and hence prevent an access of the vast majority of immunologically relevant cells. Major histocompatibility complex (MHC) class II-positive dendritic antigen-presenting Langerhans cells are present in the epithelium of the peripheral cornea and their absence from the central cornea was assumed to be a major reason for corneal immune privilege. Other dendritic cells (DCs) that are negative for markers of cell activation were recently observed in the central cornea of mice [4]. Further bone marrow-derived DC precursors or macrophage-like cells were reported in the anterior stroma and in the posterior stroma.

Conjunctiva

Morphology

The conjunctiva consists of an epithelium and an underlying loose connective tissue, known as the lamina propria; both are separated by the epithelial basement membrane. The epithelial histology is stratified non-squamous and consists of two-to-three cell layers having cuboidal morphology in most parts. The lamina propria is rich in bone marrow-derived cells that form a mucosal immune system known as the conjunctiva-associated lymphoid tissue (CALT) and of blood vessels of different kinds. Apart from capillaries and lymph vessels, specialized high endothelial venules [5] for the regulated migration of lymphoid cells are present in the conjunctiva [6]. They are a normal component of ocular lymphoid tissue, have a characteristic ultrastructure as in other lymphoid tissues, and express cell adhesion molecules.

Diffuse Leukocyte Subpopulations

Over the last decades, evidence has accumulated that leukocytes, including lymphoid cells, are normal, non-inflammatory components of the ocular surface [for review see ref. 7].

Lymphocytes and plasma cells are the main populations of leukocytes [8] and form a diffuse lymphoid tissue throughout all conjunctival zones, with predominant expression in the tarso-orbital conjunctiva [6]. Lymphocytes occur in the basal layer of the epithelium as intraepithelial lymphocytes (IEL) and more frequently in the lamina propria [8, 9] as lamina propria lymphocytes. Several lines of evidence indicate that the ocular surface has a mucosal immune system with common characteristics: CD8+ suppressor/cytotoxic T cells dominate over CD4+ T helper (Th) cells in IEL and a reverse distribution occurs in lamina propria lymphocytes [9, 10]. It is assumed that most of the CD8+ cells act in the suppressor mode and hence provide an immunosuppressive environment [9]. Conjunctival lymphocytes are activated cells (CD45Ro+ and CD25+) and express human mucosal lymphocyte antigen-1 [10, 11]. Local plasma cells regularly occur in the lamina propria [6, 11–13]. They mainly produce IgA and the joining molecule (J chain) that forms the dimeric type of IgA. Its transepithelial transporter molecule secretory component (SC) is found in the epithelium, as verified by immunohistochemistry [6] and molecular biology (RT-PCR) [14]. The conjunctiva hence produces secretory SIgA on its surface and constitutes a secretory immune system [15]. Interspersed B lymphocytes are rarely found as they are restricted to organized lymphoid follicles [6, 9, 11].

Other bone marrow-derived accessory leukocyte subpopulations exist in the conjunctiva and mainly act for the innate immune system. Macrophages enable the engulfment and destruction of pathogens and remnants of dead cells, and their potential antigen presentation to lymphocytes. They are frequent in the lamina propria but difficult to detect in conventional histological specimens. An immunohistological study reported CD68+ macrophages as the second most frequent leukocyte population in the conjunctiva [11]. Dendritic Langerhans cells, which aid in the uptake and professional presentation of antigens to lymphocytes, are regularly found [16]. They express activation markers such as MHC class II or ATPase. Depending on their maturation and migratory behavior, they are critical regulators of immunity and link innate and adaptive immune effector mechanisms [17]. Mast cells are resident accessory leukocytes in the lamina propria [18]. They produce several factors, including cytokines, which recruit other leukocytes and orchestrate inflammatory reactions for the destruction of pathogens. Although their role in physiological host defense is poorly understood, they are potentially useful cells. They are mainly known, however, for their deleterious inflammatory activity during IgE-mediated allergic disease [19]. Granulocytes of different subtypes (neutrophils, basophils, and eosinophils) emigrate from the blood circulation only if recruited. Neutrophils are occasionally observed in minor amounts or as single cells in the normal human conjunctiva [6, 8]. Eosinophils are normally lacking in the absence of inflammatory conditions such as ocular allergy [8].

Follicles

Lymphoid follicles involved in the production of lymphoid effector cells are regularly observed on normal human whole-mount conjunctivas [6, 12, 13], and in several other species [20], being mostly secondary follicles [12]. Their frequency is age dependent [13]; increased levels are noted before onset of puberty which decrease with age. About 60% of individuals in their mid-70s still have follicles in the conjunctiva, with an average number of 10 follicles per conjunctival sac [6]. Follicles show typical mucosal characteristics: they consist of B cells with parafollicular T cells and associated high endothelial venules and have an apical follicle-associated epithelium. It is thin, highly permeated by lymphocytes, and includes M cells for antigen uptake in several species [21], but lacks the IgA transporter SC.

Lacrimal Gland

The human lacrimal gland is anatomically continuous with the conjunctiva via 10–12 lacrimal excretory ducts. It is a tubulo-acinar gland with short-branched tubules that end in secretory acini [1]. Between the secretory acini is a loose connective tissue resembling that of the conjunctiva and, in fact, continuous with it along the excretory ducts. Plasma cells are more frequent than lymphocytes, IEL are fewer, and CD8+ suppressor/cytotoxic T lymphocytes are generally more frequent than CD4+ Th cells in the gland in contrast to the conjunctiva [22]. Plasma cells are mainly positive for IgA, and the acinar epithelium expresses the IgA transporter SC [23]. Therefore, the lacrimal gland is an established component of the secretory immune system and was until recently considered as the only source of IgA proteins present in the tear film [9, 24]. T cells are reported to form groups around intralobular ducts [22] but ordinary lymphoid follicles are very rarely observed and may not be physiologically relevant.

Lacrimal Drainage System

The lacrimal drainage system is continuous with the conjunctiva via the lacrimal puncta and canaliculi into the lacrimal sac and through the nasolacrimal duct into the nose. Like the conjunctiva, it represents a moist mucous membrane. The epithelium is a stratified squamous non-keratinized layer inside the canaliculi and transforms into a pseudostratified epithelium with columnar ciliated cells in the lacrimal sac and nasolacrimal duct [25]. The mucosa contains diffuse lymphoid tissue [26] that contributes to the secretory immune system, and also follicles similar to the conjunctiva [25, 27]. Its mucosa-associated lymphoid tissue was accordingly integrated as a lacrimal drainage-associated lymphoid tissue (LDALT) into the mucosal immune system [25]. The reported frequency of organized lymphoid follicles with typical morphology varies from 41 [27] to 56% in old age human populations [28].

Tear Film and Integrated Proteins

The tear film is an important functional component of immune defense in the ocular mucosal surface. Apart from a cleansing effect induced by lid wiping, it contains specific IgA antibodies that are secreted by the lacrimal gland and by the ocular mucosal surfaces. In addition, there is an ever-increasing number of reported peptides and proteins of the immune system [29]. Some of them have a direct antimicrobial effect whereas others (e.g. chemokines and cytokines) recruit and activate leukocytes, including lymphoid cells.

Historically, and due to their relative concentration, three secreted antimicrobial proteins are most important. Lysozyme destroys the bacterial cell wall, lactoferrin binds iron, and tear-specific prealbumin (lipocalin) acts as a scavenger of bacterial products; complement occurs as a transudate from the serum. Angiogenin is a newly described tear protein found at high concentrations in virtually all tear samples [29]. It appears to have primarily an antimicrobial effect within the tear film. Other multifunctional antimicrobial molecules are predominant in the closed eye during sleep, e.g. specific leukocyte protease inhibitor, elafin, and neutrophil gelatinase-associated lipocalin. CXC and CC chemokines, such as interleukin (IL)-8, epithelial neutrophil-activating peptide 78, interferon-γ-inducible protein-10, growth-regulated oncogene or macrophage chemoattractant protein-1 and macrophage inhibitory protein-1β are able to recruit leukocytes into the tear film. Inflammatory cytokines such as IL-6 and macrophage colony-stimulating factor appear to occur in every normal tear film [29]. Most of these tear proteins show an inverse correlation with the amount of aqueous tear secretion and their concentration strongly increases in the closed-eye tear film, when lacrimal secretion has almost ceased.

Mucosal Immune Defense Mechanisms at the Ocular Surface

The anatomy and leukocyte cell types clearly show that a mucosal immune system is maintained at the normal human ocular surface and mucosal adnexa.

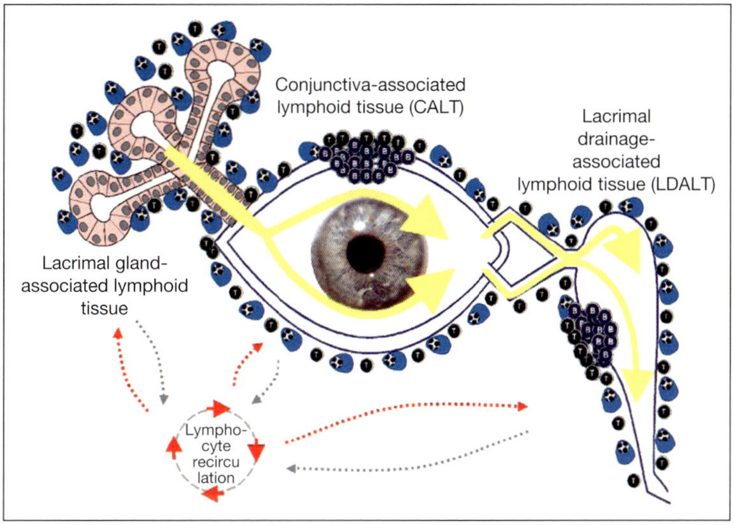

Fig. 1. The eye-associated lymphoid tissue (EALT) is the mucosa-associated lymphoid tissue for immune protection of the ocular surface and its mucosal adnexa. It is anatomically continuous from the lacrimal gland throughout the conjunctiva- and lacrimal drainage-associated lymphoid tissue (i.e. CALT and LDALT, respectively). It consists of a diffuse lymphoid tissue of T lymphocytes and IgA-secreting plasma cells, including accessory leukocyte populations in all organs and of lymphoid follicles in conjunctiva- and lacrimal drainage-associated lymphoid tissue (in the drawing, large blue cells represent plasma cells, small blue cells represent B cells and small black cells represent T cells). Protective as well as aggressive factors inside the tear film, which connects the different parts of the ocular surface and protects it from the external environment, are a major component of ocular surface immunity. The organs are also connected by lymphocyte recirculation via specialized vessels with each other and with the rest of the immune system.

It is termed 'eye-associated lymphoid tissue' (EALT) [7, 30] (fig. 1) and is integrated into the mucosal immune system of the body. Therefore, the laws of mucosal immunity apply to the ocular surface. It has certain specializations suggesting immune privilege, as discussed below. Mucosal, like systemic, immunity uses two approaches for defense, the innate and the adaptive immune system. These have almost opposing characteristics (table 1), use different effector mechanisms, and appear unrelated at first glance. Increasing knowledge has indicated, however, that they are complementary and even act in concert [31]. Together they effectively protect against a highly diverse array of non-pathogenic and pathogenic antigens combined with minimal risk of allergic and autoimmunological disease.

Table 1. Characteristics of innate and adaptive immunity

Characteristics	Innate	Adaptive
Repertoire	preexisting	acquired
Recognition	unspecific pattern	specific (to diverse epitopes)
Action	immediate	intermediate
Reaction	inflammatory	modulated (inflammation to tolerance)
Memory	–	+
Transfer	±	+

Innate Immunity at the Ocular Surface

Function of the Innate Immune System

Innate immunity is an evolutionary old system that primarily aims at the detection and destruction of microbial pathogens. To do so effectively, it relies on a limited number of conserved and genetically determined receptors that work alone or in combination with innate effector cells, mainly phagocytes. Pattern recognition receptors are able to bind to pathogen-associated molecular patterns on microbes such as lipopolysaccharides, flagellin, and CpG-DNA etc. and initiate respective immune responses.

Innate Effector Cells at the Ocular Surface

Phagocytes are important innate effector cells that contribute to defense during infection. Macrophages act almost exclusively by phagocytosis (e.g. in *Acanthamoeba* infection), but also perform antigen processing and presentation, which are necessary for the development of an acquired immune response. In dendritic Langerhans cells, as sentinels of the immune system, antigen presentation dominates phagocytosis. Neutrophil granulocytes are more effective in pathogen elimination due to the secretion of toxic mediators such as myeloperoxidase, which is able to kill pathogens such as *Acanthamoeba* cysts. Mast cells orchestrate the inflammation e.g. in *Toxoplasma gondii* infection.

Toll-Like Receptors

Different Toll-like receptors (TLR) are present in the mouse eye and induce the secretion of CXC chemokines which leads to neutrophil recruitment, a possible mechanism of corneal pathology in early stages of microbial infection [32]. Following bacterial flagellin exposure, TLR5 induces inflammation on human corneal cells. Then, cells of the ocular surface secrete inflammatory cytokines (IL-6 and IL-8) via a nuclear factor-κB-dependent pathway [33] as shown in other tissues. Other results may point into a different direction because it was found that although TLR2, TLR3 and TLR4 occur in human corneal epithelial cells, they do not induce inflammatory immune responses to lipopolysaccharides [34] as a potential mechanism to prevent constant ocular surface inflammation.

Secreted Antimicrobial Peptides

In addition to the established antimicrobial factors such as lysozyme and lactoferrin, a broad spectrum of antimicrobial peptides was recently observed in the normal human ocular surface. β-Defensin-1 to -4 were found together with liver-expressed antimicrobial peptide-1 and -2, and cathelicidin (LL37) [35]. Also, β-defensin-3 has been found to be upregulated in inflammatory conditions. Collectins, observed in human and mouse tear fluid and corneal epithelia, are able to inhibit invasion by *Pseudomonas aeruginosa* [36]. Trefoil factors TFF1 and TFF3 occur in human conjunctival goblet cells [37]. A broad spectrum of antimicrobial peptides, including different α- and β-defensins, secretory phospholipase, bactericidal permeability-increasing protein, and 37-kDa cationic antimicrobial protein, was observed in human nasolacrimal ducts with an induction of human β-defensin-2 under inflammatory conditions [38].

Specific Adaptive Immunity at the Ocular Surface

Function of the Adaptive Immune System

Similar to the innate system, the adaptive immune system is divided into cellular defense, which is mediated by direct action of T cells, and humoral defense, which is maintained by soluble antigen receptors (immunoglobulins) secreted by local mucosal plasma cells. In contrast to innate immunity, the adaptive system consists of lymphoid cells, and it offers a higher degree of specificity, variability, and immune regulation. An 'afferent' antigen uptake and processing phase must be differentiated from the 'efferent' distribution and action of effector cells. In between is the recognition of antigens by lymphocytes and their differentiation and proliferation into effector cells. The processing and presentation of antigens by phagocytes to lymphoid cells links innate and adaptive immunity.

Uptake of Antigen at the Ocular Surface

After antigen enters mucosal surfaces, it is transported by antigen presenting cells (APC) to local lymphoid follicles for its presentation to lymphocytes. Antigen can also be transported, either by APC or in a soluble form, by the efferent lymph, to follicles in regional draining lymph nodes [39]. This is shown to be an important route for processing of corneal transplantation antigens [40]. In the FAE overlying CALT and LDALT follicles, specialized M-cells take up antigen [21]. Phagocytosed antigen is degraded into small fragments and loaded onto MHC-class-II antigen presentation molecules for recognition by the cognate T-cell receptor. Ocular antigen presenting Langerhans cells, which are specialized for this purpose, are described in physiological conditions and can be altered in ocular pathology [4, 16, 41].

Immune Regulation in Follicular Lymphoid Tissue

Since lymphocytes have an enormous variety of different antigen receptor specificities, some can detect self antigens of the host, thus raising the risk of autoimmune disease [42] or allergic eye disease [43]. This is the reason that the mere recognition of an antigen by a T cell is not sufficient for its activation [31]. In contrast to lymphoid cells, innate phagocytes have the ability to recognize the microbial origin of antigens. During antigen presentation, they transmit this information by the expression of co-stimulatory molecules [31] (e.g. CD80/86, CD40, ICAM-1) that also interact with complementary lymphocyte receptors in the ocular surface immune system [44]. Additional cytokines influence the activation of Th cells that produce different cytokine profiles and hence support different immune reactions. Antigen presentation without co-stimulation results in anergy or deletion of the reactive T cells or in generation of active immunosuppressive regulatory T cells [45], both leading to non-reactivity, i.e. immune tolerance. Co-stimulation in the presence of IL-4 skews Th cells into the direction of Th2 cells, which support the differentiation of antibody-producing plasma cells that normally produce anti-inflammatory IgA. Co-stimulation in the presence of IL-12 generates Th1 cells that produce inflammatory cytokines e.g. IFN-γ or TNF-α and mount an inflammatory immune response that is detrimental to the ocular surface.

Diffuse Lymphoid Tissue with Effector Cells

After emigrating from follicular regions via the lymph eventually into the blood, effector cells recirculate in the body. They can home via specialized vessels which are also regularly present at the normal human ocular surface and are equipped with adhesion molecules. This serves for a proposed organ specificity for the same or similar tissues and is the basis for the concept of the mucosal immune system [46, 47]. The mucosal lymphoid effector cells mainly constitute the diffuse lymphoid tissue described in all parts of the eye-associated lymphoid tissue.

Table 2. Examples of strategies and mechanisms for immune privilege at the ocular surface

Strategy	Mechanisms
Ignorance	immune exclusion by secretory IgA absence of corneal lymph vessels absence of corneal lymphocytes few MHC class II on epithelium
Tolerance	immature corneal DCs potential innate corneal unresponsiveness
Immunosuppressive environment	Fas ligand on corneal epithelium factors in the tear film CD8+ IEL in the suppressor mode

Defense Strategies: One Does Not Fit for All at the Ocular Surface

The ocular surface is not only a sophistically constructed organ, but it also uses sophisticated mechanisms of immune defense to preserve its integrity. The actual approach used depends on the requirements of the situation and appears to change in a diurnal rhythm that meets the different needs of the usual open eye and of the closed eye condition during sleep.

The Immune Privilege Approach

Immune privilege (table 2) represents a state in which innate and adaptive inflammatory immune mechanisms are inhibited [42]. In terms of adaptive immune regulation, the activation of an inflammatory Th1 immune response must be avoided in favor of Th2 cells or regulatory T cells. Different strategies contribute to an immune privilege [42] such as *ignorance*, i.e. presentation of an antigen to the immune system is impeded, or the active generation of *tolerance* by regulatory T cells. Alternatively, an *immunosuppressive microenvironment* achieved by soluble factors such as transforming growth factor-β_2 or by surface-bound FAS ligand (CD95L) that eliminates CD95-positive T effector cells through apoptosis contributes to immune privilege. In the eye, this concept was primarily applied to the anterior chamber in order to explain the observed anterior chamber-associated immune deviation [48].

Some of these mechanisms of immune privilege also apply to the surface of the eye. Its immune protection is governed by the rules of the mucosal immune system which generally favors the inhibition of inflammation by tolerogenic mechanisms [49]. The generation of secretory IgA is one of the best-characterized mucosal effector mechanisms [15]. IgA is anti-inflammatory since it does not activate complement. It leads to immune exclusion because it is deposited on the ocular surface and in the tear film where it prevents the entrance of pathogens into the body and can even clear the tissue of antigens during its active SC-mediated transepithelial transport. The majority of environmental antigens and pathogens is hence ignorant to T cells. If the mucosal immune system is deregulated and the default IgA response is switched to IgE, the unresponsiveness to non-pathogenic antigens is lost and allergy occurs [43, 50]. A deregulation of the mucosal immune system with loss of physiological tolerance seems to represent a yet underestimated factor in inflammatory ocular surface conditions in general [51]. Furthermore, the central cornea is less immunogenic because the epithelial cells normally express few MHC class II antigens, it has no blood and lymph vessels and contains no resident lymphoid cells. Some characteristics of an immunosuppressive microenvironment are also present at the ocular surface because the corneal epithelium, like the corneal endothelium, expresses CD95L. In the conjunctiva and lacrimal gland, CD8+ IEL are assumed to be in the suppressor mode and may be anti-inflammatory [9, 22]. Immune tolerance is indicated by immature MHC class II-negative DCs [4] in the central cornea that are assumed to induce tolerance to the presented antigen [17]. Innate immune mechanisms may support immune tolerance because the human corneal epithelium shows innate microbial receptors, but does not necessarily show an inflammatory reaction to ubiquitous microbial stimuli such as lipopolysaccharides [34].

The Pro-Inflammatory Approach

At the ocular surface, there seems to be a unique shift of paradigms for optimal immune protection that follows a diurnal cycle [52] because the conditions and hence the requirements change dramatically when the eye is closed for 6–8 h or more overnight. During this time, lacrimal secretion has almost ceased, and entrapped microbes enjoy a 'moist chamber' at the ocular surface that is rich in nutrients, provides optimal temperatures and is devoid of its normal main protective lacrimal proteins lysozyme and lactoferrin. Therefore, the closed eye represents a very special condition that appears to be governed in particular by innate defense mechanisms [52].

The defense hence switches into a protective approach dominated by pro-inflammatory factors that are locally produced at the ocular surface. Numerous chemokines, cytokines and growth factors orchestrate a subclinical inflammatory reaction. In contrast to the open eye, leukocytes, in particular polymorphonuclear neutrophils (PMN), are increasingly recruited into the tear film. Neutrophils produce increased levels of proteases that attack microbes while the epithelial cells of the host are protected by anti-proteases. Leukocyte proteases also modulate the function of other proteins. For example, neutrophil elastase promotes a switch of angiogenin, which is abundantly present in the tear film, from its angiogenic function to an antimicrobial function. Consequently, a new equilibrium of pro- and anti-inflammatory factors is achieved on a higher level to suppress microbial growth. This appears as a more suitable approach in a highly contaminated closed eye environment than the promotion of immune privilege that is successful during daytime in the open eye.

Acknowledgments

The authors' research on the Eye-Associated Lymphoid Tissue (EALT) and the ocular surface immune system was supported by the *Gesellschaft der Freunde der Medizinischen Hochschule Hannover*, by the *Sandoz Stiftung für Therapeutische Forschung*, by the *Berufsverband der Augenärzte Deutschlands*, by travel fellowships and project funding (KN 317/11) from the *Deutsche Forschungsgemeinschaft* (*DFG*) and by the *Interne Forschungsförderung der Charité-Universitätsmedizin Berlin.*

References

1 Bron AJ, Tripathi DM, Tripati BJ: Wolff's anatomy of the eye and orbit. London, Chapman & Hall Medical, 1997.
2 Argueso P, Gipson IK: Epithelial mucins of the ocular surface: structure, biosynthesis and function. Exp Eye Res 2001;73:281–289.
3 Cursiefen C, Schlotzer-Schrehardt U, Kuchle M, Sorokin L, Breiteneder-Geleff S, Alitalo K, Jackson D: Lymphatic vessels in vascularized human corneas: immunohistochemical investigation using LYVE-1 and podoplanin. Invest Ophthalmol Vis Sci 2002;43:2127–2135.
4 Hamrah P, Zhang Q, Liu Y, Dana MR: Novel characterization of MHC class II-negative population of resident corneal Langerhans cell-type dendritic cells. Invest Ophthalmol Vis Sci 2002;43: 639–646.
5 Kraal G, Mebius RE: High endothelial venules: lymphocyte traffic control and controlled traffic. Adv Immunol 1997;65:347–395.
6 Knop N, Knop E: Conjunctiva-associated lymphoid tissue in the human eye. Invest Ophthalmol Vis Sci 2000;41:1270–1279.
7 Knop E, Knop N: The role of eye-associated lymphoid tissue in corneal immune protection. J Anat 2005;206:271–285.
8 Allansmith MR, Greiner JV, Baird RS: Number of inflammatory cells in the normal conjunctiva. Am J Ophthalmol 1978;86:250–259.
9 Sacks EH, Wieczorek R, Jakobiec FA, Knowles DM: Lymphocytic subpopulations in the normal human conjunctiva. A monoclonal antibody study. Ophthalmology 1986;93:1276–1283.
10 Dua HS, Gomes JA, Jindal VK, Appa SN, Schwarting R, Eagle RC Jr, Donoso LA, Laibson PR: Mucosa specific lymphocytes in the human conjunctiva, corneoscleral limbus and lacrimal gland. Curr Eye Res 1994;13:87–93.

11 Hingorani M, Metz D, Lightman SL: Characterisation of the normal conjunctival leukocyte population. Exp Eye Res 1997;64:905–912.
12 Kessing SV: Mucous gland system of the conjunctiva. A quantitative normal anatomical study. Acta Ophthalmol (Copenh) 1968;95(suppl):1–133.
13 Osterlind G: An investigation into the presence of lymphatic tissue in the human conjunctiva, and its biological and clinical importance. Acta Ophthalmol (Copenh) 1944;23(suppl):1–79.
14 Knop E, Claus P, Knop N: Eye-associated lymphoid tissue (EALT): RT-PCR verifies the presence of mRNA for IgA and its transporter (secretory component) in the normal human conjunctiva. Invest Ophthalmol Vis Sci 2003;44:S3801.
15 Brandtzaeg P, Farstad IN: The human mucosal B-cell system; in Ogra PL, Mestecky J, Lamm ME, Strober W, McGhee JR, Bienenstock J (eds): Handbook of Mucosal Immunology, ed 2. San Diego, Academic Press, 1999, pp 439–468.
16 Gillette TE, Chandler JW, Greiner JV: Langerhans cells of the ocular surface. Ophthalmology 1982;89:700–711.
17 Banchereau J, Steinman RM: Dendritic cells and the control of immunity. Nature 1998;392:245–252.
18 Morgan SJ, Williams JH, Walls AF, Church MK, Holgate ST, McGill JI: Mast cell numbers and staining characteristics in the normal and allergic human conjunctiva. J Allergy Clin Immunol 1991;87:111–116.
19 Stahl JL, Cook EB, Barney NP, Graziano FM: Pathophysiology of ocular allergy: the roles of conjunctival mast cells and epithelial cells. Curr Allergy Asthma Rep 2002;2:332–339.
20 Chodosh J, Nordquist RE, Kennedy RC: Comparative anatomy of mammalian conjunctival lymphoid tissue: a putative mucosal immune site. Dev Comp Immunol 1998;22:621–630.
21 Knop N, Knop E: Ultrastructural anatomy of CALT follicles in the rabbit reveals characteristics of M-cells, germinal centres and high endothelial venules. J Anat 2005;207:409–426.
22 Wieczorek R, Jakobiec FA, Sacks EH, Knowles DM: The immunoarchitecture of the normal human lacrimal gland. Relevancy for understanding pathologic conditions. Ophthalmology 1988;95: 100–109.
23 Franklin RM, Kenyon KR, Tomasi TB Jr: Immunohistologic studies of human lacrimal gland: localization of immunoglobulins, secretory component and lactoferrin. J Immunol 1973;110: 984–992.
24 Sullivan DA: Ocular mucosal immunity; in Ogra PL, Mestecky J, Lamm ME, Strober W, McGhee J, Bienenstock J (eds): Handbook of Mucosal Immunology, ed 2. San Diego, Academic Press, 1999, pp 1241–1281.
25 Knop E, Knop N: Lacrimal drainage-associated lymphoid tissue (LDALT): a part of the human mucosal immune system. Invest Ophthalmol Vis Sci 2001;42:566–574.
26 Knop E, Knop N: MALT tissue of the conjunctiva and nasolacrimal system in the rabbit and human. Vis Res 1996;36:S60.
27 Paulsen FP, Paulsen JI, Thale AB, Schaudig U, Tillmann BN: Organized mucosa-associated lymphoid tissue in human naso-lacrimal ducts. Adv Exp Med Biol 2002;506:873–876.
28 Knop E, Knop N: Human lacrimal drainage-associated lymphoid tissue (LDALT) belongs to the common mucosal immune system. Adv Exp Med Biol 2002;506:861–866.
29 Sack RA, Conradi L, Krumholz D, Beaton A, Sathe S, Morris C: Membrane array characterization of 80 chemokines, cytokines, and growth factors in open- and closed-eye tears: angiogenin and other defense system constituents. Invest Ophthalmol Vis Sci 2005;46:1228–1238.
30 Knop E, Knop N: A functional unit for ocular surface immune defense formed by the lacrimal gland, conjunctiva and lacrimal drainage system. Adv Exp Med Biol 2002;506:835–844.
31 Medzhitov R, Janeway CA Jr: Innate immunity: impact on the adaptive immune response. Curr Opin Immunol 1997;9:4–9.
32 Johnson AC, Heinzel FP, Diaconu E, Sun Y, Hise AG, Golenbock D, Lass JH, Pearlman E: Activation of Toll-like receptor (TLR)2, TLR4, and TLR9 in the mammalian cornea induces MyD88-dependent corneal inflammation. Invest Ophthalmol Vis Sci 2005;46:589–595.
33 Zhang J, Xu K, Ambati B, Yu FS: Toll-like receptor 5-mediated corneal epithelial inflammatory responses to *Pseudomonas aeruginosa* flagellin. Invest Ophthalmol Vis Sci 2003;44:4247–4254.

34 Ueta M, Nochi T, Jang MH, Park EJ, Igarashi O, Hino A, Kawasaki S, Shikina T, Hiroi T, Kinoshita S, Kiyono H: Intracellularly expressed TLR2s and TLR4s contribution to an immunosilent environment at the ocular mucosal epithelium. J Immunol 2004;173:3337–3347.
35 McIntosh RS, Cade JE, Al Abed M, Shanmuganathan V, Gupta R, Bhan A, Tighe PJ, Dua HS: The spectrum of antimicrobial peptide expression at the ocular surface. Invest Ophthalmol Vis Sci 2005;46:1379–1385.
36 Ni M, Evans DJ, Hawgood S, Anders EM, Sack RA, Fleiszig SM: Surfactant protein D is present in human tear fluid and the cornea and inhibits epithelial cell invasion by *Pseudomonas aeruginosa*. Infect Immun 2005;73:2147–2156.
37 Langer G, Jagla W, Behrens-Baumann W, Walter S, Hoffmann W: Secretory peptides TFF1 and TFF3 synthesized in human conjunctival goblet cells. Invest Ophthalmol Vis Sci 1999;40:2220–2224.
38 Paulsen FP, Pufe T, Schaudig U, Held-Feindt J, Lehmann J, Schroder JM, Tillmann BN: Detection of natural peptide antibiotics in human nasolacrimal ducts. Invest Ophthalmol Vis Sci 2001;42: 2157–2163.
39 Camelo S, Shanley A, Voon ASP, McMenamin PG: The distribution of antigen in lymphoid tissues following ist injection into the anterior chamber of the rat eye. J Immunol 2004;172:5388–5395.
40 Yamagami S, Dana MR: The critical role of lymph nodes in corneal alloimmunization and graft rejection. Invest Ophthalmol Vis Sci 2001;42:1293–1298.
41 Hazlett LD, McClellan SM, Hume EB, Dajcs JJ, O'Callaghan RJ, Willcox MD: Extended wear contact lens usage induces Langerhans cell migration into cornea. Exp Eye Res 1999;69:575–577.
42 Streilein JW: Ocular immune privilege: therapeutic opportunities from an experiment of nature. Nat Rev Immunol 2003;3:879–889.
43 Calder VL, Lackie PM: Basic science and pathophysiology of ocular allergy. Curr Allergy Asthma Rep 2004;4:326–331.
44 Dana MR, Qian Y, Hamrah P: Twenty-five-year panorama of corneal immunology: emerging concepts in the immunopathogenesis of microbial keratitis, peripheral ulcerative keratitis, and corneal transplant rejection. Cornea 2000;19:625–643.
45 Annacker O, Pimenta-Araujo R, Burlen-Defranoux O, Bandeira A: On the ontogeny and physiology of regulatory T cells. Immunol Rev 2001;182:5–17.
46 Bienenstock J, McDermott M, Befus D, O'Neill M: A common mucosal immunologic system involving the bronchus, breast and bowel. Adv Exp Med Biol 1978;107:53–59.
47 Mestecky J, McGhee JR, Michalek SM, Arnold RR, Crago SS, Babb JL. Concept of the local and common mucosal immune response. Adv Exp Med Biol 1978;107:185–192.
48 Niederkorn JY, Streilein JW: Induction of anterior chamber-associated immune deviation (ACAID) by allogeneic intraocular tumors does not require splenic metastases. J Immunol 1982;128: 2470–2474.
49 McGhee JR, Lamm ME, Strober W: Mucosal immune responses. An overview; in Ogra PL, Mestecky J, Lamm ME, Strober W, McGhee JR, Bienenstock J (eds): Handbook of Mucosal Immunology, ed 2. San Diego, Academic Press, 1999, pp 485–506.
50 Knop E, Knop N, Pleyer U: Clinical aspects of MALT; in Pleyer U, Mondino B (eds): Uveitis and Immunological Disorders, ed 1. Berlin, Springer, 2004, pp 67–89.
51 Knop E, Knop N: Influence of the eye-associated lymphoid tissue (EALT) on inflammatory ocular surface disease. Ocul Surface 2005;3:S180–S186.
52 Sack RA, Beaton A, Sathe S, Morris C, Willcox M, Bogart B: Towards a closed eye model of the pre-ocular tear layer. Prog Retin Eye Res 2000;19:649–668.

PD Dr. Erich Knop
Research Laboratory of the Eye Clinic CVK, Charité-University School of Medicine
Ziegelstrasse 5–9
DE–10117 Berlin (Germany)
Tel. +49 30 45055 4027, Fax +49 30 45055 4903, E-Mail erich.knop@charite.de

Niederkorn JY, Kaplan HJ (eds): Immune Response and the Eye.
Chem Immunol Allergy. Basel, Karger, 2007, vol 92, pp 50–57

Immune Privilege and Angiogenic Privilege of the Cornea

Claus Cursiefen

Department of Ophthalmology, Friedrich Alexander University Erlangen-Nürnberg, Erlangen, Germany
Schepens Eye Research Institute, Harvard Medical School, Boston, Mass., USA

Abstract

The cornea is the transparent window of the eye and corneal transparency is essential for good vision. Inflammatory reactions within the cornea cannot only cause tissue destruction and scar formation, but are also associated with angiogenesis and lymphangiogenesis in the cornea. Both inflammation-associated processes interfere with corneal transparency and cause corneal blindness. During evolution the cornea has developed mechanisms for preventing and modulating inflammatory and angiogenic reactions. The fact that the cornea is normally devoid of both blood and lymphatic vessels and actively maintains this avascularity has been termed 'corneal *angiogenic privilege*'. Corneal '*immune privilege*', on the other hand, indicates that the cornea is an immune-privileged site and tissue, enabling the extraordinary success of histologically incompatible corneal transplantation. Recent evidence indicates that there is considerable overlap in the molecular mechanisms maintaining corneal 'angiogenic' and 'immune privilege'.

Transparency of the cornea, the 'window of the eye', is essential for good vision [1, 2]. Therefore, evolutionarily developed strategies to interfere with processes that endanger corneal transparency can be explained teleologically. Clinically, the three entities most severely affecting corneal transparency are inflammatory reactions within the cornea, corneal neovascularization, and finally loss of corneal endothelial pump function (either due to degeneration or in the course of inflammation). Inflammation not only causes loss of transparency by the influx of inflammatory cells into the stroma, but also due to secondary changes, e.g. scar formation and destruction of endothelial pump cells. Similarly, corneal neovascularization reduces transparency not only by itself, but also due to leakage of lipids, fluid, and erythrocytes into the cornea [3, 4]. Consequently, higher animals have developed strategies for limiting and modulating the response to inflammatory stimuli in the cornea and maintaining corneal avascularity. The first strategy refers to corneal '*immune privilege*' [1, 5–7]. The normal cornea is devoid of blood and lymphatic vessels and actively maintains this avascularity; this has been termed '*angiogenic privilege*' (by Streilein), being analogous to immune privilege. This study describes the two interdependent phenomena, their overlapping molecular mechanisms and novel immunomodulatory treatment options based on antihem- and antilymphangiogenic agents, i.e. 'immune privilege through angiogenic privilege' [8].

Common Phenomenology of Corneal Immune and Angiogenic Privilege

The normal cornea is avascular and, in contrast to other tissues, does not respond with hem- or lymphangiogenesis in response to the plethora of minor inflammatory and angiogenic stimuli in the cornea, due to its anatomical position, to which it is constantly exposed. Surprisingly, tissue destruction caused by refractive laser procedures never initiates angiogenesis. This suggests active modulation and inhibition of corneal angiogenic responses to minor stimuli, which are physiologically unnecessary and would interfere with corneal transparency (i.e. '*corneal angiogenic privilege*'). By contrast, if an angiogenic response becomes necessary (e.g. in severe, eye-threatening corneal infections), both hem- and lymphangiogenesis can be initiated within hours [9, 10]. In analogy, the extraordinary success of allogeneic corneal transplantation is related to the ocular surface being an *immune-privileged site* and the cornea in addition an *immune-privileged tissue* [11]. Therefore, the cornea has mechanisms actively and passively interfering with the afferent and efferent arms of the immune reflex arc [1].

There are several parallels between these two forms of privilege: first, both are redundant. Several active and passive mechanisms are responsible for corneal immune privilege [5–7]. In analogy, the cornea uses different strategies to maintain avascularity and buffer low-grade angiogenic stimuli. Genetic removal of one or more of the endogenous inhibitors of angiogenesis does not cause spontaneous corneal neovascularization, suggesting multiple backup mechanisms [12]. Second, both forms of privilege are incomplete, i.e. they can be overcome, as shown by immune rejection after keratoplasty and neovascularization during herpetic keratitis. Third, they are actively maintained [12]. Fourth, both are essential for vision and are highly conserved evolutionary. Finally, both forms of privilege are interdependent, i.e. invasion of blood and lymphatic vessels into the cornea abrogates corneal immune privilege [13]. On the other hand, severe corneal inflammation also leads to breakdown of the angiogenic privilege [3].

Common Molecular Mechanisms of Corneal Immune and Angiogenic Privilege

Novel insights into the molecular mechanisms of hem- and lymphangiogenesis explain the close interrelations between neovascularization and immunity/inflammation. Most mediators of angiogenesis, e.g. vascular endothelial growth factor (VEGF), which have traditionally been thought of as acting solely on vascular endothelium, also have profound effects on immune and inflammatory reactions. For example, VEGF-A (via its receptor 1: VEGFR1) is a potent chemoattractant for macrophages [3, 10]. VEGF-C, in addition to being the most potent lymphangiogenic growth factor, can recruit dendritic cells via VEGFR3 [14]. Hence, endogenous anti-angiogenic mechanisms targeting these agents have anti-inflammatory effects and also promote both angiogenic and immune privilege. Alternatively, most pro-inflammatory cytokines incite hem- and lymphangiogenesis [3]. Neutralization of interleukin-1 almost completely abrogates the angiogenic response to inflammation in the corneal suture model [15]. Endogenous interleukin-1 receptor antagonist expression, therefore, promotes both angiogenic and immune privilege [1]. Indeed, both processes are so closely interrelated that it is nearly impossible to experimentally differentiate the two pathways in the cornea [10].

In addition to immunomodulation by angiogenic growth factors and angiogenesis by pro-inflammatory cytokines, inflammatory cells themselves also play paramount roles in the process of corneal angiogenesis. The immune amplification cascade leading to corneal hem- and lymphangiogenesis after corneal inflammation critically depends on the recruitment of macrophages, which in turn are potent sources for all major hem- and lymphangiogenic growth factors (VEGF-A, VEGF-C, and VEGF-D). Local depletion of macrophages can completely prevent the outgrowth of blood and lymphatic vessels [10].

From the inhibitory perspective, endogenous corneal thrombospondin-1 is an essential inhibitor and downregulator of both inflammatory and neovascular reactions in the course of corneal inflammation [12], and its deficiency leads to significantly prolonged inflammatory reactions and enhanced corneal neovascularization [12].

The close association between angiogenesis/lymphangiogenesis and immune reactions is further exemplified by findings indicating that inflammatory cells (CD11b+ macrophages), which can express the lymphatic vascular endothelial hyaluronate receptor LYVE-1 under certain pro-inflammatory conditions, cannot only release angiogenic growth factors [10], but also become *integral* components of inflammation-induced new (corneal) lymphatic vessels in the cornea [16].

Developmentally, corneal angiogenic privilege is established very early: already at fetal stages, the human cornea – in contrast to the adjacent conjunctiva – is devoid of lymphatic and blood vessels [Cursiefen et al., unpublished findings]. Whether corneal immune privilege is already fully active at these early stages is currently not known, but corneal antigen-presenting cells lacking major histocompatibility complex (MHC) class II are not present in fetal corneas before term [17].

Analogy exists between both forms of privilege regarding their anatomy; both have a transition zone at the limbus, where vascularized conjunctiva transitions into avascular cornea and where MHC class II-positive antigen-presenting cells decrease in number [18, 19].

Corneal Immune Privilege

There are numerous active and passive mechanisms that contribute to corneal immune privilege via all three aspects of the immune reflex arc [5–7]. These include: lack of blood and lymphatic vessels, reduced numbers of MHC class II-positive antigen-presenting cells, reduced corneal expression of MHC class I, expression of CD95 ligand, an immunosuppressive microenvironment (α-melanocyte-stimulating hormone and vasoactive intestinal polypeptide) and the fact that the cornea is part of the anterior chamber with its immune deviant, immunosuppressive mechanism of anterior chamber-associated immune deviation [1, 5–7]. The cornea is not only an immune-privileged *site* (as shown by low rejection rates after histologically incompatible allografting for example), it is also an immune-privileged *tissue*, which resists immune destruction, as shown by extended survival when transplanted into non-immune-privileged sites [11]. When grafted into a heterotopic site, the alloimmunogenicity of the normal cornea resides within its epithelial and stromal layers, whereas immune privilege arises from the endothelium. In analogy, the cornea is not only an angiogenically privileged *site*, but also an angiogenically privileged *tissue*, as shown by the observation that the cornea remains avascular when transplanted heterotopically to vascularized sites [11].

Corneal Angiogenic and Lymphangiogenic Privilege

Due to its normal avascularity, the cornea has been the prime in vivo model system to study the mechanisms of angiogenesis and lymphangiogenesis [3, 10].

The precise mechanisms of neovascularization in the course of corneal disease are only partly understood. In general, angiogenic growth factors (e.g. the VEGF family) induce angiogenesis by binding to their VEGF receptors on vascular endothelial cells at the limbal vascular arcade. Stimuli for the release of these factors are inflammation and hypoxia [3, 4]. How the cornea normally prevents ingrowth of blood and lymphatic vessels in response to the plethora of minor angiogenic and inflammatory stimuli has only recently gained wider attention [4, 8, 12]. As mentioned above, there seem to be several redundant mechanisms in place securing this evolutionarily important privilege. Several anti-angiogenic factors have been localized within the cornea, especially at the inner and outer basement membranes and endothelial/epithelial cells; these include thrombospondin-1, pigment epithelium-derived factor, anti-angiogenic extracellular matrix breakdown products (e.g. angiostatin and endostatin) as well as receptor antagonists, e.g. interleukin-1 receptor antagonist. In addition, aqueous humor seems to contribute to the angiogenic immune privilege of the cornea by sequestering angiogenic growth factors, e.g. by soluble VEGFR1 or heparan sulfate binding of fibroblast growth factor [20, 21]. Nevertheless, the precise mechanisms of this system of buffering low concentrations of angiogenic factors and allowing angiogenesis to occur if this threshold is passed, are still unclear.

Although at least some of the endogenous angiogenesis inhibitors are known, so far, endogenous inhibitors of lymphangiogenesis remain to be determined. The normally alymphatic cornea is an excellent model to study these unknown factors.

Immunomodulatory Effects of Antihem- and Antilymphangiogenic Therapies in the Cornea

Corneal immune privilege depends on its angiogenic privilege. Consequently, the survival of allogeneic grafts placed in an avascular 'low-risk' recipient bed is very good. By contrast, survival rates dramatically fall when grafts are placed into prevascularized corneal beds (i.e. 'high-risk' keratoplasty). Both mouse experiments [22] and clinical studies [23] have shown that preoperative corneal neovascularization (i.e. loss of angiogenic privilege) is one of the strongest predictors of subsequent immune rejections [23]. Therefore, it was hypothesized that antihem- and antilymphangiogenic therapies could have beneficial effects on corneal graft survival by interfering with the 'afferent and efferent arms' of an immune response. Several recent publications provide 'proof-of-principle' for this novel concept.

Pharmacologic neutralization of VEGF-A using novel cytokine traps completely inhibits hem- and lymphangiogenesis normally produced in the mouse model of suture-induced high-risk keratoplasty [10]. When corneal allografts are placed in these 'avascular high-risk beds', graft survival is significantly higher compared to 'vascularized high-risk beds' [Cursiefen and Streilein, in preparation], indicating an important role of the lacking *angiogenic* privilege for the high rate of graft rejections in high-risk settings. Therefore, novel anti-angiogenic drugs given during corneal inflammation might prevent the development of a high-risk bed and thereby promote graft survival if future keratoplasty becomes necessary.

If primary prevention fails, secondary prevention has to take place. The most common keratoplasties are performed in low-risk patients who have avascular graft beds. However, even in these situations, about 10% of patients reject their corneal graft and also develop corneal neovascularization postoperatively [24]. Using the mouse model of low-risk keratoplasty, we have recently shown that this mild postkeratoplasty angiogenesis is accompanied by clinically invisible lymphangiogenesis, which compromises corneal immune privilege by providing access to both the afferent and efferent arm of the immune reflex arc [9]. Indeed, in the mouse model of low-risk keratoplasty, both vessel types reached the interface within 1 week of grafting, and inhibition of this postkeratoplasty neovascularization significantly improved graft survival [9]. Moreover, even in prevascularized high-risk graft beds, inhibition of the additional, postoperatively occurring hem- and lymphangiogenesis reduces the risk of subsequent graft rejections [25].

Besides the approaches targeting primarily hem- and lymphangiogenesis, anti-angiogenic strategies targeting the immune effects of angiogenic growth factors have recently been shown to be very effective. Blocking antibodies against VEGFR3-mediated migration of dendritic cells to the regional lymph nodes significantly improves corneal graft survival [14]. Likewise, the beneficial effect of local macrophage depletion on corneal graft survival, which has previously been attributed to 'immunologic ignorance' [26], can also be explained by the antihem- and antilymphangiogenic effects of the liposome-depleting agent clodronate [10]. Furthermore, this clodronate-based, macrophage-depleting anti-angiogenic approach could even prolong graft survival in animal models of xenotransplantation [Borges et al., unpublished findings].

Angiogenesis and lymphangiogenesis tend to follow strong inflammatory processes in the cornea [27, 28]. There is evidence that corneal neovascularization, at least in some instances, is not only a result, but can also be a cause of corneal inflammation. The pathogenesis of herpetic keratitis seems to depend on corneal angiogenesis [29]. Anti-angiogenic therapies can prevent herpetic keratitis [29] and, indeed, could become part of future therapeutic regimens against corneal herpes infections.

In summary, due to its immune and angiogenic privilege, the cornea has acquired two fascinating systems to maintain transparency and to preserve vision. Further unraveling of the molecular mechanisms of these processes will not only allow better understanding of corneal function, but will also provide useful new tools for immunomodulatory and anti-angiogenic/antilymphangiogenic therapies for diseases of the eye and maybe other organs as well [30].

References

1 Streilein JW: Ocular immune privilege: therapeutic opportunities from an experiment of nature. Nat Rev Immunol 2003;3:879–889.

2 Streilein JW: Ocular immune privilege: the eye takes a dim but practical view of immunity and inflammation. J Leukoc Biol 2003;74:179–185.

3 Cursiefen C, Kruse FE: New aspects of corneal angiogenesis; in Reinhard T, Larkin F (eds): Cornea and External Eye; in Krieglstein GK, Weinreb RN (ser eds): Essentials in Ophthalmology. New York, Springer, 2006, pp 83–99.

4 Chang JH, Gabison EE, Kato T, Azar DT: Corneal neovascularization. Curr Opin Ophthalmol 2001;12:242–249.

5 Streilein JW, Yamada J, Dana MR, Ksander BR: Anterior chamber-associated immune deviation, ocular immune privilege, and orthotopic corneal allografts. Transplant Proc 1999;31:1472–1475.

6 Niederkorn JY: The immune privilege of corneal allografts. Transplantation 1999;67:503–508.

7 Streilein JW: New thoughts on the immunology of corneal transplantation. Eye 2003;17:943–948.

8 Cursiefen C, Chen L, Dana MR, Streilein JW: Corneal lymphangiogenesis: evidence, mechanisms and implications for transplant immunology. Cornea 2003;22:273–281.

9 Cursiefen C, Maruyama K, Liu Y, Chen L, Jackson D, Wiegand S, Dana MR, Streilein JW: Inhibition of hemangiogenesis and lymphangiogenesis *after* normal-risk corneal transplantation by neutralizing VEGF promotes graft survival. Invest Ophthalmol Vis Sci 2004;45: 2666–2673.

10 Cursiefen C, Chen L, Borges L, Jackson D, Cao J, Radziejewski C, D'Amore PA, Dana MR, Wiegand SJ, Streilein JW: VEGF-A stimulates lymphangiogenesis and hemangiogenesis in inflammatory neovascularization via macrophage recruitment. J Clin Invest 2004;113:1040–1050.

11 Hori J, Jouyce N, Streilein JW: Epithelium-deficient corneal allografts display immune privilege beneath the kidney capsule. Invest Ophthalmol Vis Sci 2000;41:443–452.

12 Cursiefen C, Masli S, Ng TF, Dana MR, Bornstein P, Lawler J, Streilein JW: Roles of thrombospondin 1 and 2 in regulating spontaneous and induced angiogenesis in the cornea and iris. Invest Ophthalmol Vis Sci 2004;45:1117–1124.

13 Dana MR, Streilein JW: Loss and restoration of immune privilege in eyes with corneal neovascularization. Invest Ophthalmol Vis Sci 1996;37:2485–2494.

14 Chen L, Hamrah P, Cursiefen C, Jackson D, Streilein JW, Dana MR: Vascular endothelial growth factor receptor-3 (VEGFR-3) mediates dendritic cell migration to lymph nodes and induction of immunity to corneal transplants. Nat Med 2004;10:813–815.

15 Cao J, Renard R, Song H, Ioffe E, Mosher V, Rudge JS, Koehler-Stec EM, Yancopoulos GD, Wiegand SJ: Inhibition of IL-1 blocks corneal inflammation and neovascularization. Invest Ophthalmol Vis Sci 2003;44:E823.

16 Maruyama K, Li M, Cursiefen C, Jackson DG, Keino H, Tomita M, Van Rooijen N, Takenaka H, D'Amore PA, Stein-Streilein J, Losordo DW, Streilein JW: Inflammation-induced lymphangiogenesis in the cornea arises from CD11b-positive macrophages. J Clin Invest 2005;115: 2363–2372.

17 Diaz-Araya CM, Madigan MC, Provis JM, Penfold PL: Immunohistochemical and topographic studies of dendritic cells and macrophages in human fetal cornea. Invest Ophthalmol Vis Sci 1995;36:644–656.

18 Hamrah P, Zhang Q, Liu Y, Dana MR: Novel characterization of MHC class II-negative population of resident corneal Langerhans cell-type dendritic cells. Invest Ophthalmol Vis Sci 2002;43:639–646.
19 Brisette-Storkus C, Reynolds S, Lepisto A, Hendricks RL: Identification of a novel macrophage population in the normal mouse corneal stroma. Invest Ophthalmol Vis Sci 2002;43:2264–2271.
20 Lai CM, Brankov M, Zaknich T, Lai YK, Shen WY, Constable IJ, Kovesdi I, Rakoczy PE: Inhibition of angiogenesis by adenovirus-mediated sFlt-1 expression in a rat model of corneal neovascularization. Hum Gene Ther 2001;12:1299–1310.
21 Fannon M, Forsten-Willimas K, Dowd CJ, Freedmann DA, Folkman J, Nugent MA: Binding inhibition of angiogenic factors by heparan sulfate proteoglycans in aqueous humor: potential mechanism for maintenance of an avascular environment. FASEB J 2003;17:902–904.
22 Sano Y, Ksander BR, Streilein JW: Fate of orthotopic corneal allografts in eyes that cannot support anterior chamber-associated immune deviation induction. Invest Ophthalmol Vis Sci 1995;36:2176–2185.
23 Maguire MG, Stark WJ, Gottsch JD, Stulting RD, Sugar A, Fink NE, Schwartz A; Collaborative Corneal Transplantation Studies Research Group: Risk factors for corneal graft failure and rejection in the collaborative corneal transplantation studies. Ophthalmology 1994;101:1536–1547.
24 Cursiefen C, Wenkel H, Martus P, Langenbucher A, Nguyen N, Seitz B, Küchle M, Naumann GOH: Impact of short-term versus long-term topical steroids on corneal neovascularization after non-high-risk keratoplasty. Graefes Arch Clin Exp Ophthalmol 2001;239:514–521.
25 Bachmann B, Lütjen-Drecoll E, Wiegand SJ, Streilein JW, Kruse FE, Cursiefen C: Inhibition of angiogenesis and lymphangiogenesis after high-risk keratoplasty by neutralizing VEGF-A improves corneal graft survival. Invest Ophthalmol Vis Sci 2005;46:E4743.
26 Slegers TP, van der Gaag R, van Rooijen N, van Rij G, Streilein JW: Effect of local macrophage depletion on cellular immunity and tolerance evoked by corneal allografts. Curr Eye Res 2003;26:73–79.
27 Cursiefen C, Schlötzer-Schrehardt U, Küchle M, Sorokin L, Breitender-Geleff S, Alitalo K, Jackson D: Lymphatic vessels in vascularized human corneas: immunohistochemical investigation using LYVE-1 and podoplanin. Invest Ophthalmol Vis Sci 2002;43:2127–2135.
28 Cursiefen C, Ikeda S, Nishina PM, Smith RS, Ikeda A, Jackson D, Mo JS, Chen L, Dana RM, Pytowski B, Kruse FE, Streilein JW: Spontaneous corneal hem- and lymphangiogenesis in mice with destrin-mutation depend on VEGFR3 signaling. Am J Pathol 2005;166:1367–1377.
29 Zheng M, Schwarz MA, Lee S, Kumaraguru U, Rouse BT: Control of stromal keratitis by inhibition of neovascularization. Am J Pathol 2001;159:1021–1029.
30 Cursiefen C, Chen L, Saint-Geniez M, Hamrah P, Jin Y, Rashid S, Pytowski B, Persaud K, Wu Y, Streilein JW, Dana R: Nonvascular VEGF receptor 3 expression by corneal epithelium maintains avascularity and vision. Proc Natl Acad Sci 2006;103:11405–11410.

Dr. Claus Cursiefen, FEBO
Department of Ophthalmology, Friedrich Alexander University Erlangen-Nürnberg
Schwabachanlage 6
DE–91054 Erlangen (Germany)
Tel. +49 9131 8533001, Fax +49 9131 8536401, E-Mail ccursiefen@yahoo.com

Niederkorn JY, Kaplan HJ (eds): Immune Response and the Eye.
Chem Immunol Allergy. Basel, Karger, 2007, vol 92, pp 58–70

Corneal Antigen-Presenting Cells

Pedram Hamrah, M. Reza Dana

Schepens Eye Research Institute, Massachusetts Eye and Ear Infirmary, and
Department of Ophthalmology, Harvard Medical School, Boston, Mass., USA

Abstract

Corneal antigen-presenting cells (APCs) were thought to reside exclusively in the peripheral cornea. However, recent evidence demonstrates that the central cornea is also endowed with a heterogeneous population of bone marrow-derived cells, including epithelial Langerhans cells (LCs) and anterior stromal dendritic cells (DCs), which under certain conditions can function as APCs. While the corneal periphery contains mature and immature resident bone marrow-derived DCs, the central cornea is endowed exclusively with highly immature/precursor-type DCs. During inflammation, a majority of resident DCs undergo maturation by acquiring high expression of major histocompatibility complex class II antigens and B7 (CD80/CD86) and CD40 costimulatory molecules. Further, macrophages are present in the posterior corneal stroma. In transplantation, donor-derived DCs migrate to host cervical lymph nodes and activate host T cells via the direct pathway when allografts are placed in inflamed, but not normal uninflamed, host beds. Migration of DCs to cervical lymph nodes is, in part, regulated by the vascular endothelial growth factor receptor-3 (VEGFR-3) that is expressed on corneal DCs. Blockade of the VEGFR-3 signaling significantly suppresses corneal DC trafficking to draining lymph nodes and rejection of corneal transplants. Much remains unknown about the function of these cells including their role in innate responses as well as in tolerance. Regardless, these data revise the tenet that the cornea is immune privileged due to a lack of resident lymphoreticular cells per se, but suggest that the cornea is capable of actively participating in the immune response to foreign antigens and autoantigens, rather than being a passive bystander. Additionally, one important aspect of immune privilege is likely the ocular 'imposition' of the immature phenotype on its resident bone marrow-derived cells.

Introduction and Historical Overview

Antigen-presenting cells (APCs) serve as the principal immune sentinels to the foreign world and can be divided into 'professional' and 'nonprofessional' types. While the latter are found among nonlymphoid tissues (e.g. vascular endothelial or some tissue epithelial cells), professional APCs, such as dendritic cells (DCs), epithelial Langerhans cells (LCs), macrophages, and B cells, are bone marrow (BM) derived and form an integral part of the immune system. Expression of major histocompatibility (MHC) class II antigens on APCs, whose primary function is to distinguish between self and non-self, plays an integral role in antigen recognition and presentation.

In 1868, the medical student Paul Langerhans discovered a population of DCs in the suprabasal regions of the skin epidermis by impregnating human skin with gold salts [1]. These cells that are now referred to as Langerhans cells were initially considered to be part of the nervous system. Silberberg [2] was able to link LCs to antigen presentation through the observation of a histological relationship between LCs and infiltrating lymphocytes in contact sensitivity reactions. In the cornea, the presence of atypical 'non-keratinocyte' cells was noted initially in 1867 by Engelmann [3]. The LCs of the corneal epithelium were originally thought of as wandering leukocytes that migrated from peripheral blood vessels [4, 5]. LCs are now known to be MHC class II-expressing BM-derived epithelial DCs which function as potent APCs [6, 7].

Over the last several decades, the search for corneal APCs, largely reliant on their presumed universal MHC class II expression, had led to the conclusion that BM-derived cells, which are capable of serving as APCs, are essentially absent in the corneal epithelium and the stroma [8–14]. This absence of APCs in the central cornea was assumed to be a critical component of corneal immune privilege [8, 12, 15]. This paradigm was recently modified with the demonstration of a heterogeneous population of resident corneal APCs by several laboratories [16–20]. These data have revised the tenet that the cornea is immune privileged due to the *lack* of resident lymphoreticular cells; rather, immune privilege is perhaps related to the universally immature phenotype of these resident cells as we discuss below.

Resident Antigen-Presenting Cells in the Normal Uninflamed Cornea

Dendritic Cells, Langerhans Cells and Dendritic Cell Precursors

In 1973, Steinman and Cohn [21] first isolated DCs from lymphoid tissue of mice. DCs have an extraordinary capacity to stimulate naïve T cells and initiate primary immune responses [22–24]. They are now recognized as essential regulators of both the innate and acquired arms of the immune system. DCs serve a unique role because they are the only APCs able to induce primary immune responses, thereby permitting establishment of immunological memory [6, 25].

The cardinal properties of DCs include their ability to (1) migrate selectively through tissues; (2) take up, process, and present antigen, and (3) stimulate and direct T lymphocyte-dependent responses. Recent studies suggest that DCs also play critical roles in the induction of peripheral tolerance [26–28], regulate T cell immune responses [25], and function as effector cells in innate immunity against microbes [29, 30]. The diverse functions of DCs depend on the diversity of DC subsets and lineages and on the functional plasticity of DCs at their immature stage [6, 7, 25, 31]. Similar to other cell types within the immune system, DCs are continuously produced from hematopoietic stem cells within the BM and are widely distributed as precursors or immature DCs, including LCs, within lymphoid and nonlymphoid tissues, e.g. solid organs such as the heart, liver or kidney [32–35].

Immature DCs are characterized by a high capacity for antigen capture and processing, but a low T cell-stimulatory capability [36]. In addition, immature DCs have a low to negligible amount of MHC class II expression and lack the requisite accessory (co-stimulatory) signals for T cell activation, such as CD40, CD80 (B7-1), and CD86 (B7-2) [7]. Maturation of DCs induces redistribution of MHC molecules from the intracellular endocytic compartments of DCs to the cell surface. DC maturation, which renders these cells poor in antigen capture, but potent in T cell stimulation, is either triggered by pathogens directly, or by stimuli such as pro-inflammatory cytokines [7, 24, 36].

In the eye, DCs are found in a variety of tissues including the cornea, conjunctiva, iris, and the ciliary body. Activation and recruitment of DCs in the cornea has been associated with loss of 'immune privilege' in the anterior segment [37], exacerbation of herpetic and *Pseudomonas* keratitis [38–40], and amplification of transplant immunity [41–43]. Some of the phenotypic characteristics of corneal DCs are unique and are discussed below.

Epithelial Langerhans Cells

Under non-pathological circumstances, LCs are the only cells that constitutively express MHC class II molecules in the corneal epithelium [44]. Recent examinations of normal murine corneas have revealed that both the peripheral and central areas of the epithelium contain BM-derived CD11c+ CD11b– LCs, with the density of these cells decreasing from the limbus (178 LCs/mm^2) toward the center (100 LCs/mm^2) [18]. While a large number of LCs are MHC class II positive in the periphery, a large population of MHC class II-*negative* immature/precursor LCs are present both in the periphery and the center of the epithelium, with the center being *exclusively* MHC class II negative and B7 (CD80 or CD86) negative [18]. These LCs have a classic dendritic morphology, and transmission electron microscopy of the epithelium demonstrates the presence of numerous dendritiform cells with long processes interdigitating among the corneal epithelial cells, containing the LC-specific Birbeck granules.

In addition to murine data, recent in vivo data in humans, studying 112 healthy volunteers by in vivo confocal microscopy, have confirmed the presence of LCs in the central human cornea [45]. In 30 of these volunteers, LCs were found in both the central and peripheral corneal epithelium. In the periphery of the cornea, LC density was 98 ± 8 LCs/mm^2 compared to 34 ± 3 LCs/mm^2 in the central cornea. LCs are located at a depth of 35–60 μm, mostly at the level of basal epithelial cells and the subbasal nerve plexus [45].

Corneal Stromal Dendritic Cells

Examination of the corneal stroma for APCs has been performed by several laboratories [17, 46–50]. In the initial studies by Hamrah et al. [46], murine corneas were deprived of their epithelium, stained with a series of antibodies, and studied with confocal microscopy. Staining revealed the presence of significant numbers of CD45+ CD11c+ CD11b+ CD8α– DCs in the periphery and center of the anterior stroma, therefore demonstrating myeloid DCs from a monocytic lineage. Further staining demonstrated that a population of these stromal DCs was MHC class II positive and further positive for co-stimulatory markers CD80, CD86, and CD40 in the periphery of the normal corneal stroma. The stromal center however contained *exclusively* MHC class II-negative CD80– CD86– DCs, similar to findings of the highly immature LCs in the epithelium. These ex vivo studies have further been confirmed by in vitro data by flow cytometry and immunocytochemistry.

Additional evidence for the presence of DCs in the corneal stroma has recently been demonstrated by Nakamura et al. [47] through the use of BM transplantation studies. Intravenous transplantation of BM cells and BM-derived hematopoietic stem/progenitor cells from enhanced green fluorescent protein (GFP) transgenic mice was performed into irradiated wild-type C57BL/6 mice, and the corneas were examined 4–6 months after transplantation by immunohistochemistry. GFP-positive cells gradually migrate into the cornea as soon as 2 weeks after transplantation, with distribution in the entire cornea at 2–6 months. Around 27% of all BM-derived cells in the peripheral cornea are GFP positive, while around 8% are GFP positive in the center of the corneal stroma. Between 19 and 36% of GFP-positive cells are CD11c+ in the periphery, while 15–41% are CD11c+ in the central cornea, depending on transplantation of BM cells or BM-derived hematopoietic stem/progenitor cells [47].

What is unique to the DCs of the *central* cornea is that they are universally MHC class II negative and co-stimulatory factor (CD40, CD80, CD86) negative and hence incapable of T cell priming. While highly immature APC populations have been identified in lymphoid organs and blood [7, 34, 51], no other tissue is replete with *universally* MHC class II-negative DCs.

Dendritic Cell Precursors

Most studies suggest that in addition to the immature DCs, proliferating stem cells also give rise to two types of non-proliferating DC precursors in the blood, monocytes (pre-DC1) and plasmacytoid cells (pre-DC2). During hematopoiesis, DC precursors seed lymphoid and nonlymphoid tissue as immature myeloid monocytic DCs or lymphoid DCs, respectively [24, 31, 51]. These DC precursors display many different properties. In the mouse, monocytic DC precursors express the myeloid antigens CD11b and CD11c, while lymphoid DC precursors express CD8α and CD11c, and are negative for CD11b [52]. Further, corneas that are stained for CD14, an 'immature' or precursor-type cell surface marker associated with undifferentiated DCs and other cells of the myeloid lineage, demonstrate high numbers of CD14-expressing cells in the stroma [46]. These represent a population distinct from the CD11c+ DCs described above, which are $CD14^{lo/-}$. The corneal CD14+ cells, similar to the resident DCs, are further negative for MHC class II, B7, CD40, GR-1, and CD3, and the number of CD14+ cells is by far larger than the number of CD11c+ or CD11b+ cells, indicating that the large number of CD14+ cells represent a population of undifferentiated monocytic precursor cells distinct from DC and macrophage populations [46, 53]. The presence of an undifferentiated precursor DC would be similar to the finding of DC precursors in the central nervous system [54], where these cells can be skewed toward an either DC- or macrophage-like profile in response to different factors. Thus, in contrast to other organs, where terminally differentiated populations of resident DCs and/or macrophages outnumber colonizing precursors, large numbers of DCs within the cornea remain in an undifferentiated state.

Macrophages

Macrophages are BM-derived monocytic cells that reside in virtually every tissue. They are integral to the innate immune response because of their phagocytosis of foreign material, expression of a variety of surface receptors specific for pathogens or antigens, and secretion of pro-inflammatory cytokines [55–57]. Macrophages develop from myeloid progenitor cells, enter the bloodstream as monocytes, and migrate into tissues as macrophages. Their expression of (relative to DCs, low) levels of MHC class II and co-stimulatory molecules enables them to act as APCs, albeit much less efficiently than DCs [22]. In addition, resident tissue macrophages are in general poorly responsive to activation signals [58]. Macrophages also play a role in other processes including immune regulation and suppression, tissue reorganization, and angiogenesis [59].

Until recently, resident macrophages of the ocular surface were thought to reside in the conjunctiva and limbus only [60, 61]. Recently however, resident tissue macrophages have been found by confocal microscopy in normal mouse corneas [17, 19, 46]. These macrophages are CD11c– CD11b+ cells, and are present primarily in the posterior stroma of normal cornea, and are distinct from the DCs described in the anterior stroma. Resident stromal macrophages may provide a critical first-line defense against pathogens that breach the epithelial barrier of the cornea by producing antimicrobial substances, as well as other inflammatory cytokines and chemokines to attract and activate additional macrophages, neutrophils, and DCs.

Antigen-Presenting Cells in Inflammation and Immunity

The questions arises as to whether the phenotype of corneal APCs (both those that normally reside in the cornea and those that are recruited there from the limbus) changes during inflammation. Experiments have demonstrated that a subset of resident MHC class II-negative epithelial LCs [18] and stromal DCs [17] in the center of the cornea can significantly upregulate the expression of this marker already 24 h after induction of inflammation by application of electric cautery to the central epithelium. In addition, during inflammation, the surface expression of B7 co-stimulatory molecules, CD80 and CD86 (critical for providing T cells with the 'second' activation signal), as well as CD40 is similarly increased by both peripheral corneal DCs/LCs, as well as acquired de novo by DCs/LCs in the central areas of the corneal stroma and epithelium [17, 18, 53].

The acquisition of these maturation markers by resident corneal DCs is perhaps best shown in the corneal transplantation model because the MHC of the host and donor tissues can be readily distinguished [17, 18, 53]. Staining for donor-type MHC class II of C57BL/6 mice (Ia^b) at different time points after corneal transplantation into BALB/c (Ia^d) recipients shows that the resident DCs in the donor button of the grafted corneas are MHC class II negative 12 h after surgery. While donor corneas do not stain for MHC class II immediately after grafting, by 24 h after transplantation, novel donor class II (Ia^b) expression can be detected close to the graft-host junction [17]. At the early time points, when no staining for donor MHC class II is detected, a centrifugal migration of MHC class II-negative DCs toward the graft-host border is seen. Most likely, release of pro-inflammatory cytokines, such as interleukin (IL)-1, granulocyte-macrophage colony stimulating factor, tumor necrosis factor (TNF)-α, CD40L and lipopolysaccharide, or heat-shock protein from dying cells, creates a microenvironment that activates immature APCs [62–65]. DCs themselves are also important producers of type 1 interferons, TNF-α, and IL-1β, which can act in an autocrine fashion to promote their activation and maturation [29].

In addition to the resident APC population, APCs are also recruited into the cornea from the limbal area. Studies by Dana et al. [66–68] and others [69–73] have shown that cornea-expressed IL-1 and TNF-α are upregulated after inflammation and induce migration of DCs, including LCs, into the cornea; conversely, suppression of IL-1 and TNF-α downmodulated DC/LC migration into the cornea and reestablished immune privilege in the anterior eye.

In addition to corneal DCs, corneal epithelium [74, 75], corneal keratocytes [76, 77], vascular endothelial cells [78], and macrophages may express MHC class II under conditions of inflammation. These cells may acquire the ability to present antigen and amplify immune responses [77]. Recent evidence further suggests that recruitment of macrophages into the cornea could play a crucial role in inducing inflammatory neovascularization by supplying/amplifying signals essential for pathological hemangiogenesis and lymphangiogenesis [79]. Moreover, corneal macrophages have been shown to be able to form tube-like structures during inflammation, which express markers for lymphatic vessels, indicating an important role in corneal lymphangiogenesis [80].

Antigen-Presenting Cell Trafficking and Their Role in Corneal Transplantation

Migration to Draining Lymph Nodes

Solid organ grafts (e.g. the heart, kidney, and skin) are significantly endowed with MHC class II-positive DCs, capable of migrating to host lymphoid organs and stimulating T cells directly by presenting donor-derived peptides in the context of donor MHC class II [24, 26, 81, 82]. To demonstrate the functional capacity of corneal DCs as APCs, transgenic GFP or C57BL/6 (Ia^b) mice were transplanted into BALB/c (Ia^d) hosts [20]. Initial evaluation of corneal specimens was performed at various time points after surgery to examine whether GFP-positive cells could be seen emigrating out of the grafts. As soon as 24 h after transplantation, GFP-positive cells migrate centrifugally out into the wild-type recipient beds. Lymph nodes that were harvested at various time points after corneal transplantation and examined under confocal microscopy for detection, localization, and quantification of GFP-positive cells demonstrate that there is ample traffic of donor MHC class II-positive cells to draining lymph nodes after corneal transplantation and that these donor MHC class II-positive cells co-localize strongly with GFP expression [20].

Initial clues as to the functional relevance of this traffic came when Yamagami et al. [83] and Yamagami and Dana [84] demonstrated that disruption of the eye-lymph node axis, through surgical cervical lymphadenectomy, leads to both complete abrogation of host allosensitization as well as to universal and indefinite allograft survival. These recent findings suggest that the tenet of antigenic sequestration, as it applies to the cornea, is at best a relative, and not an absolute concept, since donor cells and antigens clearly are capable of having ample access to host lymphoid tissues and in fact lead to a chimeric state as has been described for other solid organ grafts [26].

The Role of Vascular Endothelial Growth Factor Receptor-3

The data summarized above suggest that corneal APCs are capable of trafficking relatively efficiently to lymphoid organs. How does this occur? First, although the cornea is free of lymphatics, lymphatic vessels readily grow into the cornea upon significant inflammatory stimulation [85, 86]. Moreover, the conjunctiva is rich in lymphatics, and corneal APCs may readily gain access to lymphatics upon (centrifugal) migration into the limbus. Finally, it was recently determined that the same molecular mechanisms that regulate corneal *lymphangiogenesis* also mediate APC trafficking into afferent lymphatics [87–90]. This signaling is mediated by vascular endothelial growth factor receptor (VEGFR)-3 (flt-4), a receptor that is distinct from VEGFR-1 (flt-1) and VEGFR-2 (flt-2 or kdr) that regulate hemangiogenesis [91, 92]. The ligands to VEGFR-3 are VEGF-C and VEGF-D, both of which can serve as growth factors for lymphatic endothelium [93–95], and can hence result in lymphangiogenesis.

Hamrah et al. [89] recently demonstrated that VEGFR-3 overexpression by endothelial cells in response to inflammation is also accompanied by increased surface expression of VEGFR-3 by mature (but not immature) corneal DCs. Further, while VEGFR-3+ DCs in normal corneas are VEGF-C–, they express VEGF-C after induction of inflammation [89]. In corneal inflammation, the DCs/APCs that congregate around the budding lymphatics are almost all VEGFR-3+, suggesting that they may respond to the same signals (e.g. VEGF-C) that induce lymphatic growth into the cornea [88].

More recently, the functionality of VEGFR-3 by corneal DCs has been demonstrated by Chen et al. [90], through demonstration of a dose-dependent chemotactic response of corneal DCs to VEGF-C. Further, it was possible to block this chemotaxis by a VEGFR-3/immunoglobulin chimeric molecule [90]. Moreover, it was demonstrated that by blocking *local* VEGFR-3 signaling, the migration of corneal APCs to regional draining lymph nodes is profoundly suppressed. The abolished APC trafficking through blockade of VEGFR-3 after corneal transplantation diminishes the induction of allospecific delayed-type hypersensitivity significantly and leads to a significant reduction in the rate of graft rejection [90]. This functional effect of VEGFR-3 antagonism as a non-surgical strategy, targeting lymphatic drainage, has been termed 'molecular lymphadenectomy'.

Direct versus Indirect Pathway of Sensitization

The functional relevance of the graft-derived cells in mediating allorejection (and breaking the normal tolerance generated to corneal grafts) has recently been elucidated. Data by Huq et al. [96] have demonstrated that in high-risk corneal transplantation, but *not* in low-risk grafting, there is significant induction of IL-2- and interferon-γ-secreting *directly* primed CD4+ T cells well before the onset of clinical rejection, as measured in enzyme-linked immunosorbent spot assays. In addition, when the direct pathway is blocked using class II knockout donors, the frequency of rejection in high-risk (but not low-risk) grafts is significantly dampened, reflecting the role of the graft-derived APCs in mediating direct sensitization. However, blockade of the direct pathway still led to rejection rates that were higher than what is normally seen in low-risk transplants (reliant on the indirect pathway alone), emphasizing the dominant role played by the *indirect pathway* of sensitization in both the high-risk and low-risk settings [97]. Therefore, in settings of ample inflammation, corneal APCs acquire significant T cell-stimulatory capacity as they abrogate the normal tolerogenic milieu of the ocular compartment.

Implications and Future Directions

The constitutive presence of APCs, including DCs, in the cornea has important implications for a variety of pathological and immunoinflammatory responses in the ocular anterior segment, including alloimmune, autoimmune, and innate immune responses. Importantly, the recent findings focus attention on the cornea itself as a participant in immune and inflammatory responses, rather than it simply serving as a passive tissue that responds to the activity of infiltrating cells.

Many questions remain unanswered. What is the constitutive role of corneal APCs in maintaining tolerance? What factors of the ocular microenvironment promote or actively maintain their highly immature phenotype? What is the role of the resident BM-derived cells in mediating wound healing and regulating matrix-keratocyte interactions? There is little doubt that a better understanding of these issues could shed important insights into tolerance induction, autoimmunity, and allergy to name a few.

References

1 Langerhans P: Über die Nerven der menschlichen Haut. Virchows Arch Pathol Anat Physiol 1868;44:325–337.
2 Silberberg I: Apposition of mononuclear cells to Langerhans cells in contact allergic reactions. An ultrastructural study. Acta Derm Venereol 1973;53:1–12.
3 Engelmann TW: Über die Hornhaut des Auges. Leipzig, Universität Leipzig, 1867.
4 Ranvier L: Cornée; in Ranvier L (ed): Leçons d'anatomie générale faites au Collège de France. Paris, Baillière, 1881, pp 1878–1879.
5 Egorow I: Nervenelemente der Cornea im Meerschweinchenauge. Graefes Arch Ophthalmol 1934;131:531–553.
6 Liu, YJ: Dendritic cell subsets and lineages, and their functions in innate and adaptive immunity. Cell 2001;106:259–262.
7 Banchereau J, Briere F, Caux C, Davoust J, Lebecque S, Liu YJ, Pulendran B, Palucka K: Immunobiology of dendritic cells. Annu Rev Immunol 2000;18:767–811.
8 Gillette TE, Chandler JW, Greiner JV: Langerhans cells of the ocular surface. Ophthalmology 1982;89:700–711.
9 Jager MJ: Corneal Langerhans cells and ocular immunology. Reg Immunol 1992;4:186–195.
10 Peeler JS, Niederkorn JY: Antigen presentation by Langerhans cells in vivo: donor-derived Ia^+ Langerhans cells are required for induction of delayed-type hypersensitivity but not for cytotoxic T lymphocyte responses to alloantigens. J Immunol 1986;136:4362–4371.
11 Rowden G: Expression of Ia antigens on Langerhans cells in mice, guinea pigs, and man. J Invest Dermatol 1980;75:22–31.
12 Streilein JW, Toews GB, Bergstresser PR: Corneal allografts fail to express Ia antigens. Nature 1979;282:320–321.
13 Streilein JW: Regional immunity and ocular immune privilege; in Streilein JW (ed): Immune Response and the Eye. Chem Immunol Basel, Karger, 1999, vol 73, pp 11–38.
14 Pepose JS, Gardner KM, Nestor MS, Foos RY, Pettit TH: Detection of HLA class I and II antigens in rejected human corneal allografts. Ophthalmology 1985;92:1480–1484.
15 Rocha G, Deschênes J, Rowsey JJ: The immunology of corneal graft rejection. Crit Rev Immunol 1998;18:305–325.
16 Haftek M, Faure M, Schmitt D, Thivolet J: Langerhans cells in skin from patients with psoriasis: quantitative and qualitative study of T6 and HLA-DR antigen-expressing cells and changes with aromatic retinoid administration. J Invest Dermatol 1983;81:10–14.
17 Hamrah P, Liu Y, Zhang Q, Dana MR: Alterations in corneal stromal dendritic cell phenotype and distribution in inflammation. Arch Ophthalmol 2003;121:1132–1140.
18 Hamrah P, Zhang Q, Liu Y, Dana MR: Novel characterization of MHC class II-negative population of resident corneal Langerhans cell-type dendritic cells. Invest Ophthalmol Vis Sci 2002;43: 639–646.
19 Brissette-Storkus CS, Reynolds SM, Lepisto AJ, Hendricks RL: Identification of a novel macrophage population in the normal mouse corneal stroma. Invest Ophthalmol Vis Sci 2002;43: 2264–2271.
20 Liu Y, Hamrah P, Zhang Q, Taylor AW, Dana MR: Draining lymph nodes of corneal transplant hosts exhibit evidence for donor major histocompatibility complex (MHC) class II-positive dendritic cells derived from MHC class II-negative grafts. J Exp Med 2002;195:259–268.
21 Steinman RM, Cohn ZA: Identification of a novel cell type in peripheral lymphoid organs of mice. I. Morphology, quantitation, tissue distribution. J Exp Med 1973;137:1142–1162.
22 Steinman RM: The dendritic cell system and its role in immunogenicity. Annu Rev Immunol 1991;9:271–296.
23 Hart DNJ: Dendritic cells: unique leukocyte populations which control the primary immune response. Blood 1997;90:3245–3287.
24 Banchereau J, Steinman RM: Dendritic cells and the control of immunity. Nature 1998;392:245–252.
25 Lanzavecchia A, Sallusto F: The instructive role of dendritic cells on T cell responses: lineages, plasticity and kinetics. Curr Opin Immunol 2001;13:291–298.
26 Thomson AW, Lu L, Murase N, Demetris AJ, Rao AS, Starzl TE: Microchimerism, dendritic cell progenitors and transplantation tolerance. Stem Cells 1995;13:622–639.

27 Thomson AW, Lu L: Dendritic cells as regulators of immune reactivity: implications for transplantation. Transplantation 1999;68:1–8.
28 Steinman RM, Nussenzweig MC: Avoiding horror autotoxicus: the importance of dendritic cells in peripheral T cell tolerance. Proc Natl Acad Sci USA 2002;99:351–358.
29 Rescigno M, Borrow P: The host-pathogen interaction: new themes from dendritic cell biology. Cell 2001;106:267–270.
30 Palucka K, Banchereau J: How dendritic cells and microbes interact to elicit or subvert protective immune responses. Curr Opin Immunol 2002;14:420–431.
31 Liu YJ, Kanzler H, Soumelis V, Gilliet M: Dendritic cell lineage, plasticity and cross-regulation. Nat Immunol 2001;2:585–589.
32 Cella M, Sallusto F, Lanzavecchia A: Origin, maturation and antigen presentation function of dendritic cells. Curr Opin Immunol 1997;9:10–16.
33 Austyn JM: New insights into the mobilization and phagocytic activity of dendritic cells. J Exp Med 1996;183:1287–1292.
34 Austyn JM, Hankins DF, Larsen CP, Morris PJ, Rao AS, Roake JA: Isolation and characterization of dendritic cells from mouse heart and kidney. J Immunol 1994;152:2401–2410.
35 Larsen CP, Ritchie SC, Hendrix R, Lindsey PS, Hathcock KS, Hodes RJ, Lowry RP, Pearson TC: Regulation of immunostimulatory function and costimulatory molecule (B7-1 and B7-2) expression on murine dendritic cells. J Immunol 1994;152:5208–5219.
36 Mellman I, Steinman RM: Dendritic cells: specialized and regulated antigen processing machines. Cell 2001;106:255–258.
37 Dana MR, Streilein JW: Loss and restoration of immune privilege in eyes with corneal neovascularization. Invest Ophthalmol Vis Sci 1996;37:2485–2494.
38 Jager MJ, Atherton SS, Bradley D, Streilein JW: Herpetic stromal keratitis in mice: less reversibility in the presence of Langerhans cells in the central cornea. Curr Eye Res 1991;10:69–73.
39 McLeish W, Rubsamen P, Atherton SS, et al: Immunobiology of Langerhans cells on the ocular surface. II. Role of central corneal Langerhans cells in stromal keratitis following experimental HSV-1 infection in mice. Reg Immunol 1989;2:236–243.
40 Hazlett LD: Pathogenic mechanisms of P. aeruginosa keratitis: a review of the role of T cells, Langerhans cells, PMN, and cytokines. DNA Cell Biol 2002;21:383–390.
41 Niederkorn JY: The immune privilege of corneal allografts. Transplantation 1999;67: 1503–1508.
42 Niederkorn JY, Peeler JS, Ross J, Callanan D: The immunogenic privilege of corneal allografts. Reg Immunol 1989;2:117–124.
43 Streilein JW: Immunobiology and immunopathology of corneal transplantation; in Streilein JW (ed): Immune Response and the Eye. Chem Immunol. Basel, Karger, 1999, vol 73, pp 186–206.
44 Klareskog L, Forsum U, Malmnäs T, Rask L, Peterson PA: Expression of Ia antigen-like molecules on cells in the corneal epithelium. Invest Ophthalmol Vis Sci 1979;18:310–313.
45 Zhivov A, Stave J, Vollmar B, Guthoff R: In vivo confocal microscopic evaluation of Langerhans cell density and distribution in the normal human corneal epithelium. Graefes Arch Clin Exp Ophthalmol 2005;243:1056–1061.
46 Hamrah P, Liu Y, Zhang Q, Dana MR: The corneal stroma is endowed with significant numbers of resident dendritic cells. Invest Ophthalmol Vis Sci 2003;44:581–589.
47 Nakamura T, Ishikawa F, Sonoda KH, Hisatomi T, Qiao H, Yamada J, Fukata M, Ishibashi T, Harada M, Kinoshita S: Characterization and distribution of bone marrow-derived cells in the mouse cornea. Invest Ophthalmol Vis Sci 2005;46:497–503.
48 Dana MR: Corneal antigen-presenting cells: diversity, plasticity and disguise: the Cogan lecture. Invest Ophthalmol Vis Sci 2004;45:722–727.
49 Novak N, Siepmann K, Zierhut M, Bieber T: The good, the bad and the ugly – APCs of the eye. Trends Immunol 2003;24:570–574.
50 Streilein JW: Ocular immune privilege: therapeutic opportunities from an experiment of nature. Nat Rev Immunol 2004;3:879–889.
51 Inaba K, Steinman RM, Witmer Pack M, Aya H, Inaba M, Sudo T, Wolpe S, Schuler G: Identification of proliferating dendritic cell precursors in mouse blood. J Exp Med 1992;175: 1157–1167.

52 O'Keeffe M, Hochrein H, Vremec D, Scott B, Hertzog P, Tatarczuch L, Shortman K: Dendritic cell precursor populations of mouse blood: identification of the murine homologues of human blood plasmacytoid pre-DC2 and $CD11c^{+}$ DC1 precursors. Blood 2003;101:1453–1459, erratum 2003;101:3364.
53 Hamrah P, Huq SO, Liu Y, Zhang Q, Dana MR: Corneal immunity is mediated by heterogeneous population of antigen-presenting cells. J Leukoc Biol 2003;74:172–178.
54 Santambrogio L, Belyanskaya SL, Fischer FR, Cipriani B, Brosnan CF, Ricciardi-Castagnoli P, Stern LJ, Strominger JL, Riese R: Developmental plasticity of CNS microglia. Proc Natl Acad Sci USA 2001;98:6295–6300.
55 McKnight AJ, Gordon S: Membrane molecules as differentiation antigens of murine macrophages. Adv Immunol 1998;68:271–314.
56 Morrissette N, Gold E, Aderm A: The macrophage: a cell for all seasons. Trends Cell Biol 1999;9: 199–201.
57 van Rooijen N, Wijburg OL, van den Dobbelsteen GP, Sanders A: Macrophages in host defense mechanisms. Curr Top Microbiol Immunol 1996;210:159–165.
58 Unanue ER: Antigen-presenting function of the macrophage. Annu Rev Immunol 1984;2:395–428.
59 Adams DO: Macrophage activation; in Roitt IM, Delves PJ (eds): Encyclopedia of Immunology. London, Academic Press, 1992, pp 1020–1026.
60 Hingorani M, Metz D, Lightman SL: Characterization of the normal conjunctival leukocyte population. Exp Eye Res 1997;64:905–912.
61 Sacks E, Rutgers J, Jakobiec FA, Bonetti F, Knowles DM: A comparison of conjunctival and nonocular dendritic cells utilizing new monoclonal antibodies. Ophthalmology 1986;93: 1089–1097.
62 Caux C, Dezutter-Dambuyant C, Schmidt D, Banchereau J: GM-CSF and TNF-α cooperate in the generation of dendritic Langerhans cells. Nature 1992;360:258–261.
63 Cumberbatch M, Dearman RJ, Kimber I: Langerhans cells require signals from both tumor necrosis factor-α and interleukin-1β for migration. Immunology 1997;92:388–395.
64 Reis e Sousa C: Dendritic cells as sensors of infection. Immunity 2001;14:495–498.
65 Srivastava P: Interaction of heat shock proteins with peptides and antigen presenting cells: chaperoning of the innate and adaptive immune responses. Annu Rev Immunol 2002;20:395–425.
66 Dana MR, Yamada J, Streilein JW: Topical interleukin 1 receptor antagonist promotes corneal transplant survival. Transplantation 1997;63:1501–1507.
67 Dana MR, Dai R, Zhu SN, Yamada J, Streilein JW: Interleukin-1 receptor antagonist suppresses Langerhans cell activity and promotes ocular immune privilege. Invest Ophthalmol Vis Sci 1998;39:70–77.
68 Dana MR, Zhu SN, Yamada J: Topical modulation of interleukin-1 activity in corneal neovascularization. Cornea 1998;17:403–409.
69 Dekaris I, Yamada J, Streilein JW, Dana MR: Effect of topical interleukin-1 receptor antagonist (IL-1ra) on corneal allograft transplant survival in presensitized hosts. Curr Eye Res 1999;19: 456–459.
70 Dekaris I, Zhu SN, Dana MR: TNF-α regulates corneal Langerhans cell migration. J Immunol 1999;162:4235–4239.
71 Qian Y, Dekaris I, Yamagami S, Dana MR: Topical soluble tumor necrosis factor receptor type I suppresses ocular chemokine gene expression and rejection of allogeneic corneal transplants. Arch Ophthalmol 2000;118:1666–1671.
72 Yamada J, Dana MR, Zhu SN, Alard P, Streilein JW: Interleukin 1 receptor antagonist suppresses allosensitization in corneal transplantation. Arch Ophthalmol 1998;116:1351–1357.
73 Zhu S, Dekaris I, Duncker G, Dana MR: Early expression of proinflammatory cytokines interleukin-1 and tumor necrosis factor-alpha after corneal transplantation. J. Interferon Cytokine Res 1999;19:661–669.
74 Iwata M, Kiritoshi A, Roat MI, Yagihashi A, Thoft RA: Regulation of HLA class II antigen expression on cultured corneal epithelium by interferon-gamma. Invest Ophthalmol Vis Sci 1992;33:2714–2721.
75 Dreizen NG, Whitsett CF, Stulting RD: Modulation of HLA antigen expression on corneal epithelial and stromal cells. InvestOphthalmol Vis Sci 1988;29:933–939.
76 Young E, Stark WJ, Prendergast RA: Immunology of corneal allograft rejection: HLA-DR antigens on human corneal cells. Invest Ophthalmol Vis Sci 1985;26:571–574.

77 Seo SK, Gebhardt BM, Lim HY, Kang SW, Higaki S, Varnell ED, Hill JM, Kaufman HE, Kwon BS: Murine keratocytes function as antigen-presenting cells. Eur J Immunol 2001;31: 3318–3328.
78 Gerritsen M: Cytokine activation of human macro- and microvessel-derived endothelial cells. Blood Cells 1993;19:325.
79 Cursiefen C, Chen L, Borges LP, Jackson D, Cao J, Radziejewski C, D'Amore PA, Dana MR, Wiegand SJ, Streilein JW: VEGF-A stimulates lymphangiogenesis and hemangiogenesis in inflammatory neovascularization via macrophage recruitment. J Clin Invest 2004;113: 1040–1050.
80 Maruyama K, Ii M, Cursiefen C, Jackson DG, Keino H, Tomita M, Van Rooijen N, Takenaka H, D'Amore PA, Stein-Streilein, J, Losordo DW, Streilein JW: Inflammation-induced lymphangiogenesis in the cornea arises from CD11b-positive macrophages. J Clin Invest 2005;115: 2363–2372.
81 Austyn JM, Larsen CP: Migration patterns of dendritic leukocytes. Implications for transplantation. Transplantation 1990;49:1–7.
82 Roake JA, Rao AS, Morris PJ, Larsen CP, Hankins DF, Austyn JM: Systemic lipopolysaccharide recruits dendritic cell progenitors to nonlymphoid tissues. Transplantation 1995;59:1319–1324.
83 Yamagami S, Dana MR, Tsuru T: Draining lymph nodes play an essential role in alloimmunity generated in response to high-risk corneal transplantation. Cornea 2002;21:405–409.
84 Yamagami S, Dana MR: The critical role of draining lymph nodes in corneal allosensitization. Invest Ophthalmol Vis Sci 2001;42:1293–1298.
85 Collin HB: Corneal lymphatics in alloxan vascularized rabbit eyes. Invest Ophthalmol Vis Sci 1966;5:1–13.
86 Collin HB: Lymphatic drainage of ^{131}I-albumin from the vascularized cornea. Invest Ophthalmol Vis Sci 1970;9:146–155.
87 Hamrah P, Zhang Q, Dana MR: Expression of vascular endothelial growth factor receptor-3 (VEGFR-3) in the conjunctiva – a potential link between lymphangiogenesis and leukocyte trafficking on the ocular surface. Adv Exp Med Biol 2002;506:851–858.
88 Hamrah P, Chen L, Cursiefen C, Zhang Q, Joyce NC, Dana MR: Expression of vascular endothelial growth factor receptor-3 (VEGFR-3) on monocytic bone marrow-derived cells in the conjunctiva. Exp Eye Res 2004;79:553–561.
89 Hamrah P, Chen L, Zhang Q, Dana MR: Novel expression of vascular endothelial growth factor receptor (VEGFR)-3 and VEGF-C on dendritic cells in the cornea. Am J Pathol 2003;163:57–68.
90 Chen L, Hamrah P, Cursiefen C, Zhang Q, Pytowski B, Streilein JW, Dana MR: Vascular endothelial growth factor receptor-3 mediates induction of corneal alloimmunity. Nat Med 2004;10: 813–815.
91 Jussila L, Alitalo K: Vascular growth factors and lymphangiogenesis. Physiol Rev 2002;82: 673–700.
92 Veikkola T, Alitalo K: VEGFs, receptors and angiogenesis. Semin Cancer Biol 1999;9:211–220.
93 Joukov V, Pajusola K, Kaipainen A, Chilov D, Lahtinen I, Kukk E, Saksela O, Kalkkinen N, Alitalo K: A novel vascular endothelial growth factor, VEGF-C, is a ligand for the FLT4 (VEGFR-3) and KDR (VEGFR-2) receptor tyrosine kinases. EMBO J 1996;15:290–298.
94 Achen MG, Jeltsch M, Kukk E, Mäkinen T, Vitali A, Wilks AF, Alitalo K, Stacker SA: Vascular endothelial growth factor D (VEGF-D) is a ligand for the tyrosine kinases VEGF receptor 2 (Flk1) and VEGF receptor 3 (Flt4). Proc Natl Acad Sci USA 1998;95:548–553.
95 Kukk E, Lymboussaki A, Taira S, Kaipainen A, Jeltsch M, Joukov V, Alitalo K: VEGF-C receptor binding and pattern of expression with VEGFR-3 suggests a role in lymphatic vascular development. Development 1996;122:3829–3837.
96 Huq S, Liu Y, Benichou G, Dana MR: Relevance of the direct pathway of sensitization in corneal transplantation is dictated by the graft bed microenvironment. J Immunol 2004;173:4464–4469.
97 Boisgérault F, Liu Y, Anosova N, Ehrlich E, Dana MR, Benichou G: Role of $CD4^+$ and $CD8^+$ T cells in allorecognition. Lessons from corneal transplantation. J Immunol 2001;167:1891–1899.

Dr. Pedram Hamrah
Cornea Service, Mass. Eye and Ear Infirmary, Harvard Medical School
243 Charles Street, Boston, MA 02114 (USA)
Tel. +1 617 573 4300, Fax +1 617 573 4300, E-Mail pedram_hamrah@meei.harvard.edu

Niederkorn JY, Kaplan HJ (eds): Immune Response and the Eye.
Chem Immunol Allergy. Basel, Karger, 2007, vol 92, pp 71–85

Ocular Immunosuppressive Microenvironment

Andrew W. Taylor

Schepens Eye Research Institute, Harvard Medical School, Boston, Mass., USA

Abstract

Over the past 30 years, it has become evident that within the ocular microenvironment there are active mechanisms of immunoregulation and immunosuppression. The immunoregulation and immunosuppression are mediated by the constitutive presence of neuropeptides found in aqueous humor. Each of these immunosuppressive neuropeptides contributes in its own way to suppress induction of delayed-type hypersensitivity and to induce regulatory immunity. Collectively, the neuropeptides in aqueous humor suppress the activation of Th1 cells while promoting the induction of CD25+ CD4+ regulatory T cells. The central mediator of aqueous humor regulation of immunity is the neuropeptide α-melanocyte stimulating hormone (α-MSH). This ocular system of immunoregulation and immunosuppression through α-MSH not only suppresses immunogenic inflammation, but also actively manipulates immunity to make the immune response itself immunosuppressive.

Our initial criteria for calling a factor in the ocular microenvironment immunosuppressive were whether the factor suppressed the activation of Th1 cells and the induction of delayed-type hypersensitivity (DTH) [1–3]. This simple, but important, definition of the activity of ocular immunosuppressive factors has evolved into mediators of regulatory T (T_{reg}) cell activation, and regulators of the innate-adaptive immune interface. These factors are the molecular basis of immune privilege, and are the evolutionary adaptation that drives immunoregulation and immunosuppression in an active ocular system [4]. Other chapters in this volume describe the induction of a systemic immune response to antigen placed within the ocular microenvironment that leads to immune deviation; this chapter focuses on the mechanisms and the consequences by which efferent DTH immunity is suppressed within the ocular microenvironment.

Table 1. Major stages of DTH induction

APC processing and presentation of antigen (part of innate immunity)
Activation of Th1 cell proliferation and IFN-γ production
IFN-γ activation of macrophages
Macrophage production of inflammatory factors

Delayed-Type Hypersensitivity

There are several steps in the DTH response (table 1) that ultimately ends in a cytokine storm that manifests itself with the classical characteristics of inflammation (pain, heat, redness, and swelling), and if this happens in the eye, there is loss of vision and possible blindness. The initial steps involve tissue antigen-presenting cell (APC) processing, and presenting an antigen into the cleft of a type II major histocompatibility complex (MHC) molecule that is expressed on the surface of APC. The antigen presented is recognized by primed antigen-specific CD4+ T cells that express T-cell receptors that specifically recognize the antigen presented in the context of MHC class II [5]. The T cell and the APC then tightly bind to each other forming an immunological synapse [6]. Besides binding to their cognate antigen, the T cells also need additional second signals from the APC for activation. This second signal can come in the form of soluble factors or as adhesion molecules [7–11]. At this step, innate immunity, which is discussed later, has its greatest influence on the type of T-cell immunity activated. This second signal is less of a requirement for the activation of primed/memory T cells in the periphery than naive T-cell activation in the draining lymph nodes [12]. Following activation, the T cells enter the growth cycle, proliferate, and produce specific patterns of lymphokines. The T cells that mediate DTH, Th1 cells, are characterized by their lymphokine production of interferon-γ (IFN-γ) [13].

The IFN-γ produced by the Th1 cells activates macrophages and other cells in the surrounding tissue [14–16]. IFN-γ-activated macrophages begin to produce biochemical substances and other inflammatory cytokines of the cytokine storm and the observed inflammatory response. The inflammation associated with a DTH response often involves capillary break-down, fibrosis, and cell death [17–21]. There is also cellular proliferation and tissue remodeling especially upon resolution of inflammation through the mechanisms of wound repair [22]. Such tissue remodeling in the eye, a tissue that has limited regenerative potential and a dependence on a distinct structure for function, leads to loss of vision and potentially to blindness. It can be easily speculated that the evolutionary adaptation of immune privilege to suppress inflammatory immunity within the eye has a selective advantage [23].

Innate Immunity and T-Cell Activation in Delayed-Type Hypersensitivity

The accessory signals that promote the activation of DTH-mediating CD4+ T cells are from APC that are macrophages and dendritic cells, which are also effector cells of innate immunity [24]. They respond to pathogen-associated molecular patterns (PAMP), and specific intrinsic structures of bacteria, viruses, and fungi [25]. A family of Toll-like receptors (TLR) expressed by macrophages and dendritic cells bind specific PAMPs [24–26]. Depending on the PAMP and the TLR engaged, the macrophages and dendritic cells mediate specific inflammatory responses and stimulate specific effector functions of T cells [27, 28].

There are at least 11 TLR expressed on the surface and intercellular areas of macrophages and dendritic cells [29]. Each TLR has a defined set of PAMPs that they bind and initiate an intercellular signaling pathway that activates innate host defenses to fight off and clear the invading pathogens. The activation of DTH-mediating T cells is highly linked to the stimulation of TLR4 on APC [30]. TLR4 detects lipopolysaccharide (LPS) of Gram-negative bacteria [31]. Engagement of TLR4 with LPS along with several other soluble LPS-binding proteins promotes an intense inflammatory response that can lead to septic shock. It also induces macrophage and dendritic cell production of interleukin (IL)-12p70, which promotes activation of the DTH-mediating Th1 cells [30].

The intercellular signaling pathways initiated by TLR-4 involve the activation of the responsive element, common to all the TLRs, NF-κB, which mediates the activation of genes associated with inflammation, cytokines, nitric oxide synthase, reactive oxygen enzymes, and costimulatory molecules for T-cell activation [32]. In addition, TLR4 initiates a pathway shared with TLR3 (viral dsRNA detector), which activates IFN-responsive factor 3 [33], which in turn activates the promoter for type I IFN, IFN-β. In an autocrine manner, IFN-β induces IL-12p70 synthesis, which in turn promotes the activation of Th1 cells [34]. Therefore, it is possible to specifically regulate the type of adaptive immunity activated by APC (macrophages and dendritic cells) by regulating the innate immune response within the APC.

The Immunosuppressive Ocular Microenvironment

The remodeling that follows inflammation in tissues such as the skin is usually handled with complete recovery of the normal structure and cellular functions of the tissue; however, in the eye, cells rarely proliferate and the remodeling leads to an irreversible destruction of light gathering and neural signaling activities of the eye. To prevent the induction of immunogenic inflammation,

Table 2. The effects of aqueous humor on DTH induction

Suppresses innate immunity associated with Th1 cell activation
Suppresses activation of Th1 cell proliferation and IFN-γ production
Suppresses IFN-γ activation of macrophages
Promotes the activation of CD25+ CD4+ T_{reg} cells

the eye has evolutionarily adapted mechanisms of immune privilege to establish an immunosuppressive microenvironment protecting it from the induction of immunogenic inflammation and the subsequent remodeling [23].

The first example that the ocular microenvironment can manipulate immunity to antigen was demonstrated by Kaplan et al. [35] some 30 years ago. They demonstrated that immunity to an antigen placed into the eye initiates an immune response that was devoid of an immunogenic inflammatory response. They presented the possibility that the immune response to the antigen is manipulated within the ocular microenvironment. Later, Kaiser et al. [36] proposed that soluble immunosuppressive factors in aqueous humor, the fluid filling the anterior chamber of the eye, regulate immunity within the ocular microenvironment when they found that aqueous humor suppresses effector T-cell functions in vitro. Also, an efferent blockade of DTH within the anterior chamber of the eye was found by Niederkorn et al. [37]. Although placement of syngeneic tumor cells into the skin of alloantigen-immunized mice evokes a strong DTH response, placement of the tumor cells into the ocular anterior chamber of immunized mice elicited no DTH response. Recent evidence indicates that in healthy aqueous humor the ocular microenvironment constitutively expresses several soluble factors associated with the nervous system suppressing the activation of a DTH response [4].

Regulation of T-Cell Activity by Aqueous Humor

The presence of soluble immunosuppressive factors in healthy aqueous humor is demonstrated by decreased IFN-γ production in aqueous humor in vitro and reduced DTH-mediated activity in vivo by activated primed Th1 cells (table 2) [38, 39]. The aqueous humor-treated, activated, primed T cells produce less IFN-γ, IL-4, and IL-10, but abundant TGF-β_1, and they are able to proliferate [4]. These effector T cells cannot mediate DTH, even when they are transferred with antigen-pulsed APC into conventional immune tissues. Moreover, the aqueous-humor-induced, TGF-β-producing, T cells act as T_{reg} cells and suppress other

IFN-γ-producing T cells and DTH [40]. These aqueous-humor-induced T_{reg} cells suppress other cells through their production of TGF-β_1. Although this is a non-specific mechanism of suppression, the aqueous humor-induced T_{reg} cells require stimulation by their specific antigen to activate their suppressive activity [40]. These results show that the ocular microenvironment constitutively produces potent factors that do not only suppress expression of immunogenic inflammation, but also regionally coerces the immune system to respond in a manner that can be described as peripheral immune tolerance. Of the factors found in aqueous humor, TGF-β_2 and α-MSH account for the majority of aqueous humor suppression of DTH-mediating T cells and induction of T_{reg} cells [4].

In aqueous humor, the concentration of TGF-β_2 is between 1 and 10 ng/ml [1–3] and most (<10%) of the TGF-β_2 is in its latent form [41]. In healthy aqueous humor, only the TGF-β_2 isoform is expressed. This is interesting since mRNA for all three TGF-β isoforms is found in cells of the eye, but only the TGF-β_2 protein is found in aqueous humor of healthy eyes [1, 42, 43]. The isoform TGF-β_2 has also been found to be an important cytokine of other immune-privileged tissues that promote the induction of macrophages that mediate an anterior chamber-associated immune deviation (ACAID)-like immune response [44].

The effects of TGF-β_2 on APC stimulation of T cells is well documented in the ACAID literature; however, TGF-β_2 can influence APC activation of Th1 cells within the eye. TGF-β_2-treated APC are unable to activate DTH-mediating activity of T cells. The APC are impaired in their production of IL-12 and their expression of accessory signals of CD40 activation [45, 46]. The APC themselves produce TGF-β, which can directly affect T-cell activation. The TGF-β_2-treated macrophages are unable to secrete inflammatory cytokines or generate reactive oxygen intermediates making them unable to amplify the cytokine response and induce inflammation through innate immune mechanisms [47–49]. Therefore, the presence of TGF-β_2 within the ocular microenvironment alters APC (macrophages and dendritic cells) production and the expression of signals needed to activate DTH-mediating T cells, and may also prevent macrophages from being inflammatory effector cells in the DTH response.

Under serum-free culture conditions, aqueous humor does not suppress antigen-stimulated T-cell proliferation, but does suppress IFN-γ production and induces TGF-β_1 production by T cells [50]. This has been difficult to explain since TGF-β_2 treatment of cultured T cells suppresses T-cell proliferation [1], yet TGF-β_2 is normally latent in aqueous humor and needs to be activated [41]. This last finding suggests that the absence of serum proteases and cofactors [51, 52] in the serum-free conditions may slow the activation rate of TGF-β_2 to a level where it either has no affect or may regulate some other effector T-cell activity. However, TGF-β_2 contributes to aqueous humor induction of regulatory T cells [40]. Although TGF-β_2 alone is sufficient to induce T_{reg} cell activity in vitro, these T cells cannot function in vivo when adoptively transferred. The induction of T_{reg} cells by aqueous humor is dependent on the neuropeptide α-MSH, which is constitutively expressed in the immune-privileged ocular microenvironment [39, 53–55].

The neuropeptide α-MSH is a 13-amino-acid (1.6-kDa) polypeptide that is encoded within the pro-opiomelanocortin hormone (POMC) gene and is a proteolytic cleavage product of POMC [56, 57]. This neuropeptide has a fundamental role in modulating inflammatory responses in mammals by its ability to suppress innate immune-mediated inflammation and fever induced by endotoxin, IL-1, and TNF-α [58–62]. α-MSH suppresses activated macrophage generation of reactive oxygen intermediates and nitric oxide, and production of inflammatory cytokines, while they are enhanced in expressing α-MSH receptors, and producing IL-10 and more α-MSH and IL-10 [63–65]. The sources of α-MSH are centrally derived neurons, macrophages, keratinocytes, and possibly any other cell that can synthesize POMC and the specific endopeptidases that sequentially cleave POMC to α-MSH, which are expressed in the eye [63, 66–68]. There is a constitutive expression of α-MSH in healthy aqueous humor averaging 20 pM [39].

At its ocular physiological concentration, α-MSH suppresses IFN-γ production by antigen-stimulated primed T cells under serum-free conditions with no affect on proliferation [39]. Neutralization of α-MSH in whole aqueous humor also neutralizes the ability of aqueous humor to suppress IFN-γ production by the antigen-stimulated primed T cells [69]. These results further support the possibility that TGF-β_2 in aqueous humor affects T-cell activation other than suppressing proliferation. We have found that α-MSH treatment renders primed T cells resistant to the anti-proliferative activity of TGF-β_2 but not to TGF-β_1 [40].

Like whole aqueous humor, α-MSH-treated primed T cells activated by antigen-pulsed APC or with anti-T-cell-receptor antibody (anti-CD3) produce a cytokine profile that lacks IFN-γ, IL-4, and IL-10, but produces TGF-β_1 [54]. When transferred into cultures of activated Th1 cells, these T cells suppressed the production of IFN-γ by the activated Th1 cells, and this suppression can be blocked by neutralizing TGF-β_1. Moreover, α-MSH induction of these T_{reg} cells can be blocked using antibodies against the melanocortin 5 receptor (MC5r), which is the receptor for α-MSH on CD4 T cells [54]. Flow-cytometric analysis of α-MSH-treated, activated, primed T cells reveals that α-MSH induced a population of CD25+ CD4+ T_{reg} cells. These T_{reg} cells require antigen-specific reactivation of their suppressor activity, but, as described before, they are able to suppress other nearby T cells stimulated by a different antigen [54]. The ability of α-MSH to induce T_{reg} cells is enhanced by TGF-β_2 in aqueous humor [55]. When α-MSH-induced T_{reg} cells or T_{reg} cells generated with the combination of α-MSH and TGF-β_2 are made to a specific autoantigen of the eye, intraphotoreceptor retinoid binding protein, these T_{reg} cells can suppress experimental autoimmune uveitis even when a different retinal autoantigen is used to induce the disease [55]. Although TGF-β_2 can induce T_{reg} cells in vitro, it is α-MSH that mediates the induction of T_{reg} cells that function in vivo.

In the mouse model, α-MSH injection into uveitic eyes causes a rapid clearance of inflammation [53, 70–72]. Besides the possibility that α-MSH is suppressing T-cell-inflammatory activity, α-MSH may also suppress macrophage activity, and the interface between innate and adaptive immunity that drives the activation of DTH-mediating T cells. We have found that α-MSH suppression of LPS activation of macrophages is more distal to the LPS receptor TLR4 [73]. α-MSH stimulates the intracellular signaling inhibitor IRAK-M to bind IRAK-1 of the TLR4 intracellular signaling cascade. However, the mechanism by which α-MSH can mediate IRAK-M activity within the macrophage cytoplasm remains to be determined. The results of this effect of α-MSH on macrophages are quite clear. There is suppression of TLR4-mediated inflammatory activity in the macrophages, including suppression of IL-12p70 production. Also, there is no suppression of antigen presentation and T-cell activation by the macrophages except that the activated T cells do not produce IFN-γ [39]. Therefore, the ocular microenvironment constitutively contains one of the most potent anti-inflammatory neuropeptides, α-MSH, which, along with TGF-β_2, induces the activation of T_{reg} cells.

Other immunosuppressive neuropeptides that have been found in healthy aqueous humor include vasoactive intestinal peptide (VIP), calcitonin gene-related peptide (CGRP), and somatostatin (SOM) [74–76]. Immunohistochemical analysis shows that each of these neuropeptides is present in fibers innervating the eye [77–86]. Pro-SOM message has been found in the retina, suggesting that SOM is also a locally produced neuropeptide [87–91]. Unlike TGF-β_2 and α-MSH, the effects of these neuropeptides on primed T-cell activation do not mimic all the effects of aqueous humor. Each contributes, in part, to aqueous humor suppression of DTH-mediating T cells. Unlike whole aqueous humor, VIP at its aqueous humor concentration suppresses antigen-stimulated, primed T cell proliferation; however, VIP-induced suppression of T-cell proliferation is only 50% [76]. It has been suggested that VIP affects selective populations of T cells [92]. We find that CGRP targets macrophages responding to LPS by suppressing nitric oxide generation by the macrophages [74]. Antibody neutralization of CGRP in aqueous humor neutralizes some of the aqueous suppression of LPS-stimulated inflammatory activity in macrophages; however, CGRP suppresses TLR4 intracellular signaling at a level that is distal from where α-MSH suppresses TLR4 intracellular signals, and is separate from TLR4-mediated antigen-presenting activity in the macrophages [74]. Therefore, the role of CGRP in immune privilege is to regulate innate immunity. SOM induces the

Table 3. The 'incomplete' list of aqueous humor factors and their immunoregulatory and immunosuppressive activity

	Macrophage inflammatory activity (innate immunity)	APC activity	Th1 activity	Mediates activation of T_{reg} cells
TGF-β_2	S	A	S	yes[1]
α-MSH	S	A	S	yes
VIP	?	?	S	no
CGRP	S	N	N	no
SOM	N	A	S	yes[1]

S = Suppresses; N = no effect; ? = unknown; A = alters (APC do not stimulate Th1 cells).
[1] Via α-MSH.

activation of T_{reg} cells; however, this induction is mediated by SOM inducing α-MSH production by the activated primed T cells [75]. It is the autocrine effect of α-MSH induced by SOM that results in the activation of T_{reg} cells. Therefore, SOM contributes to the induction of antigen-specific T_{reg} cells, and further induces production of an immunosuppressive factor by immune cells themselves.

The presence of these immunosuppressive neuropeptides in aqueous humor is an indication of the importance of the nervous system in regulating immunity. These findings initially appear as what would be expected, redundancies in the mechanisms of immunosuppression. However, the dissimilar effects of each neuropeptide on immune cells suggests that the evolutionary adaptation of using the neuropeptides in immune privilege is to cover all levels of an immunogenic immune response from activation of innate immunity through Th1 cell activation and beyond (table 3). This is not only the suppression of immunogenic inflammation within the ocular microenvironment, but an active manipulation of immunity to make the immune response itself immunosuppressive.

The Immune Response within the Eye

The composite of immunoregulatory and immunosuppressive activity associated with the factors found in the eye suggests that if an efferent immune response occurs in the ocular microenvironment, the inflammatory response should be suppressed and regulatory immunity should emerge from this response. A method for initiating an efferent immune response within the eye is to use the experimental autoimmune uveoretinitis (EAU) disease model in mice [93]. Susceptible mouse strains do not spontaneously develop uveitis, but need to be immunized with human retinal autoantigens with an intense stimulation of innate immunity through Freund's complete adjuvant and sometimes with pertussis toxin. This results in the induction of primed Th1 cells that are specific for retinal autoantigen. These Th1 cells mediate autoimmune uveitis. Susceptible mouse strains recover from experimentally induced uveitis and do not spontaneously relapse with a second uveitic episode. This recovery is the result of the ocular microenvironment re-imposing immunoregulation and immunosuppression via the generation of MC5r (the α-MSH receptor on CD4+ T cells)-dependent, CD25+ CD4+ T_{reg} cells in the post-EAU spleen [94].

These CD25+ CD4+ T_{reg} cells are not found in naive mice or in the spleens of retinal autoantigen-immunized enucleated mice, indicating that it is the immune response in the ocular microenvironment and the ocular microenvironment itself that mediates their induction. The CD25+ CD4+ T_{reg} cells require activation by post-EAU splenic APC to mediate suppression [94]. These APC can be either macrophages or B cells found in the post-EAU spleen. Other APC from naive mice or from other tissues cannot stimulate regulatory activity in these T_{reg} cells. The presence of regulatory immunity-mediating APC suggests that ACAID has been induced. However, there are features about this post-EAU regulatory immunity that are different from the ACAID phenomenon. Unlike ACAID cells, the adoptive transfer of APC only [95, 96] or T_{reg} cells only [95, 96] does not transfer suppression. Only the transfer of APC and CD25+ CD4+ T_{reg} cells together or the transfer of only *restimulated* CD25+ CD4+ T_{reg} cells will transfer suppression of retinal inflammation in other mice immunized for EAU. In addition, in contrast to ACAID where CD4+ T_{reg} cells are afferent suppressors [97], the post-EAU CD25+ CD4+ T_{reg} cells suppress only efferent activity of the autoimmunity.

MC5r-knockout mice reveal the role of the ocular microenvironment in mediating the induction of post-EAU T_{reg} cells and their role in autoimmunity. In a soon to be published work, we have found that there is no regulatory immunity in the spleens of MC5r-knockout mice following an episode of EAU [98]. Such post-EAU mice when re-immunized with autoantigen have a rapid onset of uveitis that has a severity of inflammation that exceeds the initial episode of EAU, from simple infiltration and vasculitis to hemorrhage and retinal detachment. In comparison, re-immunized post-EAU wild-type mice have a delay of 7 days in the induction of the second episode of uveoretinitis, with the severity of inflammation not exceeding the first episode. The wild-type mice behaved as if they were naïve to the autoantigen. The adoptive transfer of spleen cells from post-EAU wild-type mice suppressed the severity of the uveoretinitis in the knockout mice, but not the onset of the second episode in the MC5r-knockout mice. These findings indicate that the ocular microenvironment, through the effects of α-MSH on the autoreactive primed T cells, contributes to the induction of T_{reg} cells that function to prevent the establishment of memory immune responses to ocular autoantigens. Therefore, an immune response within the ocular microenvironment influences systemic immunity by promoting antigen-specific immunological tolerance through CD25+ CD4+ T_{reg} cells.

Conclusions

The ocular microenvironment suppresses DTH through immunosuppressive factors constitutively produced and found in aqueous humor. Each of the immunosuppressive factors has its own distinct affects on APC, effector T cells, and inflammatory macrophages. Together they change the manner by which APC present antigen, suppress IFN-γ production by activated effector T cells, and inhibit inflammatory activity by macrophages, thus preventing the induction of immunogenic inflammation within the immune-privileged ocular microenvironment. This immunosuppressive activity is not only downregulatory, it is also promotes the induction of T_{reg} cells. These T_{reg} cells reinforce immune privilege by their ability to suppress immunity and to produce additional immunosuppressive factors into the ocular microenvironment. In addition, these induced T_{reg} cells help to maintain tolerance to ocular autoantigens and prevent induction of memory immunity to ocular autoantigens following autoimmune uveoretinitis.

Identifying factors that mediate suppression of immunogenic inflammation and induce T_{reg} cells should make it possible to treat uveitic eyes with the immunosuppressive factors to decrease inflammation, reestablish immune privilege, and induce tolerance to ocular antigens. The treatment could be accomplished through gene therapy [99–101]. Delivering vectors encoding aqueous humor immunosuppressive factors into the uveitic eye might result in sustained cytokine levels without repeated injections into the eye. The sustained production of the cytokines would suppress inflammation and re-establish immune privilege. It is possible that inducting the same ocular factors in transplanted tissues or in other inflamed tissue sites would also produce suppression of inflammation and tolerance to tissue antigens.

The ability of the ocular microenvironment to manipulate immune responses has implications about how immunity is regulated and how immune responses can be manipulated. The ocular microenvironment is an example of a tissue site that mediates the termination of inflammatory T-cell activity through specific neuropeptides. It is also a tissue site that uses the same anti-inflammatory neuropeptides to promote the development of T_{reg} cells. Since other tissues normally also express some of neuropeptides occurring in the eye, such as α-MSH in the skin [102, 103], our understanding of the role of neuropeptides in ocular immune privilege may suggest their systemic role in maintaining immunological and inflammatory homeostasis. Examination of the unique relationship between the ocular microenvironment, immune system, and the nervous system has not only given us insight into the mechanisms of immune privilege, but also paves the way for methods for regulating and tailoring an immune response in specific tissues and to specific antigens.

References

1 Cousins SW, McCabe MM, Danielpour D, Streilein JW: Identification of transforming growth factor-beta as an immunosuppressive factor in aqueous humor. Invest Ophthalmol Vis Sci 1991;32:33–43.

2 Jampel HD, Roche N, Stark WJ, Roberts AB: Transforming growth factor-β in human aqueous humor. Curr Eye Res 1990;9:963–969.

3 Granstein R, Staszewski R, Knisely TL, et al: Aqueous humor contains transforming growth factor-β and a small (<3500 daltons) inhibitor of thymocyte proliferation. J Immunol 1990;144:3021–3026.

4 Taylor A: A review of the influence of aqueous humor on immunity. Ocul Immunol Inflamm 2003;11:231–241.

5 Jorgensen JL, Reay PA, Ehrich EW, Davis MM: Molecular components of T-cell recognition. Annu Rev Immunol 1992;10:835–873.

6 Friedl P, Storim J: Diversity in immune-cell interactions: states and functions of the immunological synapse. Trends Cell Biol 2004;14:557–567.

7 Rosmarin D, Strober BE: The potential of interleukin 12 inhibition in the treatment of psoriasis. J Drugs Dermatol 2005;4:318–325.

8 Chen H, Hendricks RL: B7 costimulatory requirements of T cells at an inflammatory site. J Immunol 1998;160:5045–5052.

9 June CH, Bluestone JA, Nadler LM, Thompson CB: The B7 and CD28 receptor family. Immunol Today 1994;15:321–331.

10 Liu Y, Linsley PS: Costimulation of T-cell growth. Curr Opin Immunol 1992;4:265–270.

11 Lenschow DJ, Walunas TL, Bluestone JA: CD28/B7 system of T cell costimulation. Annu Rev Immunol 1996;14:233–258.

12 Dutton RW, Bradley LM, Swain SL: T cell memory. Annu Rev Immunol 1998;16:201–223.

13 Cher DJ, Mosmann TR: Two types of murine helper T cell clone. II. delayed-type hypersensitivity is mediated by Th1 clones. J Immunol 1987;138:3688–3694.

14 Yoneda Y, Yoshida R: The role of T cells in allografted tumor rejection: IFN-γ released from T cells is essential for induction of effector macrophages in the rejection site. J Immunol 1998;160:6012–6017.

15 Trinchieri G, Perussia B: Immune interferon: a pleiotropic lymphokine with multiple effects. Immunol Today 1985;6:131–136.

16 Farrar MA, Schreiber RD: The molecular cell biology of interferon-γ and its receptor. Annu Rev Immunol 1993;11:571–611.

17 Wangoo A, Cook HT, Taylor GM, Shaw RJ: Enhanced expression of type 1 procollagen and transforming growth factor-beta in tuberculin induced delayed type hypersensitivity. J Clin Pathol 1995;48:339–345.

18 Kimura R, Hu H, Stein-Streilein J: Delayed-type hypersensitivity responses regulate collagen deposition in the lung. Immunology 1992;77:550–555.

19 Dvorak HF, Mihm MC Jr, Dvorak AM, et al: Morphology of delayed-type hypersensitivity reactions in man. I. Quantitative description of the inflammatory response. Lab Invest 1974;31: 111–130.
20 Dvorak AM, Mihm MC Jr, Dvorak HF: Morphology of delayed-type hypersensitivity reactions in man. II. Ultrastructural alterations affecting the microvasculature and the tissue mast cells. Lab Invest 1976;34:179–191.
21 Buchanan KL, Murphy JW: Kinetics of cellular infiltration and cytokine production during the efferent phase of a delayed-type hypersensitivity reaction. Immunology 1997;90:189–197.
22 Bennett NT, Schultz GS: Growth factors and wound healing: biochemical properties of growth factors and their receptors. Am J Surg 1993;165:728–737.
23 Streilein JW, Takeuchi M, Taylor AW: Immune privilege, T-cell tolerance, and tissue-restricted autoimmunity. Hum Immunol 1997;52:138–143.
24 Akira S, Takeda K, Kaisho T: Toll-like receptors: critical proteins linking innate and acquired immunity. Nat Immunol 2001;2:675–680.
25 Akira S, Hemmi H: Recognition of pathogen-associated molecular patterns by TLR family. Immunol Lett 2003;85:85–95.
26 Akira S: Mammalian Toll-like receptors. Curr Opin Immunol 2003;15:5–11.
27 Qi H, Denning TL, Soong L: Differential induction of interleukin-10 and interleukin-12 in dendritic cells by microbial Toll-like receptor activators and skewing of T-cell cytokine profiles. Infect Immun 2003;71:3337–3342.
28 Schnare M, Barton GM, Holt AC, et al: Toll-like receptors control activation of adaptive immune responses. Nat Immunol 2001;2:947–950.
29 Bowie A, O'Neill LA: The interleukin-1 receptor/Toll-like receptor superfamily: signal generators for pro-inflammatory interleukins and microbial products. J Leukoc Biol 2000;67:508–514.
30 Re F, Strominger JL: Toll-like receptor 2 (TLR2) and TLR4 differentially activate human dendritic cells. J Biol Chem 2001;276:37692–37699.
31 Triantafilou M, Triantafilou K: Lipopolysaccharide recognition: CD14, TLRs and the LPS-activation cluster. Trends Immunol 2002;23:301–304.
32 Akira S, Takeda K: Toll-like receptor signalling. Nat Rev Immunol 2004;4:499–511.
33 Doyle S, Vaidya S, O'Connell R, et al: IRF3 mediates a TLR3/TLR4-specific antiviral gene program. Immunity 2002;17:251–263.
34 Gautier G, Humbert M, Deauvieau F, et al: A type I interferon autocrine-paracrine loop is involved in Toll-like receptor-induced interleukin-12p70 secretion by dendritic cells. J Exp Med 2005;201: 1435–1446.
35 Kaplan HJ, Streilein JW, Stevens TR: Transplantation immunology of the anterior chamber of the eye. II. Immune response to allogeneic cells. J Immunol 1975;115:805–810.
36 Kaiser C, Ksander B, Streilein J: Inhibition of lymphocyte proliferation by aqueous humor. Reg Immunol 1989;2:42–49.
37 Niederkorn JY, Benson JL, Mayhew E: Efferent blockade of delayed-type hypersensitivity responses in the anterior chamber of the eye. Reg Immunol 1991;3:349–354.
38 Cousins SW, Trattler WB, Streilein JW: Immune privilege and suppression of immunogenic inflammation in the anterior chamber of the eye. Curr Eye Res 1991;10:287–297.
39 Taylor AW, Streilein JW, Cousins SW: Identification of alpha-melanocyte stimulating hormone as a potential immunosuppressive factor in aqueous humor. Curr Eye Res 1992;11: 1199–1206.
40 Nishida T, Taylor AW: Specific aqueous humor factors induce activation of regulatory T cells. Invest Ophthalmol Vis Sci 1999;40:2268–2274.
41 Taylor AW: Immunoregulation of the ocular effector responses by soluble factors in aqueous humor. Reg Immunol 1994;6:52–57.
42 Pasquale LR, Dorman-Pease ME, Lutty GA, Quigley HA, Jampel HD: Immunolocalization of TGF-β1, TGF-1β2, and TGF-2β3 in the anterior segment of the human eye. Invest Ophthalmol Vis Sci 1993;34:23–30.
43 Knisely TL, Bleicher PA, Vibbard CA, Granstein RD: Production of latent transforming growth factor-beta and other inhibitory factors by cultured murine iris and ciliary body cells. Curr Eye Res 1991;10:761–771.

44 Wilbanks GA, Streilein JW: Fluids from immune privileged sites endow macrophages with the capacity to induce antigen-specific immune deviation via a mechanism involving transforming growth factor-beta. Eur J Immunol 1992;22:1031–1036.
45 Takeuchi M, Kosiewicz MM, Alard P, Streilein JW: On the mechanisms by which transforming growth factor-β2 alters antigen-presenting abilities of macrophages on T cell activation. Eur J Immunol 1997;27:1648–1656.
46 Takeuchi M, Alard P, Streilein JW: TGF-β promotes immune deviation by altering accessory signals of antigen-presenting cells. J Immunol 1998;160:1589–1597.
47 Tsunawaki S, Sporn M, Ding A, Nathan C: Deactivation of macrophages by transforming growth factor-β. Nature 1988;334:260–262.
48 Chantry D, Turner M, Abney E, Feldmann M: Modulation of cytokine production by transforming growth factor-β. J Immunol 1989;142:4295–4300.
49 Bogdan C, Paik J, Vodovotz Y, Nathan C: Contrasting mechanisms for suppression of macrophage cytokine release by transforming growth factor-β and interleukin-10. J Biol Chem 1992;267:23301–23308.
50 Taylor AW, Alard P, Yee DG, Streilein JW: Aqueous humor induces transforming growth factor-beta (TGF-beta)-producing regulatory T-cells. Curr Eye Res 1997;16:900–908.
51 Nunes I, Shapiro RL, Rifkin DB: Characterization of latent TGF-beta activation by murine peritoneal macrophages. J Immunol 1995;155:1450–1459.
52 Munger JS, Harpel JG, Gleizes PE, et al: Latent transforming growth factor-beta: structural features and mechanisms of activation. Kidney Int 1997;51:1376–1382.
53 Taylor AW, Yee DG, Nishida T, Namba K: Neuropeptide regulation of immunity. The immunosuppressive activity of alpha-melanocyte-stimulating hormone (alpha-MSH). Ann N Y Acad Sci 2000;917:239–247.
54 Taylor A, Namba K: In vitro induction of CD25+ CD4+ regulatory T cells by the neuropeptide alpha-melanocyte stimulating hormone (alpha-MSH). Immunol Cell Biol 2001;79:358–367.
55 Namba K, Kitaichi N, Nishida T, Taylor AW: Induction of regulatory T cells by the immunomodulating cytokines alpha-melanocyte-stimulating hormone and transforming growth factor-β2. J Leukoc Biol 2002;72:946–952.
56 Nakanishi S, Inoue A, Kita T, et al: Nucleotide sequence of cloned cDNA for bovine corticotropin-β-lipotropin precursor. Nature 1979;278:423–427.
57 Lee TH, Lerner AB, Buettner-Janusch V: The isolation and structure of α- and β-melanocyte-stimulating hormones from monkey pituitary glands. J Biol Chem 1961;236:1390–1394.
58 Watanabe T, Hiltz ME, Catania A, Lipton JM: Inhibition of IL-1β-induced peripheral inflammation by peripheral and central administration of analogs of the neuropeptide α-MSH. Brain Res Bull 1993;32:311–314.
59 Martin LW, Catania A, Hiltz ME, Lipton JM: Neuropeptide alpha-MSH antagonizes IL-6- and TNF-induced fever. Peptides 1991;12:297–299.
60 Lipton JM, Catania A: Anti-inflammatory actions of the neuroimmunomodulator α-MSH. Immunol Today 1997;18:140–145.
61 Lipton JM: Modulation of host defense by the neuropeptide α-MSH. Yale J Biol Med 1990;63:173–182.
62 Holdeman M, Khorram O, Samson WK, Lipton JM: Fever-specific changes in central MSH and CRF concentrations. Am J Physiol 1985;248:R125–R129.
63 Star RA, Rajora N, Huang J, et al: Evidence of autocrine modulation of macrophage nitric oxide synthase by α-MSH. Proc Natl Acad Sci 1995;90:8856–8860.
64 Rajora N, Ceriani G, Catania A, et al: α-MSH production, receptors, and influence on neopterin in a human monocyte/macrophage cell line. J Leukoc Biol 1996;59:248–253.
65 Chiao H, Foster S, Thomas R, Lipton J, Star RA: α-Melanocyte stimulating hormone reduces endotoxin-induced liver inflammation. J Clin Invest 1996;97:2038–2044.
66 Ortego J, Wollmann G, Coca-Prados M: Differential regulation of gene expression of neurotensin and prohormone convertases PC1 and PC2 in the bovine ocular ciliary epithelium: possible implications on neurotensin processing. Neurosci Lett 2002;333:49–53.
67 O'Donohue TL, Dorsa DM: The opiomelanotropinergic neuronal and endocrine systems. Peptides 1982;3:353–395.

68 Chakraborty AK, Funasaka Y, Slominski A, et al: Production and release of proopiomelanocortin (POMC) derived peptides by human melanocytes and keratinocytes in culture: regulation by ultraviolet B. Biochim Biophys Acta 1996;1313:130–138.
69 Taylor AW, Streilein JW, Cousins SW: Alpha-melanocyte-stimulating hormone suppresses antigen-stimulated T cell production of gamma-interferon. Neuroimmunomodulation 1994;1:188–194.
70 Nishida T, Miyata S, Itoh Y, et al: Anti-inflammatory effects of alpha-melanocyte-stimulating hormone against rat endotoxin-induced uveitis and the time course of inflammatory agents in aqueous humor. Int Immunopharmacol 2004;4:1059–1066.
71 Shiratori K, Ohgami K, Ilieva IB, et al: Inhibition of endotoxin-induced uveitis and potentiation of cyclooxygenase-2 protein expression by alpha-melanocyte-stimulating hormone. Invest Ophthalmol Vis Sci 2004;45:159–164.
72 Naveh N, Marshall J: Melanocortins are comparable to corticosteroids as inhibitors of traumatic ocular inflammation in rabbits. Graefes Arch Clin Exp Ophthalmol 2001;239:840–844.
73 Taylor AW: The immunomodulating neuropeptide alpha-melanocyte-stimulating hormone (alpha-MSH) suppresses LPS-stimulated TLR4 with IRAK-M in macrophages. J Neuroimmunol 2005;162:43–50.
74 Taylor AW, Yee DG, Streilein JW: Suppression of nitric oxide generated by inflammatory macrophages by calcitonin gene-related peptide in aqueous humor. Invest Ophthalmol Vis Sci 1998;39:1372–1378.
75 Taylor AW, Yee DG: Somatostatin is an immunosuppressive factor in aqueous humor. Invest Ophthalmol Vis Sci 2003;44:2644–2649.
76 Taylor AW, Streilein JW, Cousins SW: Immunoreactive vasoactive intestinal peptide contributes to the immunosuppressive activity of normal aqueous humor. J Immunol 1994;153:1080–1086.
77 Muscettola M, Grasso G: Somatostatin and vasoactive intestinal peptide reduce interferon gamma production by human peripheral blood mononuclear cells. Immunobiology 1990;180:419–430.
78 O'Dorisio MS, Wood CL, O'Dorisio TM: Vasoactive intestinal peptide and neuropeptide modulation of the immune response. J Immunol 1985;135:792s–796s.
79 Ottaway CA: Vasoactive intestinal peptide as a modulator of lymphocyte and immune function. Ann N Y Acad Sci 1988;527:486–500.
80 Stanisz AM, Scicchitano R, Bienenstock J: The role of vasoactive intestinal peptide and other neuropeptides in the regulation of the immune response in vitro and in vivo. Ann N Y Acad Sci 1988;527:478–485.
81 Tseng J, O'Dorisio MS: Mechanism of vasoactive intestinal peptide (VIP)-mediated immunoregulation; in Goetzl EJ, Spector NH (eds): Neuroimmune Networks: Physiology and Diseases. New York, Liss, 1989, pp 105–111.
82 Boudard F, Bastide M: Inhibition of mouse T-cell proliferation by CGRP and VIP: effects of these neuropeptides on IL-2 production and cAMP synthesis. J Neurosci Res 1991;29:29–41.
83 Ganea D, Sun L: Vasoactive intestinal peptide downregulates the expression of IL-2 but not of INF-γ from stimulated murine T lymphocytes. J Neuroimmunol 1993;47:147–158.
84 Uddman R, Alumets J, Ehinger B, et al: Vasoactive intestinal peptide nerves in ocular and orbital structures of the cat. Invest Ophthalmol Vis Sci 1980;19:878–885.
85 Terenghi G, Polak JM, Ghatei MA, et al: Distribution and origin of calcitonin gene-related peptide (CGRP) immunoreactivity in the sensory innervation of the mammalian eye. J Comp Neurol 1985;233:506–516.
86 Wright LL, Luebke JI: Somatostatin-, vasoactive intestinal polypeptide- and neuropeptide Y-like immunoreactivity in eye- and submandibular gland-projecting sympathetic neurons. Brain Res 1989;494:267–275.
87 Vasilaki A, Papadaki T, Notas G, et al: Effect of somatostatin on nitric oxide production in human retinal pigment epithelium cell cultures. Invest Ophthalmol Vis Sci 2004;45:1499–1506.
88 Cristiani R, Petrucci C, Dal Monte M, Bagnoli P: Somatostatin (SRIF) and SRIF receptors in the mouse retina. Brain Res 2002;936:1–14.
89 Larsen JN, Bersani M, Olcese J, Holst JJ, Moller M: Somatostatin and prosomatostatin in the retina of the rat: an immunohistochemical, in-situ hybridization, and chromatographic study. Vis Neurosci 1990;5:441–452.

90 Gaur VP, Yamaguchi K, Turner JE: Somatostatin in rat retina: localization by in situ hybridization histochemistry and immunocytochemistry. Tohoku J Exp Med 1990;162:121–126.
91 Yamaguchi K, Gaur VP, Spira AW, Turner JE: Cellular localization of somatostatin mRNA in rat retina. Neuropeptides 1990;17:13–16.
92 Ottaway CA: Selective effects of vasoactive intestinal peptide on the mitogenic response of murine T cells. Immunology 1987;62:291–297.
93 Caspi RR, Sun B, Agarwal RK, et al: T cell mechanisms in experimental autoimmune uveoretinitis: susceptibility is a function of the cytokine response profile. Eye 1997;11(pt 2):209–212.
94 Kitaichi N, Namba K, Taylor AW: Inducible immune regulation following autoimmune disease in the immune-privileged eye. J Leukoc Biol 2005;77:496–502.
95 Lin HH, Faunce DE, Stacey M, et al: The macrophage F4/80 receptor is required for the induction of antigen-specific efferent regulatory T cells in peripheral tolerance. J Exp Med 2005;201: 1615–1625.
96 D'Orazio TJ, Mayhew E, Niederkorn JY: Ocular immune privilege promoted by the presentation of peptide on tolerogenic B cells in the spleen. II. Evidence for presentation by Qa-1. J Immunol 2001;166:26–32.
97 Wilbanks GA, Streilein JW: Characterization of suppressor cells in anterior chamber-associated immune deviation (ACAID) induced by soluble antigen. Evidence of two functionally and phenotypically distinct T-suppressor cell populations. Immunology 1990;71:383–389.
98 Taylor AW, Kitaichi N, Biros DJ: Melanocortin 5 receptor and ocular immunity. Cell Mol Biol (Noisy-le-grand) 2006;52:53–59.
99 Song XY, Gu M, Jin WW, Klinman DM, Wahl SM: Plasmid DNA encoding transforming growth factor-beta1 suppresses chronic disease in a streptococcal cell wall-induced arthritis model. J Clin Invest 1998;101:2615–2621.
100 Croxford JL, Triantaphyllopoulos K, Podhajcer OL, et al: Cytokine gene therapy in experimental allergic encephalomyelitis by injection of plasmid DNA-cationic liposome complex into the central nervous system. J Immunol 1998;160:5181–5187.
101 Brauner R, Nonoyama M, Laks H, et al: Intracoronary adenovirus-mediated transfer of immunosuppressive cytokine genes prolongs allograft survival. J Thorac Cardiovasc Surg 1997;114:923–933.
102 Wintzen M, Gilchrest BA: Proopiomelanocortin, its derived peptides, and the skin. J Invest Dermatol 1996;106:3–10.
103 Thody AJ, Ridley K, Penny RJ, et al: MSH peptides are present in mammalian skin. Peptides 1983;4: 813–816.

Dr. Andrew W. Taylor
Schepens Eye Research Institute, Harvard Medical School
20 Staniford Street
Boston, MA 02114 (USA)
Tel. +1 617 912 7452, Fax +1 617 912 0137, E-Mail awtaylor@vision.eri.harvard.edu

Niederkorn JY, Kaplan HJ (eds): Immune Response and the Eye.
Chem Immunol Allergy. Basel, Karger, 2007, vol 92, pp 86–93

Immunosuppressive Properties of the Pigmented Epithelial Cells and the Subretinal Space

Parisa Zamiri, Sunao Sugita, J. Wayne Streilein†

Schepens Eye Research Institute, Harvard Medical School, Boston, Mass., USA

Abstract

The immune privilege of the anterior chamber of the eye has been recognized for over 100 years. However, the unique immunological properties of the pigmented epithelial (PE) cells of the eye and the subretinal space (SRS) have only recently been appreciated. The PE cells of the iris, ciliary body, and retina reside in anatomically disparate locations and serve distinctly different functions, yet share interesting immunomodulatory properties that contribute to ocular immune privilege. PE cells in the ciliary body and retina elaborate a variety of soluble factors that either directly or indirectly dampen immune-mediated inflammation; these include transforming growth factor-β, somatostatin, thrombospondin and pigment epithelial derived factor (PEDF). The constitutive expression of the immune co-stimulatory molecule, CD86, on iris PE cells not only inhibits T cell proliferation, but also promotes the generation of regulatory T cells. The SRS is now recognized as an immune-privileged site that shares many, but not all, of the properties ascribed to the anterior chamber, including the induction of systemic immune deviation. The prospect of therapeutic retinal transplantation and the possible immunologic etiology for some forms of age-related macular degeneration provides new impetus for gaining a better understanding of ocular immune privilege in the posterior regions of the eye.

Although the anterior chamber of the eye is a classic example of an immune privileged site, it is important to note that ocular immune privilege extends beyond the anterior chamber and is also manifested in the vitreous cavity and subretinal space (SRS) [1–6]. Until recently, the unique immunological properties of the pigmented epithelia (PE) of the eye and the SRS have received only modest attention. However, two important developments have recently kindled renewed interest in the immunoregulatory features of the PE and the

SRS: the prospect of therapeutic retinal transplantation and the possible immunologic etiology for some forms of age-related macular degeneration (AMD). In 2005, three separate laboratories simultaneously reported that a single nucleotide polymorphism in the human genome results in a three- to sevenfold increase in the risk of developing AMD [7–9]. The polymorphism occurs in the gene that encodes complement factor H, a key regulator of the complement cascade and inflammation. The role of complement activation and inflammation in the pathogenesis of AMD was proposed over 3 years ago by Anderson et al. [10] and fits neatly with the aforementioned reports indicating a strong association between polymorphism in the factor H gene and AMD. Thus, the immunoregulatory properties of ocular PE cells and the SRS have now taken on an even greater significance.

Immunoregulatory Properties of Pigmented Epithelial Cells in the Eye

The PE cells of the iris, ciliary body, and retina share important immunological properties, even though they reside in anatomically disparate locations and serve different functions. Cultured iris and ciliary body PE cells secrete a variety of immunosuppressive and anti-inflammatory factors [11, 12]. Retinal PE (RPE) cells also express cell membrane-bound molecules, such as FasL (CD95L), which induces apoptosis of CD95+ inflammatory cells and contributes to ocular immune privilege [13, 14].

PE cells of the iris, ciliary body, and retina not only suppress T cell activation in vitro [15], but also endow T cells with immunoregulatory properties and convert them to suppressor cells [16]. The inhibition of T cell proliferation is mediated by two distinctly different mechanisms; one is contact dependent and is mediated by iris PE cells, while the other is mediated by soluble factors secreted by ciliary body and RPE cells [17].

Using an RPE eyecup organ culture system, we have demonstrated that factors present in the supernatant of RPE eyecup organ cultures profoundly inhibit T cell proliferation and interferon-γ (IFN-γ) production in both antigen-stimulated and anti-CD3-stimulated T cells [18]. Active transforming growth factor-β (TGF-β), thrombospondin (TSP-1) and somatostatin (SOM) were found to be the main factors responsible for this T cell inhibition.

Transforming Growth Factor-β

TGF-β is a member of a family of structurally related dimeric proteins secreted by nearly all cell types. TGF-β is secreted as a biologically inactive complex consisting of latent TGF-β and the latent TGF-β binding protein. RPE cells express mRNA for TGF-β_1 and TGF-β_2, and for TGF-β binding protein [19], but predominantly secrete TGF-β_2 in the SRS. RPE cells express all of the type I TGF-β receptors and some of the type II receptors [20]. Latent TGF-β, which is present in supernatants of RPE cell cultures, does not inhibit T cell proliferation unless it is activated. However, upon activation, TGF-β suppresses T cell proliferation and IFN-γ production. Moreover, supernatant from RPE cell cultures does not inhibit activation of purified T cells taken from TGF-β receptor II dominant negative mice. TSP-1 is also produced by RPE cells and plays a central role in converting latent TGF-β into its active, immune-inhibitory form [18].

Thrombospondin-1

Thrombospondins are a family of glycoproteins that participate in cell-to-cell or cellto-matrix communications [21]. TSP-1 binds to small latent TGF-β complex (TGF-β-LAP) releasing active TGF-β, independent of the presence of proteases [22]. RT-PCR and immunoblot analysis of TSP-1 expression has shown that both human and murine RPE cell cultures contain mRNA for TSP-1 and secrete TSP-1 protein [18, 23]. Supernatants from RPE cell cultures prepared from TSP-1 null mice are ineffective in inhibiting T-cell activation. Although latent TGF-β is present in the same quantity in RPE cell supernatants from both TSP-1 null and C57BL/6 mice, active TGF-β is not present in RPE cell supernatants from TSP-1 null animals. Activation of TGF-β in vitro is achieved by treating latent TGF-β with extreme heat or pH, whereas in vivo the activation of TGF-β is largely enzymatic [22]. Although RPE cells produce plasminogen activators and express receptors for urokinase [24], RPE cells from TSP-1 null mice are unable to activate TGF-β through enzymatic mechanisms alone. Both the anterior chamber and SRS of TSP-1 null mice fail to support induction of ovalbumin-specific immune deviation [18]. Moreover, TSP-1 null mice that are immunized with interphotoreceptor binding protein to induce experimental autoimmune uveitis experience significantly enhanced uveitis that fails to resolve [18]. These results suggest that TSP-1 contributes to the immune privilege in the anterior chamber and in the SRS by promoting the induction of immune deviation.

Somatostatin

SOM is a neuropeptide with wide distribution in the body and a diverse function as a neurotransmitter, anti-secretory, and anti-proliferative agent [25]. SOM inhibits IFN-γ production by antigen-stimulated granuloma cells and splenocytes of schistosome-infected mice [26]. Transcripts for SOM and its receptors are present within the human RPE [27] and we have shown that murine RPE cells synthesize mRNA for SOM and secrete SOM protein in RPE cell cultures [28]. SOM not only suppresses IFN-γ production by activated T cells, but also induces the production of α-melanocyte stimulating hormone, which has anti-inflammatory properties and also promotes the generation of CD4+ CD25+ regulatory T cells [29].

Pigment Epithelial Derived Factor

Pigment Epithelial derived factor (PEDF) is a 50-kD protein member of the serine protease inhibitor family and is found in the RPE, ciliary body, cornea, and retina [30]. PEDF inhibits proliferation of cells of the innate immune system such as macrophages [31]. We have recently found PEDF message in RPE cells and PEDF protein in RPE cell culture supernatants [28]. Moreover, PEDF, produced by RPE cells, strongly inhibits IL-12 and nitric oxide production by lipopolysaccharide-activated macrophages, while it upregulates anti-inflammatory IL-10 cytokine [28]. PEDF is also able to significantly inhibit endotoxin-induced inflammation in the skin in vivo.

Contact-Dependent Inhibition of T Cell Proliferation by Iris Pigment Epithelial Cells

PE cells of the iris differ from ciliary body PE cells and RPE cells by their capacity to produce a contact-dependent suppression of T cell activation [32]. The constitutive expression of the immune co-stimulation molecule CD86 (B7-2) on iris PE cells enables them to alter the functional activity of T cells by transmitting inhibitory signals by engaging CD152 (cytotoxic T lymphocyte antigen-4; CTLA-4) on the T cell membrane. Although iris PE cells express both CD80 and CD86, it is the latter co-stimulation molecule that is expressed on a very high proportion of the iris PE cells and suppresses T cell activation. Mature T cells express CD28 and CTLA-4, which are the co-receptors for CD86. CD86 engagement of CTLA-4 transmits a negative signal to T cells, resulting in anergy [33], apoptosis [34], and in some cases, the generation of T regulatory cells [35–37]. Engagement of CD86 on iris PE cells not only results in the inhibition of T cell proliferation, but also promotes the generation of T regulatory cells. The demonstration of CD86 on iris PE cells is noteworthy, as this is the only report to date indicating the expression of this co-stimulation molecule on a cell of non-hematopoietic origin. Thus, the PE cells in the eye are endowed with at least three cell surface molecules that have the potential to induce contact-dependent inhibition of inflammation, CD86 [32], FasL [38], and TRAIL (tumor necrosis factor-related apoptosis-inducing ligand) [39, 40].

Immune Deviation and Immune Privilege of the Subretinal Space

The SRS is a potential space that exists between the intervagination of the outer segments of the photoreceptors with the apical surface of the RPE. This space is a remnant of the embryonic optic vesicle and is very small in the normal adult eye. However, no tissue junctions are able to form across it and it becomes open and filled with subretinal fluid in rhegmatogenous retinal detachment. The SRS is usually filled with interphotoreceptor matrix, which is composed of proteoglycans and large glycoproteins [41].

The SRS displays two important features of an immune-privileged site: it accepts allografts for prolonged intervals, and it promotes the induction of systemic immune deviation. Neonatal retinal allografts, RPE allografts, and allogeneic tumor cells placed in the SRS survive for prolonged periods of time in contrast to the fate of similar grafts placed in the subconjunctival space [1–3, 6, 42]. Moreover, the recipients of these grafts do not display donor-specific delayed-type hypersensitivity and regulatory T cells in the spleen of the recipients are able to adoptively transfer its suppression, suggesting that the SRS supports the induction of a form of immune deviation akin to anterior chamber-associated immune deviation [43]. In contrast to neonatal retinal allografts, the immune privilege of neonatal RPE allografts and allogeneic P815 tumor cells is not absolute. By day 35 following implantation into the SRS, allogeneic neonatal RPE cells lose their organization and the RPE allograft recipients display donor-specific delayed-type hypersensitivity to donor histocompatibility antigens [43]. P815 tumor cells placed in the SRS regress after day 14 leading to immune elimination. By contrast, P815 tumors placed in the anterior chamber grow progressively, metastasize extensively, and lead to the demise of the recipients. Antibody production to P815 tumor cells is also markedly diminished in the SRS in contrast to the anterior chamber [44]. These findings demonstrate that although immune privilege exists in the SRS, it is not absolute and the mechanisms for this privilege differ from the immune privilege in the anterior chamber.

The factors contributing to immune privilege of the SRS include: (a) the presence of blood-retinal barriers (BRB); (b) the absence of lymphatic drainage, and (c) the presence of an immunosuppressive microenvironment. The neuroretina is separated from the circulation by the BRB, which is comprised of two distinct components: the inner BRB is made by the retinal vascular endothelia and the outer BRB is formed by the tight junctions between RPE cells [45]. The zonula adherens that exists between Müller cells and photoreceptors at the base of the outer segment contributes to the barrier function by limiting the movement of large molecules [46]. Together, these cellular barriers control the passage of molecules and cells into and from the retinal tissues and are essential in maintaining homeostasis of the ocular environment.

The immunosuppressive microenvironment of SRS is primarily produced by the RPE monolayer that forms the outer limit of the SRS. In addition, Müller cells have also been shown to inhibit T cell proliferation [47]. The RPE is interposed between the choroid and the neural retina and contributes to immune privilege in the SRS by forming the outer BRB and by elaborating soluble factors (described above). Secretion of prostaglandin E_2 and surface expression of CD95L by RPE are also implicated in the ability of RPE to dampen the immune response [38, 48].

Conclusions

The immune properties of the SRS and the PE cells of the eye have been largely neglected until recently. However, an emerging body of data indicates that PE cells dampen immune-mediated inflammation by contact-dependent signals transmitted by the immune system co-stimulation molecule CD86 and contact-independent mechanisms mediated by soluble anti-inflammatory cytokines. Recent findings suggesting a possible immune-mediated etiology for some forms of AMD add a sense of urgency for us to learn more about the immunological properties of the retina and the cells of the posterior regions of the eye.

References

1 Jiang LQ, Jorquera M, Streilein JW: Subretinal space and vitreous cavity as immunologically privileged sites for retinal allografts. Invest Ophthalmol Vis Sci 1993;34:3347–3354.

2 Jiang LQ, Jorquera M, Streilein JW: Immunologic consequences of intraocular implantation of retinal pigment epithelial allografts. Exp Eye Res 1994;58:719–728.

3 Jiang LQ, Streilein JW: Immune privilege extended to allogeneic tumor cells in the vitreous cavity. Invest Ophthalmol Vis Sci 1991;32:224–228.

4 Sonoda KH, Sakamoto T, Qiao H, Hisatomi T, Oshima T, Tsutsumi-Miyahara C, Exley M, Balk SP, Taniguchi M, Ishibashi T: The analysis of systemic tolerance elicited by antigen inoculation into the vitreous cavity: vitreous cavity-associated immune deviation. Immunology 2005;116: 390–399.

5 Wenkel H, Chen PW, Ksander BR, Streilein JW: Immune privilege is extended, then withdrawn, from allogeneic tumor cell grafts placed in the subretinal space. Invest Ophthalmol Vis Sci 1999;40:3202–3208.

6 Wenkel H, Streilein JW: Analysis of immune deviation elicited by antigens injected into the subretinal space. Invest Ophthalmol Vis Sci 1998;39:1823–1834.

7 Klein RJ, Zeiss C, Chew EY, Tsai JY, Sackler RS, Haynes C, Henning AK, SanGiovanni JP, Mane SM, Mayne ST, Bracken MB, Ferris FL, Ott J, Barnstable C, Hoh J: Complement factor H polymorphism in age-related macular degeneration. Science 2005;308:385–389.

8 Edwards AO, Ritter R 3rd, Abel KJ, Manning A, Panhuysen C, Farrer LA: Complement factor H polymorphism and age-related macular degeneration. Science 2005;308:421–424.

9 Haines JL, Hauser MA, Schmidt S, Scott WK, Olson LM, Gallins P, Spencer KL, Kwan SY, Noureddine M, Gilbert JR, Schnetz-Boutaud N, Agarwal A, Postel EA, Pericak-Vance MA:

Complement factor H variant increases the risk of age-related macular degeneration. Science 2005;308:419–421.
10 Anderson DH, Mullins RF, Hageman GS, Johnson LV: A role for local inflammation in the formation of drusen in the aging eye. Am J Ophthalmol 2002;134:411–431.
11 Knisely TL, Bleicher PA, Vibbard CA, Granstein RD: Production of latent transforming growth factor-beta and other inhibitory factors by cultured murine iris and ciliary body cells. Curr Eye Res 1991;10:761–771.
12 Streilein JW, Bradley D: Analysis of immunosuppressive properties of iris and ciliary body cells and their secretory products. Invest Ophthalmol Vis Sci 1991;32:2700–2710.
13 Griffith TS, Ferguson TA: The role of FasL-induced apoptosis in immune privilege. Immunol Today 1997;18:240–244.
14 Jorgensen A, Wiencke AK, la Cour M, Kaestel CG, Madsen HO, Hamann S, Lui GM, Scherfig E, Prause JU, Svejgaard A, Odum N, Nissen MH, Ropke C: Human retinal pigment epithelial cell-induced apoptosis in activated T cells. Invest Ophthalmol Vis Sci 1998;39:1590–1599.
15 Yoshida M, Takeuchi M, Streilein JW: Participation of pigment epithelium of iris and ciliary body in ocular immune privilege. 1. Inhibition of T-cell activation in vitro by direct cell-to-cell contact. Invest Ophthalmol Vis Sci 2000;41:811–821.
16 Yoshida M, Kezuka T, Streilein JW: Participation of pigment epithelium of iris and ciliary body in ocular immune privilege. 2. Generation of TGF-beta-producing regulatory T cells. Invest Ophthalmol Vis Sci 2000;41:3862–3870.
17 Ishida K, Panjwani N, Cao Z, Streilein JW: Participation of pigment epithelium in ocular immune privilege. 3. Epithelia cultured from iris, ciliary body, and retina suppress T-cell activation by partially non-overlapping mechanisms. Ocul Immunol Inflamm 2003;11:91–105.
18 Zamiri P, Masli S, Kitaichi N, Taylor AW, Streilein JW: Thrombospondin plays a vital role in the immune privilege of the eye. Invest Ophthalmol Vis Sci 2005;46:908–919.
19 Tanihara H, Yoshida M, Matsumoto M, Yoshimura N: Identification of transforming growth factor-beta expressed in cultured human retinal pigment epithelial cells. Invest Ophthalmol Vis Sci 1993;34:413–419.
20 Obata H, Kaji Y, Yamada H, Kato M, Tsuru T, Yamashita H: Expression of transforming growth factor-beta superfamily receptors in rat eyes. Acta Ophthalmol Scand 1999;77:151–156.
21 Lawler J: The functions of thrombospondin-1 and -2. Curr Opin Cell Biol 2000;12:634–640.
22 Murphy-Ullrich JE, Poczatek M: Activation of latent TGF-beta by thrombospondin-1: mechanisms and physiology. Cytokine Growth Factor Rev 2000;11:59–69.
23 Miyajima-Uchida H, Hayashi H, Beppu R, Kuroki M, Fukami M, Arakawa F, Tomita Y, Kuroki M, Oshima K: Production and accumulation of thrombospondin-1 in human retinal pigment epithelial cells. Invest Ophthalmol Vis Sci 2000;41: 561–567.
24 Elner SG: Human retinal pigment epithelial lysis of extracellular matrix: functional urokinase plasminogen activator receptor, collagenase, and elastase. Trans Am Ophthalmol Soc 2002;100: 273–299.
25 Patel YC: Somatostatin and its receptor family. Front Neuroendocrinol 1999;20:157–198.
26 Blum AM, Metwali A, Mathew RC, Cook G, Elliott D, Weinstock JV: Granuloma T lymphocytes in murine schistosomiasis mansoni have somatostatin receptors and respond to somatostatin with decreased IFN-gamma secretion. J Immunol 1992;149:3621–3626.
27 Klisovic DD, O'Dorisio MS, Katz SE, Sall JW, Balster D, O'Dorisio TM, Craig E, Lubow M: Somatostatin receptor gene expression in human ocular tissues: RT-PCR and immunohistochemical study. Invest Ophthalmol Vis Sci 2001;42: 2193–2201.
28 Zamiri P, Masli S, Streilein JW, Taylor AW: Pigment epithelial growth factor suppresses inflammation by modulating macrophage activation. Invest Ophthalmol Vis Sci 2006;47:3912–3918.
29 Taylor AW, Yee DG: Somatostatin is an immunosuppressive factor in aqueous humor. Invest Ophthalmol Vis Sci 2003;44:2644–2649.
30 Karakousis PC, John SK, Behling KC, Surace EM, Smith JE, Hendrickson A, Tang WX, Bennett J, Milam AH: Localization of pigment epithelium derived factor (PEDF) in developing and adult human ocular tissues. Mol Vis 2001;7:154–163.

31 Cohen J, Sugita Y, Chader GJ, Schwartz JP: Recombinant forms of the neurotrophic factor pigment epithelium-derived factor activate cellular metabolism and inhibit proliferation of the RAW macrophage cell line. Neuroimmunomodulation 2000;7:51–58.
32 Sugita S, Streilein JW: Iris pigment epithelium expressing CD86 (B7-2) directly suppresses T cell activation in vitro via binding to cytotoxic T lymphocyte-associated antigen 4. J Exp Med 2003;198: 161–171.
33 Greenwald RJ, Boussiotis VA, Lorsbach RB, Abbas AK, Sharpe AH: CTLA-4 regulates induction of anergy in vivo. Immunity 2001;14:145–155.
34 Scheipers P, Reiser H: Fas-independent death of activated $CD4^+$ T lymphocytes induced by CTLA-4 crosslinking. Proc Natl Acad Sci USA 1998;95:10083–10088.
35 Levings MK, Sangregorio R, Sartirana C, et al: Human CD25+CD4+ T suppressor cell clones produce transforming growth factor beta, but not interleukin 10, and are distinct from type 1 T regulatory cells. J Exp Med 2002;196:1335–1346.
36 Read S, Malmstrom V, Powrie F: Cytotoxic T lymphocyte-associated antigen 4 plays an essential role in the function of $CD25^+CD4^+$ regulatory cells that control intestinal inflammation. J Exp Med 2000;192:295–302.
37 Takahashi T, Tagami T, Yamazaki S, et al: Immunologic self-tolerance maintained by $CD25^+CD4^+$ regulatory T cells constitutively expressing cytotoxic T lymphocyte-associated antigen 4. J Exp Med 2000;192:303–310.
38 Griffith TS, Brunner T, Fletcher SM, Green DR, Ferguson TA: Fas ligand-induced apoptosis as a mechanism of immune privilege. Science 1995;270:1189–1192.
39 Lee HO, Herndon JM, Barreiro R, Griffith TS, Ferguson TA: TRAIL: a mechanism of tumor surveillance in an immune privileged site. J Immunol 2002;169:4739–4744.
40 Wang S, Boonman ZF, Li HC, et al: Role of TRAIL and IFN-gamma in CD4+ T cell-dependent tumor rejection in the anterior chamber of the eye. J Immunol 2003;171:2789–2796.
41 Mieziewska K: The interphotoreceptor matrix, a space in sight. Microsc Res Tech 1996;35: 463–471.
42 Wenkel H, Streilein JW: Evidence that retinal pigment epithelium functions as an immune-privileged tissue. Invest Ophthalmol Vis Sci 2000;41:3467–3473.
43 Streilein JW, Ma N, Wenkel H, Ng TF, Zamiri P: Immunobiology and privilege of neuronal retina and pigment epithelium transplants. Vision Res 2002;42:487–495.
44 Kaplan HJ, Tezel TH, Berger AS, Del Priore LV: Retinal transplantation; in Streilein JW (ed): Immune Response and the Eye. Chem Immunol. Basel, Karger, 1999, vol 73, pp 207–219.
45 Ashton N: Bowman lecture. The blood-retinal barrier and vaso-glial relationships in retinal disease. Trans Ophthalmol Soc UK 1965;85:199–230.
46 Marmor MF: Mechanisms of fluid accumulation in retinal edema. Doc Ophthalmol 1999;97: 239–249.
47 Caspi RR, Roberge FG: Glial cells as suppressor cells: characterization of the inhibitory function. J Autoimmun 1989;2:709–722.
48 Liversidge J, McKay D, Mullen G, Forrester JV: Retinal pigment epithelial cells modulate lymphocyte function at the blood-retina barrier by autocrine PGE2 and membrane-bound mechanisms. Cell Immunol 1993;149:315–330.

Dr. Parisa Zamiri
Advanced Microscopy Program
Wellman Center for Photomedicine
CPZN8238, 185 Cambridge Street
Boston, MA 02114 (USA)
Tel. +1 617 726 4236, Fax +1 617 724 2075, E-Mail pzamiri@partners.org

Niederkorn JY, Kaplan HJ (eds): Immune Response and the Eye.
Chem Immunol Allergy. Basel, Karger, 2007, vol 92, pp 94–104

Major Histocompatibility Complex Molecules on Parenchymal Cells of the Target Organ Protect against Autoimmune Disease

Hui Shao, Henry J. Kaplan, Deming Sun

Department of Ophthalmology and Visual Sciences, Kentucky Lions Eye Center, University of Louisville, Louisville, Ky., USA

Abstract

Parenchymal cells of the autoimmune organ may only express major histocompatibility complex (MHC) molecules during the disease process. In this paper, we hypothesize that the appearance of MHC molecules on parenchymal cells may augment the activation of invading autoreactive T cells and either exacerbate or suppress local inflammation. It is speculated that like many biological responses this is a two-edge sword – namely, the expression of modest levels of MHC molecules may inhibit the activation of invading T cells, whereas overexpression of these molecules may promote activation of autoimmune T cells, enhancing the inflammatory cascade, thus leading to tissue damage.

Autoreactive T cells are found in healthy people [1] and non-immunized animals [2]; however, most people do not develop autoimmune disease and the induction of autoimmune disease in animals requires specific treatment regimens and the use of particular genetic strains. It appears that autoimmune reactions are normally suppressed and that autoimmune disease results from breakdown of this suppression. Thus, a complete understanding of the pathogenesis of autoimmune uveitis requires knowledge of the suppressive mechanisms that are normally operative, but fail during disease. Additionally, pathogenic T cells may have attributes that are lacking in their non-pathogenic counterparts. One such protective mechanism is the ability of parenchymal cells of the target organ to inhibit autoreactive T cells. Indeed, an 'intrinsic abnormality of the target organs' has been previously proposed to explain the mechanism(s) by which autoreactive T cells mediate diseases [3, 4].

Experimental autoimmune uveitis (EAU), an autoimmune disease induced in experimental animals [5–8], has been, for many years, a popular laboratory model of human uveitis and even, to some extent, other T cell-mediated autoimmune diseases. EAU can be induced either by immunization of susceptible strains of rodents with a defined autoantigen or by adoptive transfer of autoreactive antigen-specific T cells.

Active Experimental Autoimmune Uveitis

By definition, active EAU is initiated by injection of ocular antigen in an immunogenic form, usually as an emulsion in complete Freund's adjuvant. This elicits a peripheral immune response, and, in susceptible animals, ocular inflammation of the eye. Generally, symptoms of uveitis in the rat appear by the 8th–10th day following immunization, persist for a little over a week, then subside. Antigen is taken up and processed into smaller peptide fragments that become complexed to major histocompatibility complex (MHC) molecules expressed on the surface of antigen-presenting cells (APCs). For example, when interphotoreceptor retinoid-binding protein (IRBP) is used as the eliciting antigen in the C57BL/6 mouse, a large portion of the immune response is directed against the 20-mer peptide containing residues 1–20 of the protein (GPTHLFQPSLVLDMAKVLLD) [9, 10].

Adoptive Transfer of Experimental Autoimmune Uveitis

Somewhat simpler than active EAU, this begins with the transfer of lymphocytes from already immunized donors to recipients [10, 11]. Thus, the initial stages of immunization, including adjuvant effects and the activation of disease-causing T cell subsets, do not occur in the recipients. T cells prepared from the lymph nodes of animals undergoing active EAU are restimulated in culture and adoptively transferred to syngeneic animals in which they cause inflammation in the eye and consequent tissue damage. Disease onset is more rapid than in active EAU, beginning on day 4 in rats [5, 12] and days 8–10 in mice [10, 11]. Adoptive transfer of a few million newly activated syngeneic autoreactive T cells to a naïve animal can readily induce disease, suggesting the pathogenic role of autoreactive T cells in disease. The mechanism by which an organ-specific autoimmune disease can be adoptively transferred by a few million autoreactive T cells, of which only a fraction enters the autoimmune organ, remains unclear. It is hypothesized that the entry of the pathogenic T cells provokes MHC expression on parenchymal cells and release of chemoattractant factors, which, in turn, recruit inflammatory cells.

Autoreactive T Cell Lines and Clones

To characterize the mechanism by which autoreactive T cells initiate autoimmune disease and to determine the various structural and functional features that distinguish between subsets of autoreactive T cells and other antigen-specific, non-pathogenic T cells, enriched T cell populations have been prepared to determine the requirements for T cell activation [12] and the usage of the T cell antigen receptor [13–15] and accessory molecules [16, 17], as well as to assess the various cell-interacting cytokines produced by these cells [18–20]. The need for the characterization of the structure and function of autoreactive T cells by isolating antigen-specific T cell lines and clones became especially apparent when it is realized that limiting dilution analysis indicates that the number of autoreactive T cells in immunized rodents or in humans suffering from multiple sclerosis rarely exceeds 1 in 10,000 T cells [21, 22] and that the overwhelming majority of activated T cells associated with disease development are nonspecifically expanded [23].

Retinal Pigment Epithelium

Retinal pigment epithelial (RPE) cells, situated at a crucial interface between the choroidal blood supply and the photoreceptor cell layer of the neural retina, contribute to the immune-privileged status of the eye as part of the blood-eye barrier[24] by secretion of immunosuppressive factors inside the eye [25–28] and by expression of Fas ligand on their cell surface [29–31]. RPE cells may also assist in the development of intraocular inflammation [27, 32–34] and can respond to a variety of inflammatory cytokines [32, 35] and produce a myriad of molecules that can induce inflammation. For example, RPE cells can produce cytokines, such as tumor necrosis factor-α, interleukin-15 [36], and nitric oxide [37], and express cell surface MHC molecules and co-stimulatory molecules [38, 39]. In addition, RPE cells also express a number of uveitogenic antigens, such as soluble retinal antigen and IRBP, and could therefore become targets for uveitogenic T cells, leading to autoimmune reactions in the eye. While there is strong evidence that RPE cells can express MHC II molecules after activation [39, 40], the role of these molecules in the eye remains unclear.

Expression of Major Histocompatibility Complex Molecules by Retinal Pigment Epithelium

One of the seminal findings of immunology is that the recognition of T cells is strictly restricted by antigens encoded by the MHC [41]. Based on this dogma, it is believed that only those parenchymal cells in the autoimmune organ capable of expressing MHC molecules can directly interact with the invading autoreactive T cells.

Under physiological conditions, RPE do not express appreciable levels of MHC II molecules [42] but do so during disease [43] or when they are activated in vitro by pro-inflammatory cytokines, such as interferon-γ [44–46]. In the eye, aberrant expression of MHC molecules on RPE cells is therefore believed to alter disease susceptibility [47]. These cells, which can be induced to express MHC molecules and thus support T cell activation [44] in the eye, could be likely candidates for auto-attack.

The questions arise why parenchymal cells of the autoimmune organ retain the ability to express MHC II molecules but only do so during disease, and whether the appearance of MHC molecules in the autoimmune organ augments the activation of invading autoreactive T cells, and thus, exacerbates disease or, alternatively, restricts the intensification of local inflammation. It is speculated that like many biological responses this is a two-edge sword; whereas the expression of modest levels of MHC II molecules inhibits the activation of invading T cells, overexpression of these molecules promotes activation.

Thus, in early studies researchers tried to find evidence to support their hypothesis that the expression of MHC II molecules might render RPE able to stimulate autoreactive T cells [44]. Our studies have shown that depending on their state of activation, RPE cells can either inhibit or activate IRBP-specific T cells. In contrast to peripheral APCs, which elicit full activation (proliferation and cytokine release) of autoreactive T cells, RPE cells elicit only partial activation (tumor necrosis factor-α and interferon-γ production, but not proliferation) [44].

Retinal Pigment Epithelial Cells Expressing Major Histocompatibility Complex II Partially Activate Autoreactive T Cells and Drive These T Cells into a Refractory Phase

The mere presence of MHC II molecules and appropriate antigen is not sufficient to induce T cell activation, and the presence of co-stimulatory molecules on MHC II-expressing cells is crucial [48, 49]. MHC II-expressing cells that lack accessory molecules may not only fail to function effectively as APCs, but can also result in unresponsiveness of T cells [49]. Conceivably, too low a density of accessory molecules on RPE cells may result in inhibition of T cell activation. We are currently investigating this possibility.

The availability of MHC II molecules in the autoimmune organ may cause the invading T cell to be activated. However, T cell biology studies tell us that two biological features of T cells have a closer relationship with the pathogenic activity of the autoreactive T cell. Firstly, the T cell can be activated to various degrees [50–53]. So-called ‘partial activation’ means that the T cells are activated, but only some of the activation-related T cell functions are turned on. Given that the damaging effect of autoreactive T cells is more closely correlated to the degree of activation than the number of T cells, partially activated T cells may have only limited pathogenic activity, possibly because they produce a lower pathogenic amount of damaging factors and are less cytotoxic. Secondly, and more importantly, both fully and partially activated T cells can enter a refractory phase. T cells are cycling cells and, once activated, can only been re-activated after a lag period. For both rat and mouse T cells, the duration of this cycle is approximately 5–7 days. Thus, immediately after entry into the autoimmune organ or before severe inflammation has been initiated, the expression of MHC II molecules allows the parenchymal cell to interact with the invading T cells. This interaction renders the invading T cells partially activated and they then enter a refractory phase; as a result, when professional APCs arrive at the peak of the inflammation, the refractory T cells cannot be reactivated. In this sense, the ability to express MHC molecules gives the parenchymal cell a protective capability, restricting the intensity of inflammation. This assumption has been tested in in vitro assays. Thus, we have examined whether the interaction of T cells and RPE affects T cell responsiveness to subsequent antigenic challenge by first treating T cells with autoantigen in the presence or absence of RPE, then assessing their response to professional APCs. The results showed that pretreatment of T cells with RPE greatly decreased the ability of the T cells to respond to subsequent antigenic challenge [19, 44].

This assumption is also supported by the results of an in vitro experiment comparing the antigen-presenting activity of interferon-γ-activated RPE with that of professional APCs. We have observed that although RPE can activate autoreactive T cells, they are only 5–10% as effective as professional APCs. More importantly, T cells exposed to RPE expressing maximal levels of MHC II molecules produce only part of their cytokine repertoire compared to the same T cells stimulated by professional APCs. These observations led to the conclusion that unlike professional APCs, MHC II-expressing activated RPE can evoke only some of the functional properties of a T cell population [44].

Tissue damage provoked by invasion of autoreactive T cells appears to involve cascading responses in which the generation of cytokines and the recruitment of inflammatory cells reciprocally stimulate each other. Clearly, regulatory mechanisms are needed to control the intensity of inflammation and avoid tissue damage. It is hypothesized that the entry of autoreactive T cells elicits the release of cytokines or chemokines which then cause massive infiltration of inflammatory cells. Among the infiltrating cells are tissue-damaging cells, such as natural killer (NK) cells and macrophages, and others with antigen-presenting activity, such as dendritic cells and macrophages, resulting in further activation of the invading autoreactive T cells, leading to augmented infiltration and a cascading response.

Our studies have shown that MHC II molecule expression by parenchymal cells of the autoimmune organ plays a regulatory role in autoreactive T cell activation, and thus, the formation of an inflammatory response and tissue damage. This is because the activation of autoreactive T cells by the parenchymal MHC II-expressing cells is only 'partial' and the production of pro-inflammatory cytokines is lower than pathogenic levels. Furthermore, this pre-activation renders the invading T cell refractory when potent professional APCs become available during the later phases of inflammation. In short, the expression of MHC molecules by the parenchymal cell of the autoimmune organ induces the invading T cell to become anergic after producing limited amounts of pro-inflammatory cytokines. It is also likely that the expression of MHC class I molecules protects glial cells from NK cell cytotoxic effects, as MHC-negative target cells are more vulnerable to cytolysis by NK cells [54]. Indeed, studies have shown that among the cells infiltrating the target organ during inflammation, a significant proportion possess an NK-like phenotype and cytotoxic activity [55].

Thus, the expression of MHC class II molecules by the parenchymal cell of the autoimmune organ is probably more beneficial than detrimental to the host in terms of preventing the full activation and expansion of potentially pathogenic T cells. Nevertheless, the production of incremental amounts of cytokines by T cells that are partially activated may also facilitate disease progression.

Reciprocal Interaction between Autoreactive T Cells and Parenchymal Cells of the Eye

We have previously shown that autoreactive T cells vary greatly in disease-inducing capacity [56, 57]. Unfortunately, this is not always reflected by differences in the fine specificity of the cell response or the cytokine-producing pattern of the maximally activated T cells. Because of this, researchers are searching for other cellular and molecular features showing a better correlation with the pathogenic nature of the cells. For example, studies in our laboratory have shown that the degree to which an autoreactive T cell is activated and its pattern of cytokine production are not innate to the cell and are not solely determined by the type of T cell receptor ligand that induces T cell activation, as the source of the APCs and the dose of antigen available are also important [58]. Given that the major MHC-expressing cells, such as glial cells in the central nervous system and astrocytes and RPE cells in the eye, may differ from professional APCs in the periphery in terms of antigen processing or accessory molecule expression, it is of interest to know whether activation of autoreactive T cells inside the autoimmune organ differs from T cell activation in the periphery, particularly in the presence of suboptimal doses of antigen, assuming that optimal in vitro doses would not always be available in vivo. It is possible, for example, that autoreactive T cell subsets capable of responding to limited antigen doses may pose a greater threat in vivo than other T cells with the same antigenic specificity, but activated only by larger doses of antigen.

Autoreactive T cell subsets differ greatly in their ability to interact with parenchymal cells [59, 60]. This finding appears to be consistent with the previous observation that not all IRBP-reactive T cells produce a similar degree of tissue damage in the eye [12]. It remains to be determined whether the ability of T cells to interact with parenchymal cells of the autoimmune organ correlates with their pathogenic activity and whether pathogenic T cells have an enhanced or decreased ability to interact with parenchymal cells of the organ.

Conclusion

Although the physiological role of MHC molecules on parenchymal cells of the autoimmune organ is still poorly understood, it seems implausible that this expression of MHC II molecules during the genesis of autoimmune disease favors the reactivation of the invading autoreactive T cell. Since disease is always preceded by inflammation of the diseased organ, a reaction that recruits large numbers of peripheral APCs which may cause stronger activation of the invading autoimmune T cell, it is assumed that expression of limited amounts of MHC II molecules by parenchymal cells should render the invading autoreactive T cells unresponsive to the infiltrating APCs by promoting their entry into a refractory phase of the cell cycle.

By their ability to express variable amounts of MHC molecules, parenchymal cells of the autoimmune organ, such as astrocytes and RPE cells, have the ability to control the degree of T cell activation in the organ. Thus, T cells entering the autoimmune organ and in contact with cells expressing low levels of MHC class II molecules downregulate their T cell receptor and become minimally activated and hyporesponsive. These observations support the premise that the primary role of MHC II-expressing cells in the autoimmune organ is to diminish or block full T cell activation in the organ, and thereby, prevent the release of harmful cytokines. It is possible that, during massive T cell infiltration or infection, the local cells then express higher levels of MHC molecules, promoting greater T cell activation with the accompanying production of pro-inflammatory cytokines.

Circumstantial evidence indicates that interactions between autoreactive T cells and the parenchymal cells of the autoimmune organ are highly versatile. For example, only activated encephalitogenic T cells are able to penetrate the blood-brain barrier [61] and cause experimental autoimmune encephalomyelitis [62]. The levels of MHC antigens expressed on parenchymal cells determines not only the activation of invading autoreactive T cells, but also the survival of these parenchymal cells faced with the cytolytic activity of autoaggressive T cells [62]. In addition, the availability of T cell-specific antigen is critical for the cell-cell interaction [62] and for the persistence of the invading T cell in the organ [63, 64]. Further studies should provide a better understanding of the pathogenesis of autoimmune ocular disease.

Acknowledgment

This study was supported by grants EY014366 (D.S.), EY12974, EY14599 (H.S.) and R24 EY015636 from the National Institutes of Health and the Research to Prevent Blindness Endowment Fund, New York, N.Y., USA.

References

1 Burns J, Rosenzweig A, Zweiman B, et al: Isolation of myelin basic protein-reactive T-cell lines from normal human blood. Cell Immunol 1983;81:435–440.
2 Schlüsener HJ, Wekerle H: Autoaggressive T lymphocyte lines recognizing the encephalitogenic region of myelin basic protein: in vitro selection from unprimed rat T lymphocyte populations. J Immunol 1985;135:3128–3133.
3 Massa PT, ter Meulen V, Fontana A: Hyperinducibility of Ia antigen on astrocytes correlates with strain-specific susceptibility to experimental autoimmune encephalomyelitis. Proc Natl Acad Sci USA 1987;84:4219–4223.
4 Chung IY, Norris JG, Benveniste EN: Differential tumor necrosis factor α expression by astrocytes from experimental allergic encephalomyelitis-susceptible and -resistant rat strains. J Exp Med 1991;173:801–811.
5 Shao H, Sun SL, Kaplan HJ, et al: Characterization of rat CD8+ uveitogenic T cells specific for interphotoreceptor retinal-binding protein 1177–1191. J Immunol 2004;173:2849–2854.
6 Donoso LA, Merryman CF, Sery T, et al: Human interstitial retinoid binding protein: a potent uveitopathogenic agent for the induction of experimental autoimmune uveitis. J Immunol 1989;143: 79–83.

7 Chan CC, Nussenblatt RB, Wiggert B, et al: Immunohistochemical analysis of experimental autoimmune uveoretinitis (EAU) induced by interphotoreceptor retinoid-binding protein (IRBP) in the rat. Immunol Invest 1987;16:63–74.
8 Caspi RR: Experimental autoimmune uveoretinitis – rat and mouse; in Cohen IR (ed): Animal Models for Autoimmune Diseases: A Guidebook. New York, Academic Press, 1994, p 57.
9 Silver PB, Rizzo LV, Chan CC, et al: Identification of a major pathogenic epitope in the human IRBP molecule recognized by mice of the H-2r haplotype. Invest Ophthalmol Vis Sci 1995;36: 946–954.
10 Shao H, Peng Y, Liao T, et al: A shared epitope of the interphotoreceptor retinoid-binding protein recognized by the CD4+ and CD8+ autoreactive T cells. J Immunol 2005;175:1851–1857.
11 Shao H, Liao T, Ke Y, et al: Severe chronic experimental autoimmune uveitis (EAU) of the C57BL/6 mouse induced by adoptive transfer of IRBP1-20-specific T cells. Exp Eye Res 2006;82:323–331.
12 Shao H, Song L, Sun SL, et al: Conversion of monophasic to recurrent autoimmune disease by autoreactive T cell subsets. J Immunol 2003;171:5624–5630.
13 Sun D, Hu X, Le J, et al: Characterization of brain-isolated rat encephalitogenic T cell lines. Eur J Immunol 1994;24:1359–1364.
14 Sun D, Le J, Coleclough C: Diverse T cell receptor β chain usage by rat encephalitogenic T cells reactive to residues 68–88 of myelin basic protein. Eur J Immunol 1993;23:494–498.
15 Sun D, Gold DP, Smith L, et al: Characterization of rat encephalitogenic T cells bearing non-V_b8 T cell receptors. Eur J Immunol 1992;22:591–594.
16 Shao H, Fu YX, Song L, et al: LTbR-Ig treatment blocks actively induced, but not adoptively transferred, uveitis in Lewis rats. Eur J Immunol 2003;33:1743.
17 Shao H, Fu Y, Liao T, et al: Anti-CD137 mAb treatment inhibits experimental autoimmune uveitis by limiting expansion and increasing apoptotic death of uveitogenic T cells. Invest Ophthalmol Vis Sci 2005;46:596–603.
18 Sun D, Hu X, Shah R, et al: Production of tumor necrosis factor-α as a result of glia-T-cell interaction correlates with the pathogenic activity of myelin basic protein-reactive T cells in experimental autoimmune encephalomyelitis. J Neurosci Res 1996;45:400–409.
19 Sun D, Coleclough C, Whitaker JN: Nonactivated astrocytes downregulate T cell receptor expression and reduce antigen-specific proliferation and cytokine production of myelin basic protein (MBP)-reactive T cells. J Neuroimmunol 1997;78:69–78.
20 Sun D, Hu XZ, Liu XH, et al: Expression of chemokine genes in rat glial cells: the effect of myelin basic protein-reactive encephalitogenic T cells. J Neurosci Res 1997;48:192–200.
21 Olsson T, Sun J, Hillert J, et al: Increased numbers of T cells recognizing multiple myelin basic protein epitopes in multiple sclerosis. Eur J Immunol 1992;22:1083–1087.
22 Sun D, Wilson DB, Cao L, et al: The role of regulatory T cells in Lewis rats resistant to EAE. J Neuroimmunol 1998;81:177–183.
23 Werdelin O, McCluskey RT: The nature and the specificity of mononuclear cells in experimental autoimmune inflammations and the mechanisms leading to their accumulation. J Exp Med 1971;133:1242–1263.
24 Zinn KM, Benjamin-Henkind JV: Anatomy of the human retinal pigment epithelium; in Zinn KM, Marmor MF (eds): The retinal pigment epithelium. Cambridge, Harvard University Press, 2002, pp 3–31.
25 Farrokh-Siar L, Rezai KA, Semnani RT, et al: Human fetal retinal pigment epithelium suppresses the activation of $CD4^+$ and $CD8^+$ T-cells. Graefes Arch Clin Exp Ophthalmol 1999;237:934–939.
26 Faure V, Courtois Y, Goureau O: Inhibition of inducible nitric oxide synthase expression by TNF α and β in bovine retinal pigmented epithelial cells. J Biol Chem 1997;272:32169–32175.
27 Holtkamp GM, Kijlstra A, Peek R, et al: Retinal pigment epithelium-immune system interactions: cytokine production and cytokine-induced changes. Prog Retin Eye Res 2001;20:29–48.
28 Liversidge J, Forrester JV: Antigen processing and presentation in the eye: a review. Curr Eye Res 1992;11:49–58.
29 Griffith TS, Brunner T, Fletcher SM, et al: Fas ligand-induced apoptosis as a mechanism of immune privilege. Science 1995;270:1189–1192.
30 Griffith TS, Ferguson TA: The role of FasL-induced apoptosis in immune privilege. Immunol Today 1997;18:240–244.

31 Jorgensen A, Wiencke AK, la Cour M, et al: Human retinal pigment epithelial cell-induced apoptosis in activated T cells. Invest Ophthalmol Vis Sci 1998;39:1590–1599.
32 Crane IJ, Kuppner MC, Mckillop-Smith S, et al: Cytokine regulation of RANTES production by human retinal pigment epithelial cells. Cell Immunol 1998;184:37–44.
33 Crane IJ, Wallace CA, Mckillop-Smith S, et al: Control of chemokine production at the blood-retina barrier. Immunology 2000;101:426–433.
34 Devine L, Lightman S, Greenwood J: Lymphocyte migration across the anterior and posterior blood-retinal barrier in vitro. Cell Immunol 1996;168:267–275.
35 Jaffe GJ, Van Le L, Valea F, et al: Expression of interleukin-1 alpha, interleukin-1 beta, and an interleukin-1 receptor antagonist in human retinal pigment epithelial cells. Exp Eye Res 1992;55:325–335.
36 Kumaki N, Anderson DM, Cosman D, et al: Expression of interleukin-15 and its receptor by human fetal retinal pigment epithelial cells. Curr Eye Res 1996;15:876–882.
37 Liversidge J, Grabowski P, Ralston S, et al: Rat retinal pigment epithelial cells express an inducible form of nitric oxide synthase and produce nitric oxide in response to inflammatory cytokines and activated T cells. Immunology 1994;83:404–409.
38 Hamel CP, Detrick B, Hooks JJ: Evaluation of Ia expression in rat ocular tissues following inoculation with interferon-gamma. Exp Eye Res 1990;50:173–182.
39 Osusky R, Dorio RJ, Arora YK, et al: MHC class II positive retinal pigment epithelial (RPE) cells can function as antigen-presenting cells for microbial superantigen. Ocul Immunol Inflamm 1997;5:43–50.
40 Percopo CM, Hooks JJ, Shinohara T, et al: Cytokine-mediated activation of a neuronal retinal resident cell provokes antigen presentation. J Immunol 1990;145:4101–4107.
41 Zinkernagel R, Doherty PC: H-2-compatibility requirement for T cell-mediated lysis of target cells infected with lymphocytic choriomeningitis virus: different cytotoxic T cell specificities are associated with structures from H-2K or H-2D. J Exp Med 1975;141:1427–1436.
42 Wong GMW, Bartlett PF, Clark-Lewis I, et al: Inducible expression of H-2 and Ia antigens on brain cells. Nature 1984;310:688–691.
43 Traugott U, Scheinberg LC, Raine CS: On the presence of Ia-positive endothelial cells and astrocytes in multiple sclerosis lesions and its relevance to antigen presentation. J Neuroimmunol 1985;8:1.
44 Sun D, Enzmann V, Lei S, et al: Retinal pigment epithelial cells activate uveitogenic T cells when they express high levels of MHC class II molecules, but inhibit T cell activation when they express restricted levels. J Neuroimmunol 2003;144:1–8.
45 Benson MT, Shepherd L, Cottam D, et al: The expression of class I major histocompatibility antigens by human retinal pigment epithelium in vitro. Graefes Arch Clin Exp Ophthalmol 1992;230:184–187.
46 Detrick B, Newsome DA, Percopo CM, et al: Class II antigen expression and gamma interferon modulation of monocytes and retinal pigment epithelial cells from patients with retinitis pigmentosa. Clin Immunol Immunopathol 1985;36:201–211.
47 de KY, Naud MC, Bellot J, et al: Differential tumor necrosis factor expression by resident retinal cells from experimental uveitis-susceptible and -resistant rat strains. J Neuroimmunol 1994;55: 1–9.
48 Schwartz RH: Costimulation of T lymphocytes: the role of CD28, CTLA-4, and B7/BB1 in interleukin-2 production and immunotherapy. Cell 1992;71:1065–1068.
49 Jenkins MK, Schwartz R: Antigen presentation by chemically modified splenocytes induces antigen-specific T cell unresponsiveness in vitro and in vivo. J Exp Med 1987;165:302–310.
50 Cao WX, Tykodi SS, Esser MT, et al: Partial activation of $CD8^+$ T cells by a self-derived peptide. Nature 1995;378:295–298.
51 Evavold BD, Allen PM: Separation of IL-4 production from Th cell proliferation by an altered T cell receptor ligand. Science 1991;252:1308–1310.
52 Sloan-Lancaster J, Shaw AS, Rothbard JB, et al: Partial T cell signaling: altered phospho-zeta and lack of zap70 recruitment in APL-induced T cell anergy. Cell 1994;79:913–922.
53 Sousa CRE, Levine EH, Germain RN: Partial signaling by $CD8^+$ T cells in response to antagonist ligands. J Exp Med 1996;184:149–157.

54 Orihuela M, Margulies DH, Yokoyama WM: The natural killer cell receptor Ly-49A recognizes a peptide-induced conformational determinant on its major histocompatibility complex class I ligand. Proc Natl Acad Sci USA 1996;93:11792–11797.
55 Shao H, Van Kaer L, Sun SL, et al: Infiltration of the inflamed eye by NKT cells in a rat model of experimental autoimmune uveitis. J Autoimmun 2003;21:37–45.
56 Sun D, Coleclough C, Hu X: Heterogeneity of rat encephalitogenic T cells elicited by variants of the MBP (68–88) peptide. Eur J Immunol 1995;25:1687–1692.
57 Sun D, Hu X, Shah R, et al: The pattern of cytokine gene expression induced in rat T cells specific for myelin basic protein depends on the type and quality of antigenic stimulus. Cell Immunol 1995;166:1–8.
58 Sun D, Le J, Yang S, et al: Major role of antigen-presenting cells in the response of rat encephalitogenic T cells to myelin basic proteins. J Immunol 1993;151:111–118.
59 Tabi Z, McCombe PA, Pender MP: Apoptotic elimination of $Vb8.2^+$ cells from the central nervous system during recovery from experimental autoimmune encephalomyelitis induced by the passive transfer of $Vb8.2^+$ encephalitogenic T cells. Eur J Immunol 1994;24:2609–2617.
60 Pender M, McCombe PA, Yoong G, et al: Apoptosis of $\alpha\beta$ T lymphocytes in the nervous system in experimental autoimmune encephalomyelitis: its possible implications for recovery and acquired tolerance. J Autoimmun 1992;5:401–410.
61 Wekerle H, Linington C, Lassmann H, et al: Cellular immune reactivity within the CNS. Trends Neurosci 1986;9:271–277.
62 Sun D, Wekerle H: Ia-restricted encephalitogenic T lymphocytes mediating EAE lyse autoantigen-presenting astrocytes. Nature 1986;320:70–72.
63 Kawakami N, Odoardi F, Ziemssen T, et al: Autoimmune CD4+ T cell memory: lifelong persistence of encephalitogenic T cell clones in healthy immune repertoires. J Immunol 2005;175: 69–81.
64 Flugel A, Berkowicz T, Ritter T, et al: Migratory activity and functional changes of green fluorescent effector cells before and during experimental autoimmune encephalomyelitis. Immunity 2001;14:547–560.

Dr. Henry J. Kaplan
Department of Ophthalmology and Visual Science, University of Louisville
301 East Muhammad Ali Boulevard
Louisville, KY 40202 (USA)
Tel. +1 502 852 5466, Fax +1 502 852 4595, E-Mail hank.kaplan@louisville.edu

Niederkorn JY, Kaplan HJ (eds): Immune Response and the Eye.
Chem Immunol Allergy. Basel, Karger, 2007, vol 92, pp 105–114

Complement, Innate Immunity and Ocular Disease

Jeong-Hyeon Sohn[b], Puran S. Bora[a], Prushottam Jha[a], Tongalp H. Tezel[b], Henry J. Kaplan[b], Nalini S. Bora[a]

[a]Department of Ophthalmology, Jones Eye Institute, University of Arkansas for Medical Sciences, Little Rock, Ark., [b]Department of Ophthalmology and Visual Science, Kentucky Lions Eye Center, University of Louisville, Louisville, Ky., USA

Abstract

The complement system is a major component of innate immunity. During an inflammatory reaction, the eye is potentially threatened by homologous complement attack, and unregulated complement activation could lead to tissue damage and vision loss. The complement system is continuously activated at low levels in the normal eye, and intraocular complement-regulatory proteins (CRPs) tightly regulate this spontaneous complement activation so that there is elimination of potential pathogens without the induction of destructive intraocular inflammation. The presence of a complement activation product (iC3b) during the early phase of antigen and antigen-presenting cell contact is essential for the induction of systemic tolerance to antigen injected into the anterior chamber of the eye and the establishment of ocular immune privilege. The complement system and complement-regulatory proteins control intraocular inflammation in autoimmune anterior uveitis and may play an important role in the development of age-related macular degeneration. Thus, in the eye, complement functions as a double-edged sword – on one hand it provides innate immunity against pathogens while simultaneously instructing the adaptive immune response to develop tolerance to such pathogens to avoid inadvertent tissue damage in a critical organ.

Complement is a major component of innate immunity and consists of approximately 30 fluid phase and cell membrane proteins [1]. The complement system can be activated via three well-defined pathways: namely, the classical, lectin and alternative pathways. Because of its potent pro-inflammatory and destructive capabilities, the host must be protected from the inadvertent activation of complement on its own tissues during an inflammatory response. Several complement-regulatory proteins (CRPs) serve to regulate the complement cascade and provide a recognition system to distinguish self from non-self, thus, preventing damage to host tissue during an inflammatory reaction [1]. Foreign surfaces (such as invading pathogens) lacking CRPs are attacked and destroyed by complement.

The importance of complement as a component of the innate immune system is well established. Inappropriate activation of complement is crucial to the pathogenesis of various diseases [1]. In recent years it has become increasingly evident that complement is also involved in the antigen-specific immune response and plays a role in antigen processing/presentation, T cell proliferation/differentiation, B cell activation [2, 3] and systemic tolerance induced by the introduction of antigen into an immune-privileged site, such as the anterior chamber (AC) of the eye [4].

Complement and the Eye

Role in the Induction of Anterior Chamber-Associated Immune Deviation

The unique immunologic and anatomic features of the eye prevent the induction and expression of conventional immunity – a phenomenon known as 'immune privilege'. Immune privilege in the eye is a dynamic state in which the systemic immune response to antigens introduced intraocularly is aberrant, resulting in antigen-specific suppression of the delayed-type hypersensitivity response – a phenomenon referred to as AC-associated immune deviation (ACAID) or ocular tolerance [5]. Sohn et al. [4] reported that complement plays a critical role in the induction of ocular tolerance in rodents. Depletion of complement prevented the in vivo induction of ACAID to a soluble protein antigen, ovalbumin (OVA). The importance of C3, the third component of complement, was demonstrated by the inability to induce ACAID to OVA in C3-deficient mice. The administration of neutralizing anti-rat CR3 (iC3b receptor; OX-42) antibody prior to the induction of ACAID prevented the development of tolerance to OVA. In the in vitro model of ACAID, iC3b was required for the suppression of the delayed-type hypersensitivity response, as tolerance was abrogated by the addition of OX-42 to the culture. Furthermore, iC3b induced the secretion of transforming growth factor (TGF)-β_2 and interleukin (IL)-10 (with TGF-β_2 upregulated first) by antigen-presenting cells, while IL-12 was downregulated. In the presence of OX-42 this effect was abolished. Finally, neutralizing antibodies to IL-10 or TGF-β_2 reversed iC3b-induced tolerance. Thus, Sohn et al. [4] concluded that the ligation of iC3b by CR3 on antigen-presenting cells resulted in the sequential production of TGF-β_2 and IL-10 by antigen-presenting cells and was essential for the induction of ocular tolerance and the maintenance of ocular immune privilege (fig. 1).

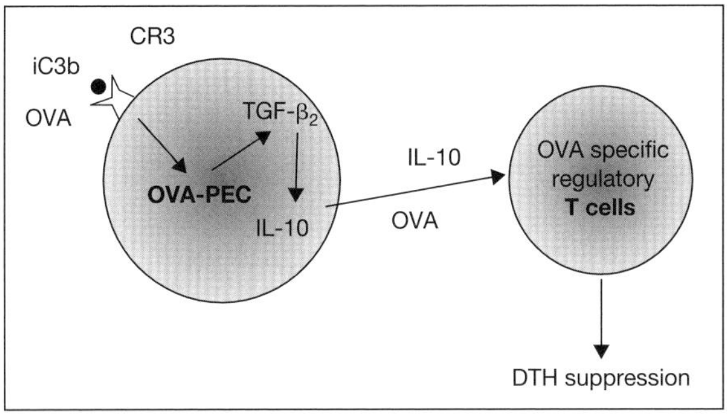

Fig. 1. Role of complement, specifically iC3b binding to CR3 on antigen-presenting cells (OVA-PEC), in the development of ACAID to OVA. DTH = Delayed-type hypersensitivity; PEC = Peritoneal exudate cells.

Chronic Activation of the Complement Cascade in the Anterior Chamber

Various complement components and CRPs, which regulate the activation of the complement system, have been detected in the human eye [6–8]. In 2000, Sohn et al. [9] reported that complement activation products, iC3b and membrane attack complex (MAC), were present in the normal rat eye. Additionally, in this report, both membrane-bound and soluble CRPs were identified in the normal rat eye. AC injection of zymosan, a well-known activator of the alternative pathway of complement, induced severe anterior uveitis. These results suggested that the complement system is continuously active, at a low level, in the normal eye. The authors suggested that this low level of complement activation is tightly regulated by intraocular CRPs, as Lewis rats injected with a neutralizing monoclonal antibody against CRPs developed a severe anterior uveitis, with increased formation of iC3b and MAC. These observations suggested that complement activation products are required for the maintenance of ocular immune privilege and that a regulatory system exists in the eye to protect ocular cells from destruction by these products during intraocular inflammation.

Complement and Ocular Diseases

In uveitis and age-related macular degeneration (AMD) there is a breakdown of the blood-aqueous or blood-retinal barriers, which leads to at least the transient loss of immune privilege in the AC and subretinal space, respectively.

Autoimmune Uveitis

The role of complement in autoimmune uveitis is not well understood. Complement activation products such as C3b and C4b are present in the eyes of patients with anterior uveitis [10]. In experimental autoimmune uveoretinitis caused by retinal S-antigen, complement activation is important for inflammation [11]. Recently, a rodent model of experimental autoimmune anterior uveitis (EAAU) was used to explore the role of complement and CRPs in the pathogenesis of ocular autoimmune disease. EAAU is an autoimmune disease of the eye and is an animal model of idiopathic human anterior uveitis [12]. This report demonstrated that the induction and progression of autoimmune uveitis is complement restricted. The expression of cytokines, chemokines and adhesion molecules necessary for the development of EAAU required complement activation. Furthermore, the local (i.e. intraocular) activation of complement was required to induce EAAU. It was also shown that various ocular tissues upregulate the expression of CRPs to avoid self-injury during intraocular inflammation, and these CRPs play an active role in the resolution of EAAU by downregulating complement activation in vivo. Thus, the local activation of complement may serve as a mechanism to target the inflammatory response to a specific organ, i.e. the eye.

Age-Related Macular Degeneration

Of the 44 million annual visits to ophthalmologists, more than half are by elderly (>65) persons [13]. This elderly population will grow from 34.4 million in 2000 to 70.3 million by 2030, with the number of persons older than 85 years growing slightly faster – from 4.1 to 8.9 million [14]. Among the elderly, AMD is the leading cause of vision loss in the United States and Western Europe [15]. Nearly 2 million Americans over the age of 55 are diagnosed with AMD each year. Approximately 230,000 of those affected have been declared legally blind. Between 1991 and 1999, the prevalence of AMD among the elderly increased from 5 to 25.6%, and with the aging of the 'baby boomer' generation, AMD is projected to affect the sight of over 6 million people [16].

AMD is the end stage of specific age-related structural fundus changes collectively called *age-related maculopathy*. The hallmark lesion of age-related maculopathy is small subretinal deposits called *drusen*. Depending on their appearances, drusen can be classified in several ways. Small (<63 μm), hard drusen are white-yellow subretinal deposits with sharp borders. They are present in almost 90% of the Caucasian population above 40 years old [17], and, classically, are not known to indicate any risk for progression to AMD [18]. However, they can occasionally evolve to form large, soft drusen or result in cell death of retinal pigment epithelium (RPE) and pigment dispersion, both of which are known to be associated with the development of AMD [19]. The prevalence and confluence of soft drusen increases with age. Large, soft drusen (>125 μm) can be seen in 2% of the population aged 43–54 years, and increases up to 24% among individuals above 75 years old [18]. These eyes are six times more likely to develop AMD [20], which is characterized by the development of two distinct lesions: geographic atrophy and subretinal neovascularization.

Geographic atrophy, a discrete area of retinal depigmentation due to loss of RPE and choriocapillaris, is at least 175 μm in diameter, with a sharp border and visible choroidal vessels without any evidence of subretinal neovascularization.

Subretinal neovascularization may result in a hemorrhagic or serous detachment of the RPE or sensory retina, subretinal fibrosis or RPE atrophy [21].

It is estimated that of the 1.75 million individuals in the United States that have AMD, 1.22 million have subretinal neovascularization in at least one eye and 973,000 have geographic atrophy [22]. Similar to age-related maculopathy, the prevalence of AMD increases with age [22]. Racial factors may also effect the presentation of the disease phenotype. For example, geographic atrophy is more common than subretinal neovascularization in Icelanders, Norwegians and Inuits; among blacks, subretinal neovascularization is less prevalent than in whites despite the frequency of predisposing lesions such as large drusen and pigmentary abnormalities [23]. Such differences can be attributed to genetic and environmental factors, as well as to the different methodology employed in various epidemiological studies.

Other risk factors for the development of AMD include family history and smoking. Single nucleotide polymorphism variants of the genes for factors H and B, as well as *LOC387715* [24], are associated with a 10.3-fold increased risk for the development of subretinal neovascularization in individuals with a sibling with exudative AMD. A positive family history also carries an important risk factor for non-exudative AMD. For example, the odds of developing RPE atrophy increases 8.2 times with a positive history in a sibling [25]. Smoking may effect the incidence of AMD via a reduction in macular carotenoids [26], adverse effects on RPE drug detoxification mechanisms, or a decrease in choroidal blood flow and antioxidant levels [27, 28].

High-dose supplements of vitamin C (500 mg), vitamin E (400 IU), β-carotene (15 mg), and zinc (80 mg) with 2 mg copper may delay the progression of intermediate AMD (large drusen >125 μm or noncentral geographic atrophy) to advanced AMD lesions, such as subretinal neovascularization or geographic atrophy [29]. Study participants were put on these supplements for an average of 6.3 years. However, delayed progression from earlier stages of AMD to intermediate or advanced AMD was not observed.

Clinically, AMD has been classified into two types: non-exudative or 'dry' (geographic atrophy only) and exudative or 'wet'. The latter is characterized by choroidal neovascularization and occurs in as many as 200,000 patients each year in the United States. Without treatment, most patients progress to a visual acuity of 20/200 or worse in less than 2 years [30]. Non-exudative AMD comprises up to 85% of AMD cases and in approximately 10–20% of patients eventually progresses to the exudative type. There is no effective treatment for the severe loss of central vision that occurs in dry AMD. Several modalities have been shown to be of benefit in the treatment of exudative AMD, including photodynamic therapy and thermal laser photocoagulation [31, 32]. Thermal laser coagulates choroidal new vessels at the cost of sacrificing central vision [33]. Even so, <20% of the patients with exudative AMD are eligible for laser photocoagulation, and half of them develop persistent or recurrent neovascularization and require multiple treatment sessions [34]. Photodynamic treatment reduces the rate of visual loss due to well-defined choroidal neovascularization but does not lead to significant visual improvement in most individuals [32]. Moreover, cost-utility models proved these palliative treatments to be highly cost-ineffective, since it requires USD 73,984–86,721 to gain one quality-of-life-adjusted year after photodynamic treatment [35] and USD 16,117–49,766 after laser photocoagulation [36]. Alternative treatment modalities, such as systemic interferon [37], radiotherapy [38], subfoveal membranectomy [39], macular translocation [40], and anti-angiogenic pharmacological agents, e.g. anti-vascular endothelial growth factor (VEGF) antibody [41], anti-VEGF aptamer [42], triamcinolone [43] and anecortave acetate [44], all aim to obliterate new choroidal vessels and/or decrease plasma leakage. Identification of VEGF as the main player in the development of ocular neovascularization by promoting angiogenesis and vascular permeability has resulted in the introduction of anti-VEGF agents into clinical use. One such agent is pegaptanib, an anti-VEGF oligonucleotide conjugated with polyethylene glycol (Macugen; EyeTech Pharmaceuticals), that binds and blocks the biologic activity of the major human soluble VEGF isoform (VEGF165). Pegaptanib has been shown to stabilize or improve vision up to 2 years. However, this effect is temporary, requires multiple injections and the long-term safety and efficacy are still not known. The risk of infectious endophthalmitis and other intravitreal injection-related complications is of concern in light of the modest benefit of treatment. Most recently, anti-VEGF antibodies, bevacizumab (Avastin) and ranibizumab (Lucentis; both Genetech), have shown increased efficacy for the return of central vision compared to the other methods of treatment [45–47]. However, the same reservations exist as for pegaptanib since frequent intravitreal injections are required.

It is obvious that current treatments are not curative, but rather remain palliative measures. They often require multiple treatment sessions due to recurrences and usually result in only slowing visual deterioration with little significant improvement in lost central vision. Eventually, persistent exudation from the subretinal fibrovascular tissue leads to fibrovascular scar formation with continuing disruption of the relationship between choriocapillaris, RPE

Complement activation in the posterior segment of the eye → MAC formation and deposition of sublytic MAC on RPE cells → Non-lethal transient changes in the membrane permeability of RPE cells

→ Induction and release of angiogenic growth factors by RPE cells → Access of released growth factors to choroidal endothelial cells → Abnormal proliferation of choroidal endothelial cells leading to the development of CNV

Fig. 2. Role of complement in the development of choroidal neovascularization (CNV).

and photoreceptors with subsequent photoreceptor cell death, and, ultimately, the loss of central vision [33].

The pathogenesis of new choroidal vessel formation is poorly understood. Only recently it has become apparent that complement is important in AMD. Vitronectin, C5 and MAC have been shown to be components of drusen in humans [48, 49]. Recently, Bora et al. [50] described a direct role of complement activation and MAC formation in the laser-induced model of choroidal angiogenesis in the rodent. They demonstrated that MAC formation and deposition was critical for the increased intraocular production of growth factors – VEGF, β-fibroblast growth factor, and TGF-β_2 – which eventually led to the development of choroidal neovascularization. The authors proposed that complement activation in the posterior segment of the eye led to the increased formation/deposition of MAC on RPE and/or choroid. This resulted in transient changes in membrane permeability followed by the induction and release of angiogenic growth factors. These growth factors cause the abnormal proliferation of choroidal endothelial cells leading to the development of choroidal neovascularization in AMD (fig. 2).

References

1 Atkinson JP, Farries T: Separation of self from non-self in the complement system. Immunol Today 1987;8:212–215.
2 Dempsey PW, Allison MED, Akkaraju S, Goodnow CC, Fearon DT: C3d of complement as a molecular adjuvant: bridging innate and acquired immunity. Science 1996;271:348–350.
3 Carroll MC: The complement system in regulation of adaptive immunity. Nat Immunol 2004;5:981–986.
4 Sohn JH, Bora PS, Suk HJ, Molina H, Kaplan HJ, Bora NS: Tolerance is dependent on complement C3 fragment iC3b binding to antigen-presenting cells. Nat Med 2003;9:206–212.
5 Streilein JW: Immunologic privilege of the eye. Springer Semin Immunopathol 1999;21:95–111.

6 Mondino BJ, Rao H: Hemolytic complement activity in aqueous humor. Arch Ophthalmol 1983;101:465–468.
7 Bora NS, Gobleman CL, Atkinson JP, Pepose JS, Kaplan HJ: Differential expression of the complement regulatory proteins in the human eye. Invest Ophthalmol Vis Sci 1993;34:3579–3584.
8 Sohn JH, Kaplan HJ, Suk HJ, Bora PS, Bora NS: Complement regulatory activity of normal human intraocular fluid is mediated by MCP, DAF, and CD59. Invest Ophthalmol Vis Sci 2000;41: 4195–4202.
9 Sohn JH, Kaplan HJ, Suk HJ, Bora PS, Bora NS: Chronic low level complement activation within the eye is controlled by intraocular complement regulatory proteins. Invest Ophthalmol Vis Sci 2000;41:3492–3502.
10 Mondino BJ, Glovsky MM, Ghekiere L: Activated complement in inflamed aqueous humor. Invest Ophthalmol Vis Sci 1984;25:871–873.
11 Marak GE, Wacker WB, Rao NA, Jack R, Ward PA: Effects of complement depletion on experimental allergic uveitis. Ophthalmic Res 1979;11:97–107.
12 Bora NS, Sohn JH, Kang SG, et al: Type I collagen is the autoantigen in experimental autoimmune anterior uveitis. J Immunol 2004;172:7086–7094.
13 Javitt JC, Chiang YP: Preparing for managed competition. Utilization of ophthalmologic services varies by state. Arch Ophthalmol 1993;111:1469–1470.
14 US Census Bureau: National population projections. I. Summary files. 2002, http://www.census.gov/population/www/projections/natsum-T3.html
15 West SK: Looking forward to 20/20: a focus on the epidemiology of eye diseases. Epidemiol Rev 2000;22:64–70.
16 Lee PP, Feldman ZW, Ostermann J, Brown DS, Sloan FA: Longitudinal prevalence of major eye diseases. Arch Ophthalmol 2003;121:1303–1310.
17 Klein R, Klein BE, Moss SE: Relation of smoking to the incidence of age-related maculopathy. The Beaver Dam Eye Study. Am J Epidemiol 1998;147:103–110.
18 Klein R, Klein BE, Tomany SC, Meuer SM, Huang GH: Ten-year incidence and progression of age-related maculopathy: the Beaver Dam Eye Study. Ophthalmology 2002;109:1767–1779.
19 Bressler NM, Munoz B, Maguire MG, et al: Five-year incidence and disappearance of drusen and retinal pigment epithelial abnormalities. Waterman study. Arch Ophthalmol 1995;113: 301–308.
20 Wang JJ, Foran S, Smith W, Mitchell P: Risk of age-related macular degeneration in eyes with macular drusen or hyperpigmentation: the Blue Mountains Eye Study cohort. Arch Ophthalmol 2003;121:658–663.
21 Bird AC, Bressler NM, Bressler SB, et al: An international classification and grading system for age-related maculopathy and age-related macular degeneration. The International ARM Epidemiological Study Group. Surv Ophthalmol 1995;39:367–374.
22 Friedman DS, O'Colmain BJ, Munoz B, et al: Prevalence of age-related macular degeneration in the United States. Arch Ophthalmol 2004;122:564–572.
23 Klein R, Peto T, Bird A, Vannewkirk MR: The epidemiology of age-related macular degeneration. Am J Ophthalmol 2004;137:486–495.
24 Marx J: Genetics. A clearer view of macular degeneration. Science 2006;311:1704–1705.
25 Klein BE, Klein R, Lee KE, Moore EL, Danforth L: Risk of incident age-related eye diseases in people with an affected sibling: the Beaver Dam Eye Study. Am J Epidemiol 2001;154: 207–211.
26 Stryker WS, Kaplan LA, Stein EA, Stampfer MJ, Sober A, Willett WC: The relation of diet, cigarette smoking, and alcohol consumption to plasma beta-carotene and alpha-tocopherol levels. Am J Epidemiol 1988;127:283–296.
27 Bettman J, Fellows V, Chao P: The effect of cigarette smoking on the intraocular circulation. Arch Ophthalmol 1958;59:481–488.
28 Friedmann E: Choroidal blood flow: pressure-flow relationships. Arch Ophthalmol 1970;83:95–99.
29 Age-Related Eye Disease Study Research Group: A randomized, placebo-controlled, clinical trial of high-dose supplementation with vitamins C and E, beta carotene, and zinc for age-related macular degeneration and vision loss: AREDS report No. 8. Arch Ophthalmol 2001;119: 1417–1436.

30 Macular Photocoagulation Study Group: Laser photocoagulation of subfoveal neovascular lesions of age-related macular degeneration. Updated findings from two clinical trials. Arch Ophthalmol 1993;111:1200–1209.
31 Macular Photocoagulation Study Group: Laser photocoagulation of subfoveal neovascular lesions in age-related macular degeneration. Results of a randomized clinical trial. Arch Ophthalmol 1991;109:1220–1231.
32 American Academy of Ophthalmology: Photodynamic therapy with verteporfin for age-related macular degeneration. Ophthalmology 2000;107:2314–2317.
33 Tezel TH, Del Priore LV, Flowers BE, et al: Correlation between scanning laser ophthalmoscope microperimetry and anatomic abnormalities in patients with subfoveal neovascularization. Ophthalmology 1996;103:1829–1836.
34 Moisseiev J, Alhalel A, Masuri R, Treister G: The impact of the macular photocoagulation study results on the treatment of exudative age-related macular degeneration. Arch Ophthalmol 1995;113:185–189.
35 Sharma S, Brown GC, Brown MM, Hollands H, Shah GK: The cost-effectiveness of photodynamic therapy for fellow eyes with subfoveal choroidal neovascularization secondary to age-related macular degeneration. Ophthalmology 2001;108:2051–2059.
36 Busbee BG, Brown MM, Brown GC, Sharma S: CME review: a cost-utility analysis of laser photocoagulation for extrafoveal choroidal neovascularization. Retina 2003;23:279–287, quiz 443–444.
37 Poliner LS, Tornambe PE, Michelson PE, Heitzmann JG: Interferon alpha-2a for subfoveal neovascularization in age-related macular degeneration. Ophthalmology 1993;100:1417–1424.
38 Ciulla TA, Danis RP, Klein SB, et al: Proton therapy for exudative age-related macular degeneration: a randomized, sham-controlled clinical trial. Am J Ophthalmol 2002;134:905–906.
39 Rao PK, Thomas MA: Update on surgical removal of choroidal neovascularization. Curr Opin Ophthalmol 2000;11:180–185.
40 Lai JC, Lapolice DJ, Stinnett SS, et al: Visual outcomes following macular translocation with 360-degree peripheral retinectomy. Arch Ophthalmol 2002;120:1317–1324.
41 Krzystolik MG, Afshari MA, Adamis AP, et al: Prevention of experimental choroidal neovascularization with intravitreal anti-vascular endothelial growth factor antibody fragment. Arch Ophthalmol 2002;120:338–346.
42 TES TESG: Anti-vascular endothelial growth factor therapy for subfoveal choroidal neovascularization secondary to age-related macular degeneration: phase II study results. Ophthalmology 2003;110:979–986.
43 Penfold PL, Wen L, Madigan MC, Gillies MC, King NJ, Provis JM: Triamcinolone acetonide modulates permeability and intercellular adhesion molecule-1 (ICAM-1) expression of the ECV304 cell line: implications for macular degeneration. Clin Exp Immunol 2000;121: 458–465.
44 D'Amico DJ, Goldberg MF, Hudson H, et al: Anecortave acetate as monotherapy for the treatment of subfoveal lesions in patients with exudative age-related macular degeneration (AMD): interim (month 6) analysis of clinical safety and efficacy. Retina 2003;23:14–23.
45 Rich RM, Rosenfeld PJ, Puliafito CA, Dubovy SR, Davis JL, Flynn HW, Gonzalez F, Feuer WJ, Lin RC, Lalwani GA, Nguyen JK, Dumar G: Short-term safety and efficacy of intravitreal bevacizumab (Avastin) for neovascular age-related macular degeneration. Retina 2006;26: 495–511.
46 Spaide RF, Laud K, Fine HF, Klancnik JM, Meyerle CB, Yannuzzi LA, Sorenson J, Slakter J, Fisher Yl, Cooney MJ: Intravitreal bevacizumab treatment of choroidal neovascularization secondary to age-related macular degeneration. Retina 2006;26:383–390.
47 Rosenfeld PJ, Heier JS, Hantsbarger G, Shams N: Tolerability and efficacy of multiple escalating doses of ranibizumab (Lucentis) for neovascular age-related macular degeneration. Ophthalmology 2006;113:632.
48 Mullins RF, Russell SR, Anderson DH, Hageman GS: Drusen associated with aging and age-related macular degeneration contain proteins common to extracellular deposits associated with atherosclerosis, elastosis, amyloidosis, and dense deposit disease. FASEB J 2000;14: 835–846.

49 Anderson DH, Mullins RF, Hageman GS, Johnson LV: A role for local inflammation in the formation of drusen in the aging eye. Am J Ophthalmol 2002;134:411–431.
50 Bora PS, Sohn JH, Cruz JM, Jha P, et al: Role of complement and complement membrane attack complex in laser-induced choroidal neovascularization. J Immunol 2005;174:491–497.

Dr. Nalini S. Bora
Department of Ophthalmology
Pat and Willard Walker Eye Research Centre
Jones Eye Insitute
University of Arkansas for Medical Sciences
4301 West Markham, 523, Little Rock, AR 72205–7199 (USA)
Tel. +1 501 686 8293, Fax +1 502 686 8316, E-Mail NBora@UAMS.edu

Niederkorn JY, Kaplan HJ (eds): Immune Response and the Eye.
Chem Immunol Allergy. Basel, Karger, 2007, vol 92, pp 115–130

Cross Talk among Cells Promoting Anterior Chamber-Associated Immune Deviation

Joan Stein-Streilein, Christine Watte

Schepens Eye Research Institute, Department of Ophthalmology,
Harvard School of Medicine, Boston, Mass., USA

Abstract

The visual axis of the eye focuses light images precisely on the retina. The retina is intolerant of distortion that might be induced by innate or immune inflammation. In addition, the corneal endothelium and the neurosensory retina are unable to regenerate if injured by trauma or inflammation. Within the environment of this visual organ a phenomenon called ocular immune privilege provides the eye with the necessary immune protection against infectious agents by allowing the expression of the least deleterious immune effector mechanisms. Moreover, the mechanisms of immune privilege are multiple, overlapping, and include both active and passive suppression of innate and immune inflammation. At the very basis of an effective immune response are cellular interactions and their cross talk. Central to the ability of cells to communicate are the intercellular channels that are established to isolate signals and movement of proteins between cells. Within this secure nano-environment, cells signal each other and even exchange proteins. Studies reviewed here are centered on knowledge and exploration of the *tolerogenic synapse* rather than the immunogenic synapse. The unique cells (invariant natural killer T cells, F4/80+ antigen-presenting cells, and T and B lymphocytes) that cluster within the marginal zone following injection of antigen in the anterior chamber (AC) express a phenotype of cell surface molecules that that seem to be uniquely critical for the development of AC-associated immune deviation. How these cell surface molecules behave during the cellular interactions that result in the development of regulatory T cells and peripheral tolerance induced through the eye is discussed.

The eye is directly exposed to environmental pathogens on its surface and to blood-borne pathogens in the internal compartments. Similar to the brain, the eye resides behind blood-tissue barriers that are formed by endothelial cell-tight junctions and other structural specialization, such as tight junctions among ocular pigment epithelial layers. While these barriers reduce the possibility of pathogens endangering the eye, they are not absolute and all types of infectious agents are known to cause eye disease. Thus, like other tissues and organs of the body, the eye needs to be defended by innate and adaptive immunity [1].

On the other hand, the visual axis of the eye focuses light images precisely on the retina which is intolerant of distortion that might be induced by innate or immune inflammation. In addition, the corneal endothelium [2] and the neurosensory retina [3] are unable to regenerate if injured by trauma or inflammation. However, a phenomenon called ocular immune privilege provides the eye with the necessary immune protection against infectious agents by allowing the expression of the least deleterious immune effector mechanisms [1]. Immune-privileged sites are defined operationally as sites in the body where foreign tissue grafts are capable of surviving for extended or indefinite periods of time. Of the ocular compartments that have been studied for immune privilege, tumor cell and antigen inoculation into the anterior chamber (AC) has been analyzed the most, but immune privilege extends to most if not all compartments of the eye [4–6]. Immune privilege was originally explained simplistically as the absence of lymphatic drainage and the creation of immunological ignorance for the organ [7]. However, the mechanisms of immune privilege are multiple and overlapping, and include both active and passive suppression of innate and immune inflammation.

At the very basis of an effective immune response are cellular interactions and their cross talk. Central to the ability of cells to communicate is the synapse or channel established that isolates the signals and movement of proteins between cells. Within this nano-environment, cells signal each other and even exchange proteins through cell surfaces. The process is often referred to as 'immunologic synapse' (in the case of immune activation) or 'inhibitory synapse' (in the case of immune regulation). Our studies pave the way for exploration of the tolerogenic synapse that will show how molecules behave during the cellular cross talk that occurs during the development of regulatory T (T_{reg}) cells and peripheral tolerance induced through the eye. At the basis of the immunologic tolerogenic synapse are the cells that interact and the molecules that are critical for the development of efferent CD8+ T_{reg} cells and peripheral tolerance during the induction of ACAID.

Pivotal to both immune response induction and the induction of tolerance (the outcome of immune privilege) is the antigen-presenting cell (APC). Compared to the APC that presents antigen for the induction of an immune response, there are major differences (table 1). The co-receptors and cytokines that are needed for inflammatory responses are downregulated, and new and novel cytokines have been associated with the generation of T_{reg} cells in models of peripheral tolerance.

The APC in eye-induced tolerance has been well studied in an animal model called AC-associated immune deviation (ACAID). In brief, 7 days after

Table 1. Comparison of an immune APC and a tolerogenic APC: characteristics that are differentially expressed during induction of immune response versus ACAID

Characteristics	Immunogenic APC	Tolerogenic APC
Co-receptors	express co-receptors, CD40, CD80/86	lack some co-receptors: CD40−, CD80/86+
Cytokines/chemokines	IL-12	TGF-β, MIP-2
Homing	home to T and B cell areas	home to MZ of the spleen
Chemokine receptors	CCR7	CCR7−, CCR7+
CD1d	moderate CD1d	high CD1d
Antigen presentation	present antigen to T cell with MHC class II and class I	present antigen to T cell with MHC class I

Some activating co-receptors (CD40), normally expressed by mature APC, are downregulated on tolerogenic APC, but others are expressed (CD80/86). Immunosuppressive cytokines (TGF-β and IL-10) are upregulated in the tolerogenic APC. Homing patterns and chemokine receptors differ for the two types of APC, and each subset of APC migrates to different compartments of the spleen. For tolerogenic APC, a role for CD1d-restricted NKT cells is critical, and protein antigen is cross-presented by MHC class I (instead of MHC class II during immune responses) for the induction of CD8+ T_{reg} cells.

inoculation of antigen into the AC of the eye, afferent CD4+ T_{reg} and efferent CD8+ T_{reg} cells can be harvested from the spleen. The antigen is known to be carried by the F4/80+ APCs, indigenous to the eye, to the marginal zone (MZ) of the spleen where they interact and orchestrate the development of the T_{reg} cells that effect peripheral tolerance. Equally important to this process are the other bone marrow-derived cells that are recruited to the MZ to participate in the cross talk for tolerance.

Characteristics of the Antigen-Presenting Cell in Anterior Chamber-Associated Immune Deviation

In general, the dendritic cell (DC) subset of APCs that is uniquely equipped for antigen presentation is regarded as the sentinel of the immune response [8]. T cells recognize antigens through interaction with APCs that most of the time process as well as present antigen. APCs include a heterogeneous family of cells that are able to process both exogenous and endogenous antigens into 10–20 amino acid peptides, load them onto major histocompatibility complex (MHC) molecules, which then traffic to the cell membrane where they can be recognized by the antigen-specific T cell receptor [9]. APCs are further classified into professional APCs (bone marrow-derived DCs) that are capable of activating and inducing clonal expansion of both naïve and memory T cells and non-professional APCs (B lymphocytes, monocytes, macrophages, and endothelial cells) that are able to stimulate memory T cells, but are poorly equipped to stimulate naïve cells. Within the tissues, the DC phenotype is immature, but is capable of maturation if presented with 'danger' signals [10, 11]. Besides expression of co-receptors (CD80, CD86, Ox40 ligand, and CD40), mature DC exhibit decreased endocytosis of extracellular antigens, translocate the peptide-loaded MHC molecules into the plasma membrane and display a long-lasting peptide-MHC complex. Mature DC also display increased membrane expression of chemokine receptor CCR7 [9] that responds to the stromal chemokines from the T cell areas of the secondary lymphoid organs. Immune-privileged sites like the eye regulate immune activation in part by interfering with the maturation of the DC and by altering the indigenous APCs toward the induction of tolerance. It appears that the APCs in the eye downregulate their chemokine receptors that direct them to the tissue; once this happens, they become mobile, dendritic in morphology, and move toward the draining lymphoid organ (in this case, the spleen). The eye-derived APCs, however, are inefficient in their upregulation of CCR7 [12] and appear to never make it to the T cell areas of the spleen, but remain in clusters in the MZ [13]. Thus, the eye-derived APC is specialized in its expression of chemokine receptors contributing to its unique function in the induction of peripheral tolerance. A comparison of the specialized characteristics of an immune APC and a tolerogenic APC is shown in table 1.

The requirement for protection against immune inflammation in the eye contributes to the need for regional specialization of the local eye-residing APCs [14]. In the eye, as within other tissues, the initiation of the immune response or immune regulation begins with the indigenous APC that picks up the antigen and carries it to the draining secondary lymphoid organ where it may present the antigen or pass off its antigen to the APCs in the region of the lymphoid organ where it finds itself. It is believed that the local APCs not only transport antigen away from the tissue but also orchestrate the outcome of antigenic insult to the eye. In this chapter, the specialized characteristics of the ACAID APCs and other bone marrow-derived cells that are critical to the peripheral tolerance outcome following antigen introduction into the eye are discussed. We address how their cross talk within their aggregates may lead to novel molecular interactions between the tolerance-inducing cells. Mechanisms used by APCs and the cells within such an immunologically tolerogenic synapse may be shared by APCs in tissues within the organism other than immune-privileged sites and, therefore, may be relevant to the induction/maintenance of self tolerance in the adult and the prevention of autoimmunity.

Why Antigen-Presenting Cells in the Eye Are Tolerogenic

It is known that the intraocular fluids of the eye [aqueous humor (AH) and vitreous humor] contain biologically relevant concentrations of various immunosuppressive neuropeptides, cytokines, growth factors, and soluble cell surface receptors that interfere with the development of immune reactivity [15]. AH inhibits innate immune effector cells [16, 17], but most important for our discussion, AH modulates the antigen-presenting capacity of the APC in eye [18–21]. Experiments have shown that ocular fluids remain immunosuppressive and anti-inflammatory even in eyes that are inflamed and under autoimmune attack; however, the spectrum of factors shifts [22–24]. The fluids from the non-inflamed eye contain an abundance of latent TGF-β_2, while the fluids from the inflamed eye contain activated TGF-β_2. This is in part because 'danger' signals (TNF-α and IL-1) from the inflammation upregulate IL-6 production by the parenchymal cells that in turn activates macrophages and the molecules that convert latent TGF-β to its active form [24]. An eye-derived APC exposed to a virtual mixture of immunosuppressive compounds takes on a unique phenotype that differs from both the immature and mature phenotypes described for DC.

Dendritic Cells and Antigen-Presenting Cells in the Anterior Chamber

In the ACAID model for immune privilege, the indigenous F4/80+ cells from the iris and ciliary body pick up antigens administered to the front of the eye by AC inoculation [1]. Recently, Camelo et al. [25] reported that the type of APC that carried antigen from the eye of the rat after intracameral injection of antigen, similar to the mouse, was predominantly resident macrophages negative for class II, but appeared to be on histological examination not only in the iris, but in all tissues lining the AC of the eye. The APCs reside mainly within the iris and ciliary body and perhaps in the cornea. Following AC inoculation, the resident F4/80+ population takes up the antigen, moves out through the trabecular meshwork into the blood, and travels to the spleen. In fact, removal of the spleen prevents the induction of tolerance (ACAID) through the eye [26]. Dullforce et al. [27] confirmed the generally accepted notion that AC-inoculated antigen was taken up by APCs that traveled to the spleen by showing that eye-derived APCs did not travel to the lymph nodes. Since lymphatics or nascent lymphatics are normally present only in the conjunctiva [28, 29] or in the inflamed cornea [30, 31], it is not surprising that antigen-transporting APCs do not travel to the draining lymph nodes.

Only a small amount of antigen is carried to the spleen by the local APCs of the eye, and 98% of the antigen inoculated into the AC goes directly into the blood. Since monocytes in the blood do not process antigen, blood-borne antigen must be presented by cells other than monocytes, and most likely are processed by APCs in the spleen. Several studies have reported that if the same amount of antigen is introduced directly into the blood, ACAID-like tolerance is not induced [13, 32, 33]. Thus it can be said that ACAID and intravenous tolerance differ in the kind of APCs that present the antigen. Sonoda et al. [34] demonstrated that mechanisms that induce ACAID allow for prolonged corneal graft survival in a mouse model. Supposedly, transplanted allogeneic corneas that abut the AC would have their antigens picked up by eye-derived APC and/or delivered to the spleen by donor APC in a similar manner. Again, this tolerance is induced by antigen transported by specialized APCs rather than leakage of antigen into the blood vessels.

As stated above, AH is an immunosuppressive fluid in the AC and, therefore, it is not surprising the APCs bathed in immunosuppressive molecules would have a distinct phenotype [18, 21]. Characteristically, the 'eye-derived' APCs share markers with DCs and macrophages. It is not clear if the APC indigenous to the anterior uveal tract is a DC with a special phenotype, or a macrophage with a special phenotype. The local APC resembles a macrophage when it is viewed in the tissue, but once it leaves the tissue, like other tissue macrophages, it takes on DC characteristics.

The ACAID-inducing APC is distinguished by its expression of F4/80 protein. F4/80 protein is a molecule that has long been regarded as a marker of tissue macrophages, but in the case of ACAID, Wilbanks et al. [35] and Wilbanks and Streilein [36] showed that the F4/80 cell was the cell-associated signal from the eye that traveled through the blood to the spleen to induce ACAID. The F4/80+ cell lacks class II, does not express traditional co-receptors for immune activation (CD40 and IL-12), and produces IL-10 and activated TGF-β [1, 37–39] (table 1). Both IL-10 and TGF-β are monokines capable of inducing their own secretion, thereby contributing to the forceful influence that eye-derived F4/80 cells have on the functional phenotype of APC/DC encountered in the periphery.

Another distinguishing characteristic of the ACAID F4/80+ cell is that it produces unique inflammatory chemokine profiles. The F4/80+ APC produces MIP-2, but not other inflammatory chemokines [13, 40]. MIP-2 is capable of recruiting CXCR2+ NKT cells to the spleen. Furthermore, it is remarkable that the ACAID F4/80+ cell must express CD1d to function in the induction of ACAID [41]. It is a requirement for the F4/80+ APC to interact with the invariant T cell receptor (TCR) on the NKT cell via its CD1d molecule if ACAID and peripheral tolerance are to be the outcome.

Since it is next to impossible to obtain sufficient resident F4/80+ eye-derived APCs, the expression of genes in ACAID-like APCs has been analyzed with surrogate ACAID F4/80+ APCs [19, 41] by two laboratories [43, 44]. Masli et al. [44] studied macrophage hybridoma 59 treated with TGF-β and antigen, and Zhang-Hoover [12] explored the genes in bone marrow-derived F4/80+ APCs generated with L929 supernatants which contain macrophage colony-stimulating factor. They found that the genes that support IFN-γ- and NFκB-dependent immune reactivity were downregulated, while the genes that promote or are involved in TGF-β function were upregulated. The F4/80+ ACAID APCs most likely do not move into the T cell areas because the critical chemokine receptor that is required for moving into the T cell area, CCR7, is expressed at only very low levels or not at all [12]. However, the F4/80+ ACAID APC also lacks the chemokine receptor that identifies immature APCs in the tissues (CCR6). Thus, studies of modulated genes in ACAID-like APCs have contributed novel and different information about APCs in immune-privileged sites, such as the eye.

Mechanisms of Anterior Chamber-Associated Immune Deviation in the Spleen

Functional studies involving the APCs in the uveal tract have been a product of the investigations on mechanisms of immune privilege and ACAID (fig. 1). As stated above, ACAID is a deviant state of immunity that is responsible for the induction of peripheral tolerance to both self and foreign antigens that occur in the eye [1, 45]. While Wilbanks et al. [35] demonstrated that the F4/80+ cell carried the tolerogenic signal to the spleen, and Niederkorn and Mayhew [46] and D'Orazio and Niederkorn [47] reported the importance of B cells in ACAID induction, Sonoda et al. [41] were the first to evidence that the 'eye-derived' APCs not only interacted (in the spleen) with the T cells that were to become T_{reg} cells, but necessarily interacted with a rare lymphocyte called the invariant NKT (iNKT) cell (fig. 1). The iNKT cell bears markers of both NK cells and the traditional T cell. Eighty-five percent of the NKT cells express the invariant Vα14Jα18 TCR that preferentially binds a few Vβ chains. The murine iNKT cell has a counter part in the human that expresses the Vα24JQα [48–50]. The TCR on the NKT cell is oligoclonal and interacts (presumably) with foreign or self lipids presented by the class I-like molecule called CD1d1 [50–53]. In the mouse, the iNKT cell may be either CD4+ or double negative, and it is suggested that the CD4+ iNKT cell produces IL-4 and IFN-γ while the double negative cells are mainly producers of Th1-type cytokines [54]. We know that during ACAID induction, the required iNKT cell is CD4+ [55] and secretes IL-10 but not IL-4 [56].

The eye-derived APCs that transport antigen to the spleen also recruit iNKT cells to their splenic destination by the release of MIP-2 [13]. Gene array

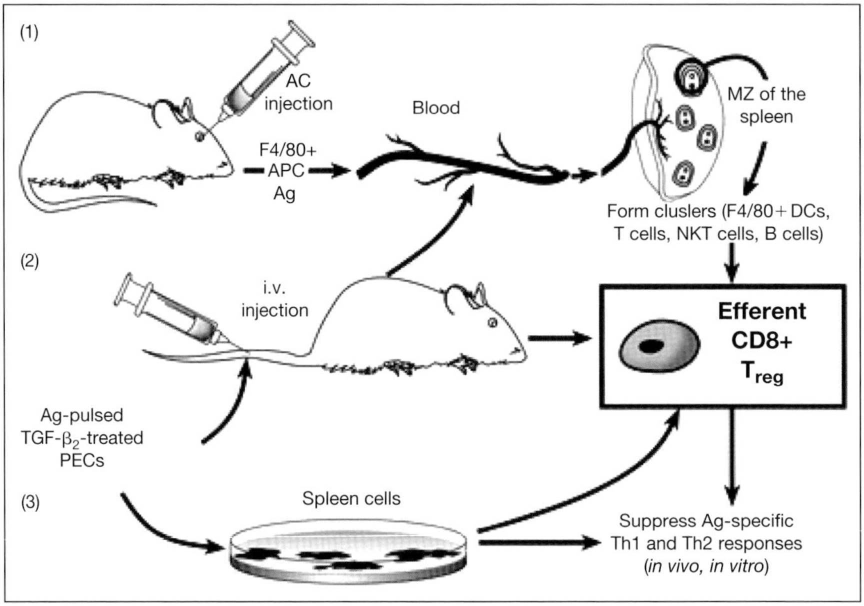

Fig. 1. Three ways to generate ACAID efferent CD8+ T_{reg} cells. (1) ACAID efferent CD8+ T_{reg} cells are generated in the MZ of the spleen 7 days after AC inoculation of antigen. (2) The inoculation of the eye may be bypassed by intravenous inoculation of in vitro generated tolerogenic APCs, previously treated with TGF-β and antigen. (3) CD8+ T_{reg} cells may be generated entirely in vitro by culturing in vitro generated tolerogenic APCs (TGF-β and antigen treated) with spleen cells for 7 days. PEC = Peritoneal exudate cells; Ag = antigen.

analyses have confirmed the increase in MIP-2 during ACAID induction [44]. During an adaptive immune response, CCR7+ APCs and other CCR7+ precursor cells that arrive in the spleen via the blood are 'poured' from the central arteriole into the MZ, but leave within 4–6 h to follow their chemokine gradient to the T cell areas. Other cells that are CCR7 negative move into the red pulp and are degraded. Faunce et al. [13] convincingly showed that the aggregates that contain the F4/80+ APCs, T cells, and NKT cells are in place in the MZ as late as 7 days after AC injection (fig. 2). B cells are also required for the induction of ACAID [38, 47]. Sonoda and Stein-Streilein [57] specified that the subset of B cells required for ACAID is the CD1d+ MZ B cell. Niederkorn's group suggested that the antigen transporting APC from the eye may 'hand over' its antigen to B cells in the spleen for a required antigen presentation by the B cell via Qa-1 (an MHC class 1-B molecule) [58] to the CD8 T cell [59, 60].

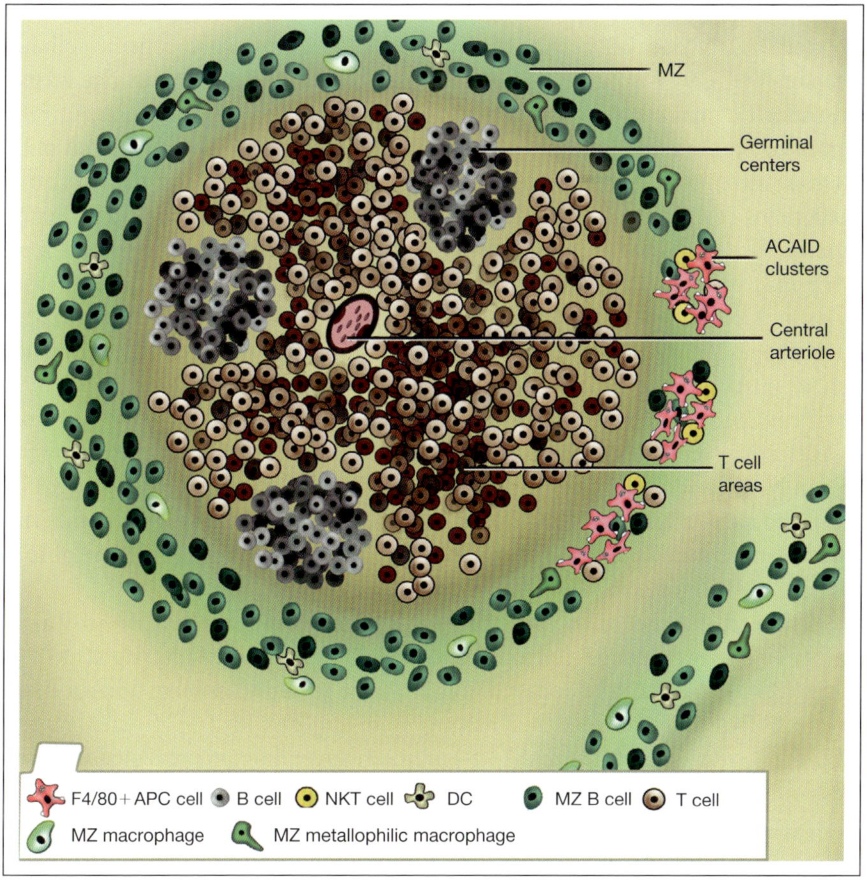

Fig. 2. Cell clusters in the splenic MZ during induction of ACAID. Artist's rendition of F4/80+ APCs aggregating with bone marrow cells in the MZ of the spleen and interacting to generate efferent CD8+ T cells.

The Role of the F4/80 Protein in Anterior Chamber-Associated Immune Deviation

F4/80 is the molecule that is recognized by an antibody that was developed by Austyn and Gordon [61] 20 odd years ago. F4/80 is a prototypic member of the EGF-TM7 receptor family that includes EMR1, EMR2, EMR3, EMR4, ETL, and CD97 [62, 63]. A dual adhesion and signaling function has thus been suggested for the EGF-TM7 molecules where the extracellular region is involved in protein-protein interaction with other cell surface proteins and/or extracellular matrix proteins, triggering intracellular signaling through the TM7 domain. Consistent with this hypothesis, specific cellular ligands for the EGF-TM7 receptors have been reported. CD55 (decay-accelerating factor) was identified as the cognate cellular receptor for CD97 [64]. The F4/80 molecule has been established as one of the most specific markers for murine macrophages. F4/80 is highly and constitutively expressed on most resident tissue macrophage populations such as the red pulp macrophages in the spleen, microglia in the brain, Kupffer cells in the liver, and Langerhans cells in the skin [63]. Furthermore, the expression of F4/80 is tightly regulated according to the physiological status of the cells. Thus, the precursor of tissue macrophages, the blood monocyte, is known to express less F4/80 than its mature counterparts [65]. F4/80 is expressed at lower levels on activated macrophages isolated from bacillus Calmette-Guérin-infected animals in comparison to unstimulated resting macrophages [66]. Similarly, F4/80 expression is downregulated on macrophages in response to interferon-γ [67]. F4/80 expression on Langerhans cells decreases after they take up antigens and become migrating DCs in lymph nodes and spleens. Since F4/80 is detected only on macrophages in T cell-independent areas [65], the fact that the ACAID cells aggregate in the MZ rather than the T cell areas of the spleen is not surprising. These studies point to a specialized function for F4/80 protein on tissue macrophages.

The early studies involving the ACAID model showed that F4/80 was a marker of the eye-derived cell that carried the tolerance-inducing signal to the spleen [35]. ACAID can be induced in naïve mice with the adoptive transfer of as few as 20 F4/80+ APC generated in vitro by treatment with TGF-β_2 and antigen [20]. Early studies indicated that F4/80 antibody given in vivo prevented the suppression of delayed hypersensitivity (ACAID) in experimental mice [35, 36]. However, the mechanism of the antibody treatment or the role of F4/80 protein in the model was not studied further until recently [68]. AC inoculation of antigen leads to the suppression of a delayed hypersensitivity response in part because of splenic CD8+ efferent T_{reg} cells that develop following AC inoculation of antigen. The efferent T_{reg} cell is capable of suppressing both effector T cell antigen-specific Th1 [1] and Th2 responses [69]. With the advent of the F4/80 knockout (KO) mouse, the function of the F4/80 protein was testable. When the splenic T cells were harvested from the AC-treated mice, the T cells from the wild-type mice were able to suppress adoptively transferred delayed hypersensitivity responses, but the T cells from the F4/80 KO mice were not. Therefore, it was concluded that peripheral tolerance (ACAID) that developed subsequent to AC inoculation of antigen failed in F4/80−/− mice due to a lack of CD8+ efferent T_{reg} cell development [68]. Thus, the F4/80 protein plays a role in the development of ACAID in part by facilitating the development of the CD8+ T_{reg} cell. Similar to the ACAID model, a low-dose oral tolerance model in mice also generates CD8+ T_{reg} cells capable of suppressing Th1 effector functions [70]. In addition, like the indigenous cells in the eye, some indigenous macrophages in Peyer's patches express the F4/80 antigen [71]. Due to the similarities in generation of efferent CD8+ T_{reg} cells in two tolerance models, Lin et al. [68] postulated a direct role for the F4/80 molecule in the induction of peripheral tolerance and showed that F4/80 expression was also required for the induction of CD8+ T_{reg} in an ovalbumin model of oral tolerance.

Role of the Ly49 Molecule

Ly49 molecules are generally known as inhibitory molecules on NK, NKT, and some T cells. They function when ligated to their corresponding self MHC I molecule to downregulate their production of IFN-γ and lytic pathways. Under conditions of a normal immune response, engagement of Ly49 receptors inhibits cytokine production by NKT cells [72, 73], NKT cell proliferation [74, 75], and cytotoxic activity [76]. However, since our studies with NKT cells and tolerance began [41, 77], we knew that the subset of NKT cells involved in tolerance expressed Ly49C/I. Critical subpopulations of NKT cells could be collected and enriched by either positive or negative selection with the use of monoclonal antibody 5E6, which is specific for Ly49C/I. We thought that Ly49C/I on NKT cells might participate in the downregulation of NKT cell-derived IFN-γ. Indeed, when the cross talk between iNKT cells and APC was blocked by interfering with the ligation of Ly49C/I by its MHC ligand, the production of CD8+ T_{reg} cells and peripheral tolerance after AC inoculation was prevented. Mechanistically, blocking Ly49C/I not only allowed for the production of IFN-γ by the NKT cell but also prevented their efficient production of IL-10. Knowing that IL-10 cross regulates IFN-γ production, we propose that engagement of Ly49C/I may downregulate IFN-γ production and lytic function in part by inducing the production of IL-10, a potent mediator of immunosuppression [manuscript in preparation].

Similarity of Anterior Chamber-Associated Imune Deviation with Other Models of Tolerance

Since there are similarities of ACAID with peripheral tolerance induced through the brain (immune privileged) [78] and through the gut (not immune privileged) [68], one might extrapolate that the cellular mechanisms that occur within the MZ of the spleen during ACAID induction might cause the induction of CD8+ T_{reg} cells and peripheral tolerance in general.

On the other hand, cells and molecules that might be involved in the induction of peripheral tolerance in a tumor model of tolerance [79] are not involved in the induction of CD8+ T_{reg} in ACAID. In the tumor model, CD1d is required, but the iNKT cell produces IL-13; during the induction of ACAID, traditional CD4+ T cells, MHC class II cells [55], IL-4, IL-13, or STAT-6 [80] are not needed for the generation of efferent CD8+ T_{reg} cells. To our knowledge, the role of these molecules and cells in the generation of afferent CD4+ T_{reg} cells has not been studied.

In support of the mechanisms we describe for the induction of peripheral tolerance through the eye being directly related to the development of efferent CD8+ T_{reg} cells, it is important to mention that we have noted that models of tolerance that are not dependent on CD1d-restricted NKT cells also do not generate efferent CD8+ T_{reg} cells. For example, an efferent CD8+ T_{reg} cell is not generated during induction of intravenously induced tolerance and intravenous tolerance can be induced in CD1d KO mice and iNKT cell-deficient mice (Jα18 KO) [13, 41]. Additionally, a model of tolerance induction where antigen was applied to the skin was also shown not to be dependent on NKT cells and regulation appeared to be mediated by an antigen-nonspecific CD4+ CD8+ T cell and not an efferent CD8+ T_{reg} cell.

Summary and Conclusion

Here we have defined the cells that leave the eye after antigen exposure to traffic to the MZ (not the T cell areas) of the spleen. By studying the cells that aggregate and cross talk in the spleen following antigen injection into the AC, we discovered that regional specialization of the indigenous F4/80+ cells in the eye allows them to recruit and educate other cells toward tolerance. During ACAID induction, specialized cells interact with each other in the MZ using select molecules and cytokines. Two kinds of APCs promote tolerance in the MZ: the F4/80+ APC and the MZ B cell. Both communicate with iNKT cells via the CD1d molecule expressed on their membrane. The ligation of the TCR on the iNKT cell with the CD1d molecule leads to the synthesis and release of a select chemokine (RANTES) that recruits more APCs and T cells to the MZ 'chat' room. MHC class I and Qa-1 on APCs also seem to be involved in the cross talk for tolerance and interact with the antigen-specific T cell to develop into a T_{reg} cell [59]. In addition, it is now known that the F4/80 protein, previously known only as a marker of tissue macrophages, is crucial for the outcome of the MZ cross talk in the aggregates. F4/80 KO mice are unable to develop CD8+ T_{reg} cells in ACAID and low-dose oral tolerance [68]. More recently, we determined that the CD4+ iNKT cell involved in ACAID expresses Ly49C/I [unpubl. findings]. Even though this NK cell-inhibitory molecule is expressed on only a minor population of CD4+ iNKT cells, it is required for the development of CD8+ T_{reg} cells.

The model of tolerance induced through the eye facilitates the study of the cellular cross talk required for peripheral tolerance induction by exploring the surface molecules that interact. In future studies, the movement and exchange of the proteins within the immunologic tolerogenic synapse will be investigated. Studying the mechanisms of ACAID is important for (1) determining the type of cells that are involved in the cross talk in the MZ that leads to tolerance; (2) analyzing the crucial molecules involved in the cross talk, and (3) determining how the molecules synergize to promote active tolerance and T_{reg} cells.

References

1 Streilein JW: Ocular immune privilege: therapeutic opportunities from an experiment of nature. Nat Rev Immunol 2003;3:878–889.

2 Matsubara M, Tanishima T: Wound-healing of corneal endothelium in monkey: an autoradiographic study. Jpn J Ophthalmol 1983;27:444–450.

3 Streilein JW: Regional immunity and ocular immune privilege; in Streilein JW (ed): Immune Response and the Eye. Chem Immunol. Basel, Karger, 1999, vol 73, pp 11–38.

4 Niederkorn J, Streilein JW, Shadduck JA: Deviant immune responses to allogeneic tumors injected intracamerally and subcutaneously in mice. Invest Ophthalmol Vis Sci 1980;20:355–363.

5 Jiang LQ, Jorquera M, Streilein JW: Subretinal space and vitreous cavity as immunologically privileged sites for retinal allografts. Invest Ophthalmol Vis Sci 1993;34:3347–3354.

6 Wenkel H, Chen PW, Ksander BR, Streilein JW: Immune privilege is extended, then withdrawn, from allogeneic tumor cell grafts placed in the subretinal space. Invest Ophthalmol Vis Sci 1999;40:3203–3208.

7 Medawar PB: Immunity to homologous grafted skin. III. The fate of skin homografts transplanted to the brain, to subcutaneous tissue and to the anterior chamber of the eye. Br J Exp Pathol 1948;29:58–69.

8 Morelli AE, Thomson AW: Dendritic cells: regulators of alloimmunity and opportunities for tolerance induction. Immunol Rev 2003;196:125–146.

9 Banchereau J, Briere F, Caux C, Savoust J, Lebecque S, Lie YJ, Pulendran B, Palucka K: Immunobiology of dendritic cells. Annu Rev Immunol 2000;18:761–811.

10 Matzinger P: Tolerance, danger, and the extended family. Annu Rev Immunol 1994;12:991–1045.

11 Matzinger P: An innate sense of danger (review). Semin Immunol 1996;10:399–415.

12 Zhang-Hoover J, Finn P, Stein-Streilein J: Modulation of ovalbumin-induced airway inflammation and hyperreactivity by tolerogenic APC. J Immunol 2005;175:7117–7124.

13 Faunce DE, Sonoda KH, Stein-Streilein J: MIP-2 recruits NKT cells to the spleen during tolerance induction. J Immunol 2001;166:313–321.

14 Streilein JW, Stein-Streilein J, Head J: Regional specialization in antigen presentation; in: The Reticuloendothelial System. New York, Plenum, 1986, pp 37–93.

15 Taylor AW, Yee DG, Streilein JW: Suppression of nitric oxide generated by inflammatory macrophages by calcitonin gene-related peptide in aqueous humor. Invest Ophthalmol Vis Sci 1998;39:1372–1378.

16 Apte RS, Niederkorn JY: Isolation and characterization of a unique natural killer cell inhibitory factor present in the anterior chamber of the eye. J Immunol 1996;156:2667–2673.

17 Streilein JW, Stein-Streilein J: Does innate immune privilege exist? J Leukoc Biol 2000;67:479–487.

18 Cousins SW, McCabe MM, Danielpour D, Streilein JW: Identification of transforming growth factor-beta as an immunosuppressive factor in aqueous humor. Invest Ophthalmol Vis Sci 1991;32:2201–2211.

19 Streilein JW, Bradley D: Analysis of immunosuppressive properties of iris and ciliary body cells and their secretory products. Invest Ophthalmol Vis Sci 1991;32:2700–2710.
20 Hara Y, Caspi RR, Wiggert B, Dorf M, Streilein JW: Analysis of an in vitro-generated signal that induces systemic immune deviation similar to that elicited by antigen injected into the anterior chamber of the eye. J Immunol 1992;149:1531–1538.
21 Wilbanks GA, Streilein JW: Fluids from immune privileged sites endow macrophages with the capacity to induce antigen-specific immune deviation via a mechanism involving transforming growth factor-beta. Eur J Immunol 1992;22:1031–1036.
22 Ohta K, Wiggert B, Yamagami S, Taylor AW, Streilein JW: Analysis of immunomodulatory activities of aqueous humor from eyes of mice with experimental autoimmune uveitis. J Immunol 2000;164:1185–1192.
23 Ohta K, Yamagami S, Taylor AW, Streilein JW: IL-6 antagonizes TGF-beta and abolishes immune privilege in eyes with endotoxin-induced uveitis. Invest Ophthalmol Vis Sci 2000;41:2591–2599.
24 Mo JS, Streilein JW: Immune privilege persists in eyes with extreme inflammation induced by intravitreal LPS. Eur J Immunol 2001;31:3806–3815.
25 Camelo S, Shanley A, Voon AS, McMenamin PG: The distribution of antigen in lymphoid tissues following its injection into the anterior chamber of the rat eye. J Immunol 2004;172: 5388–5395.
26 Streilein JW, Niederkorn JY: Induction of anterior chamber-associated immune deviation requires an intact, functional spleen. J Exp Med 1981;153:1058–1067.
27 Dullforce PA, Garman KL, Seitz GW, Fleischmann RJ, Crespo SM, Planck SR, Parker DC, Rosenbaum JT: APCs in the anterior uveal tract do not migrate to draining lymph nodes. J Immunol 2004;172:6701–6708.
28 Franklin RM, Remus LE: Conjunctival-associated lymphoid tissue: evidence for a role in the secretory immune system. Invest Ophthalmol Vis Sci 1984;25:181–187.
29 Zierhut M, Elson CO, Forrester JV, Kijlstra A, Kraehenbuhl JP, Sullivan DA: Mucosal immunology and the eye. Immunol Today 1998;19:148–150.
30 Hamrah P, Huq SO, Liu Y, Zhang Q, Dana MR: Corneal immunity is mediated by heterogeneous population of antigen-presenting cells. J Leukoc Biol 2003;74:172–178.
31 Cursiefen C, Schlotzer-Schrehardt U, Kuchle M, Sorokin L, Breiteneder-Geleff S, Alitalo K, Jackson D: Lymphatic vessels in vascularized human corneas: immunohistochemical investigation using LYVE-1 and podoplanin. Invest Ophthalmol Vis Sci 2002;43:2127–2135.
32 Wilbanks GA, Streilein JW: The differing patterns of antigen release and local retention following anterior chamber and intravenous inoculation of soluble antigen. Evidence that the eye acts as an antigen depot. Reg Immunol 1989;2:390–398.
33 Streilein JW, Wilbanks GA: Evidence that anterior chamber and intravenous antigen injections have distinctly different systemic immune consequences. Ocular Immunol Today 1990, pp 255–258.
34 Sonoda KH, Taniguchi M, Stein-Streilein J: Long-term survival of corneal allografts is dependent on intact CD1d-reactive NKT cells. J Immunol 2002;168:2028–2034.
35 Wilbanks GA, Mammolenti M, Streilein J: Studies on the induction of anterior chamber-associated immune deviation (ACAID). II. Eye-derived cells participate in generating blood-borne signals that induce ACAID. J Immunol 1991;146:3018–3024.
36 Wilbanks GA, Streilein JW: Studies on the induction of anterior chamber-associated immune deviation (ACAID). I. Evidence that an antigen-specific, ACAID-inducing, cell-associated signal exists in the peripheral blood. J Immunol 1991;146:2610–2617.
37 Flugel C, Kinne RW, Streilein JW, Lutjen-Drecoll E: Distinctive distribution of HLA class II presenting and bone marrow derived cells in the anterior segment of human eyes. Curr Eye Res 1992;11:1173–1183.
38 D'Orazio TJ, Niederkorn JY: A novel role for TGF-β and IL-10 in the induction of immune privilege. J Immunol 1996;160:2089–2098.
39 Streilein JW: Ocular immune privilege: the eye takes a dim but practical view of immunity and inflammation. J Leukoc Biol 2003;74:179–185.
40 Faunce DE, Stein-Streilein J: NKT cell-derived RANTES recruits APCs and $CD8^+$ T cells to the spleen during the generation of regulatory T cells in tolerance. J Immunol 2002;169:31–38.

41 Sonoda KH, Exley M, Snapper S, Balk S, Stein-Streilein J: CD1-reactive natural killer T cells are required for development of systemic tolerance through an immune-privileged site. J Exp Med 1999;190:1215–1225.
42 Hara Y, Okamoto S, Rouse B, Streilein JW: Evidence that peritoneal exudate cells cultured with eye-derived fluids are the proximate antigen-presenting cells in immune deviation of the ocular type. J Immunol 1993;151:5162–5171.
43 Kuchroo VK, Minami M, Diamond B, Dorf ME: Functional analysis of cloned macrophage hybridomas. VI. Differential ability to induce immunity or suppression. J Immunol 1988;141: 10–16.
44 Masli S, Turpie B, Hecker KH, Streilein JW: Expression of thrombospondin in TGFß-treated APCs and its relevance to their immune deviation-promoting properties. J Immunol 2002;168: 2264–2273.
45 Stein-Streilein J, Streilein JW: Anterior chamber associated immune deviation (ACAID); regulation, biological relevance, and implications for therapy. Int Rev Immunol 2002;21:123–152.
46 Niederkorn JY, Mayhew E: Role of splenic B cells in the immune privilege of the anterior chamber of the eye. Eur J Immunol 1995;25:2783–2787.
47 D'Orazio TJ, Niederkorn JY: Splenic B cells are required for tolerogenic antigen presentation in the induction of anterior chamber-associated immune deviation (ACAID). Immunology 1998;95: 47–55.
48 Lantz O, Bendelac A: An invariant T cell receptor alpha chain is used by a unique subset of major histocompatibility complex class I-specific $CD4^+$ and $CD4{-}8^-$ T cells in mice and humans. J Exp Med 1994;180:1097–1106.
49 Bendelac A: Mouse $NK1^+$ T cells. Curr Opin Immunol 1995;7:367–374.
50 Exley M, Garcia J, Balk SP, Porcelli S: Requirements for CD1d recognition by human invariant $V\alpha24^+$ $CD4^-$ $CD8^-$ T cells. J Exp Med 1997;186:109–120.
51 Brutkiewicz RR, Bennink JR, Yewdell JW, Bendelac A: TAP-independent, β_2-microglobulin-dependent surface expression of functional mouse CD11. J Exp Med 1995;182:1913–1919.
52 Joyce S, Woods AS, Yewdell JW, Bennink JR, De Silva AD, Boesteanu A, Balk SP, Cotter RJ, Brutkiewicz RR: Natural ligand of mouse CD1d1: cellular glycosylphosphatidylinositol. Science 1998;279:1541–1544.
53 Nishimura T, Kitamura H, Iwakabe K, Yahata T, Ohta A, Sato M, Takeda K, Okumura K, Van Kaer L, Kawano T, Taniguchi M, Nakui M, Sekimoto M, Koda T: The interface between innate and acquired immunity: glycolipid antigen presentation by CD1d-expressing dendritic cells to NKT cells induces the differentiation of antigen-specific cytotoxic T lymphocytes. Int Immunol 2000;12:987–994.
54 Gumperz JE, Miyake S, Yamamura T, Brenner MB: Functionally distinct subsets of CD1d-restricted natural killer T cells revealed by CD1d tetramer staining. J Exp Med 2002;195:625–636.
55 Nakamura T, Sonoda KH, Faunce DE, Gumperz J, Yamamura T, Miyake S, Stein-Streilein J: $CD4^+$ NKT cells, but not conventional $CD4^+$ T cells, are required to generate efferent $CD8^+$ T regulatory cells following antigen inoculation in an immune privileged site. J Immunol 2003;171:1266–1271.
56 Sonoda KH, Faunce DE, Taniguchi M, Exley M, Balk S, Stein-Streilein J: NKT cell-derived IL-10 is essential for the differentiation of antigen-specific T regulatory cells in systemic tolerance. J Immunol 2001;166:42–50.
57 Sonoda KH, Stein-Streilein J: CD1d on antigen-transporting APC and splenic marginal zone B cells promotes NKT cell-dependent tolerance. Eur J Immunol 2002;32:848–857.
58 Niederkorn JY, Chiang EY, Ungchusri T, Stroynowski I: Expression of a nonclassical MHC class Ib molecule in the eye. Transplantation 1999;68:1790–1799.
59 D'Orazio TJ, Mayhew E, Niederkorn JY: Ocular immune privilege promoted by the presentation of peptide on tolerogenic B cells in the spleen. II. Evidence for presentation by Qa-1. J Immunol 2001;166:26–32.
60 Niederkorn JY: Immune privilege in the anterior chamber of the eye. Crit Rev Immunol 2002;22: 13–46.
61 Austyn JM, Gordon S: F4/80, a monoclonal antibody directed specifically against the mouse macrophage. Eur J Immunol 1981;11:805–815.

62 McKnight AJ, Gordon S: EGF-TM7: a novel subfamily of seven-transmembrane-region leukocyte cell-surface molecules. Immunol Today 1996;17:283–287.
63 McKnight AJ, Gordon S: The EGF-TM7 family: unusual structures at the leukocyte surface. J Leukoc Biol 1998;63:271–280.
64 Hamann J, Vogel B, van Schijndel GM, van Lier RA: The seven-span transmembrane receptor CD97 has a cellular ligand (CD55, DAF). J Exp Med 1996;184:1185–1189.
65 Gordon S, Lawson L, Rabinowitz S, Crocker PR, Morris L, Perry VH: Antigen markers of macrophage differentiation in murine tissues. Curr Top Microbiol Immunol 1992;181:1–37.
66 Ezekowitz RAB, Austyn JM, Stahl PD, Gordon S: Surface properties of BCG-activated mouse macrophages. Reduced expression of mannose-specific endocytosis, Fc receptors, and antigen F4/80 accompanies induction of Ia. J Exp Med 1981;154:60–76.
67 Ezekowitz RA, Gordon S: Down-regulation of mannosyl receptor-mediated endocytosis and antigen F4/80 in bacillus Calmette-Guérin-activated mouse macrophages. Role of T lymphocytes and lymphokines. J Exp Med 1982;155:1623–1637.
68 Lin HH, Faunce DE, Stacey M, Terajewicz A, Nakamura T, Zhang-Hoover J, Kerley M, Mucenski ML, Gordon S, Stein-Streilein J: The macrophage F4/80 receptor is required for the induction of antigen-specific efferent regulatory T cells in peripheral tolerance. J Exp Med 2005;201:1615–1625.
69 Katagiri K, Zhang-Hoover J, Mo JS, Stein-Streilein J, Streilein JW: Using tolerance induced via the anterior chamber of the eye to inhibit Th2-dependent pulmonary pathology. J Immunol 2002;169:84–89.
70 Chen Y, Inobe J, Weiner HL: Induction of oral tolerance to myelin basic protein in CD8-depleted mice: both CD4+ and CD8+ cells mediate active suppression. J Immunol 1995;155:910–916.
71 Makala LHC, Reyes JCS, Nishikawa Y, Tsushima Y, Xuan X, Huang X, Battsetseg B, Matsuo T, Nagasawa H: Phenotype and function of murine discrete Peyer's patch macrophage derived-dendritic cells. J Vet Med Sci 2003;65:491–499.
72 Ikarashi Y, Mikami R, Bendelac A, Terme M, Chaput N, Terada M, Tursz T, Angevin E, Lemonnier FA, Wakasugi H, Zitvogel L: Dendritic cell maturation overrules H-2D-mediated natural killer T (NKT) cell inhibition: critical role for B7 in CD1d-dependent NKT cell interferon gamma production. J Exp Med 2001;194:1179–1186.
73 Maeda M, Lohwasser S, Yamamura T, Takei F: Regulation of NKT cells by Ly49: analysis of primary NKT cells and generation of NKT cell line. J Immunol 2001;167:4180–4186.
74 Skold M, Cardell S: Differential regulation of Ly49 expression on CD4+ and CD4– CD8– (double negative) NK1.1+ T cells. Eur J Immunol 2000;30:2488–2496.
75 Held W, Cado D, Raulet DH: Transgenic expression of the Ly49A natural killer cell receptor confers class I major histocompatibility complex (MHC)-specific inhibition and prevents bone marrow allograft rejection. J Exp Med 1996;184:2037–2041.
76 Ortaldo JR, Winkler-Pickett R, Mason AT, Mason LH: The Ly-49 family: regulation of cytotoxicity and cytokine production in murine CD3+ cells. J Immunol 1998;160:1158–1165.
77 Asea A, Stein-Streilein J: Signalling through NK1.1 triggers NK cells to die but induces NKT cells to produce interleukin-4. Immunology 1998;93:296–305.
78 Wenkel H, Streilein JW, Young MJ: Systemic immune deviation in the brain that does not depend on the integrity of the blood-brain barrier. J Immunol 2000;164:5125–5131.
79 Terabe M, Matsui S, Noben-Trauth N, Chen H, Watson C, Donaldson DD, Carbone DP, Paul WE, Berzofsky JA: NKT cell mediated repression of tumor immunosurveillance by IL-13 and the IL-4R-STAT6 pathway. Nat Immunol 2000;1:515–520.
80 Nakamura T, Terajewicz A, Stein-Streilein J: Mechanisms of peripheral tolerance following intracameral inoculation are independent of IL-13 or STAT6. J Immunol 2005;175:2643–2646.

Dr. Joan Stein-Streilein
Schepens Eye Research Institute, Harvard School of Medicine
20 Staniford Street
Boston, MA 02114 (USA)
Tel. +1 617 912 7494, Fax +1 617 912 0105, E-Mail jstein@vision.eri.harvard.edu

Niederkorn JY, Kaplan HJ (eds): Immune Response and the Eye.
Chem Immunol Allergy. Basel, Karger, 2007, vol 92, pp 131–139

Regulatory T Cells and the Eye

Jerry Y. Niederkorn

Department of Ophthalmology, University of Texas Southwestern Medical Center, Dallas, Tex., USA

Abstract

Immune-mediated inflammation can be tolerated in many organs, however in the eye it has devastating consequences, as many of the tissues in the visual axis have limited or no capacity for regeneration. Multiple mechanisms and anatomical adaptations limit the expression of immune-mediated inflammation in the eye. Among these is the generation of regulatory T (T_{reg}) cells, which act to prevent the induction and expression of T cell inflammation. At least four different pathways exist for the development of ocular T_{reg} cells. The redundancy in the generation of T_{reg} cells is a testament to their importance in restricting intraocular inflammation and preserving vision.

The immune privilege of the anterior chamber (AC) has been recognized for over a century. It is now well established that immune privilege is also expressed in the vitreous cavity, subretinal space, and cornea [1–5]. Multiple factors contribute to ocular immune privilege. Blood-tissue barriers in the retinal pigment epithelium and within the microvasculature of the retina limit inflammatory cell traffic [6]. The aqueous humor (AH) contains a myriad of anti-inflammatory and immunosuppressive molecules that inhibit lymphoproliferative responses, restrict the generation of pro-inflammatory chemokines and cytokines, and extinguish immune-mediated inflammation (table 1). The AH also contains complement regulatory proteins, which limit the expression and function of the complement system [7–9]. Tight regulation of the complement cascade within the eye is crucial. Although it is important for resistance to microbial infections, complement components and the inflammatory granulocytes that they recruit can inflict extensive injury to innocent bystander cells within the eye.

Table 1. Immunosuppressive and anti-inflammatory factors in AH

Factor	Effect
TGF-β	suppresses activation of T cells, NK cells, and macrophages induces tolerance-inducing APC
VIP	inhibits T cell activation and proliferation inhibits DTH
CGRP	inhibits elaboration of pro-inflammatory factors by macrophages
α-MSH	inhibits DTH and the elaboration of pro-inflammatory factors by macrophages inhibits activation of neutrophils induces generation of CD4+ CD25+ T_{reg} cells
Somatostatin	suppresses IFN-γ production by activated T cells induces production of α-MSH
MIF	suppresses NK cell activity
FasL	suppresses neutrophil recruitment and activation
Thrombospondin	induces APC to activate latent TGF-β, which is needed for the generation of ACAID suppresses APC expression of IL-12 and CD40
Complement-regulatory proteins	inhibit complement cascade
Idoleamine dioxygenase	depletes tryptophan and 'starves' T cells

CGRP = Calcitonin gene-related peptide; MIF = macrophage migration inhibitory factor; VIP = vasoactive intestinal peptide.

Cells that line the AC are bathed in AH and benefit from the buffering effects that it has on inflammation. However, ocular cells that are not in direct contact with the AH are potentially vulnerable to immune-mediated injury. To compensate for this, many ocular cells display cell membrane-bound molecules that either neutralize or delete inflammatory cells and inflammatory molecules. Chief among these is Fas ligand (FasL, CD95L), which is widely expressed throughout the eye and is capable of inducing programmed cell death in neutrophils and activated T cells [10]. In addition to their presence in the AH, complement-regulatory proteins are expressed as cell membrane-bound molecules on numerous ocular cells [7, 9].

One of the unique features that the eye shares with the brain is the feeble expression or frank absence of MHC molecules. Corneal endothelial cells and many of the cellular elements of the retina express little or no conventional class Ia major histocompatibility complex (MHC) molecules [1, 2]. MHC class I molecules serve as restricting elements that facilitate cytolysis of virus-infected cells by cytotoxic T lymphocytes (CTL). CTL-mediated killing of virus-infected cells is an effective mechanism for resolving viral infections in many organs. However, corneal endothelial cells and retinal cells cannot regenerate, and CTL-mediated elimination of these cells would lead to blindness. Thus, the absence or low expression of MHC class Ia molecules on these ocular cells prevents their unwitting immune elimination and, as a result, preserves vision. However, this strategy has a blind spot. Natural killer (NK) cells perceive cells that lack MHC class I molecules as foreign and are prompted to kill such cells. This is the basis for the 'missing self' hypothesis, which proposes that MHC class I molecules transmit 'off' or inhibitory signals to NK cells [11, 12]. To compensate for this blind spot, cells in the cornea and retina express nonclassical class Ib molecules, such as Qa-2 in the mouse and HLA-G in humans [13, 14]. In addition to inhibiting NK cell-mediated lysis, HLA-G also inhibits transendothelial migration of NK cells, suppresses CD4+ T cell proliferation, and can shift the immune response from a Th1 to a Th2 pathway [15].

Ocular-Induced Regulatory T Cells

Immune-mediated ocular inflammation is also inhibited by T_{reg} cells that are induced within the eye. There are at least four different pathways whereby T_{reg} cells can be generated following ocular exposure to antigens. The first pathway is evoked when antigens are introduced into the AC and it culminates in the antigen-specific downregulation of delayed-type hypersensitivity (DTH) – a phenomenon termed AC-associated immune deviation (ACAID) [5]. The second pathway occurs when CD4+ T cells come into contact with the pigmented epithelial cells of the iris and ciliary body [16]. The third route for inducing ocular T_{reg} cells occurs when T cells are exposed to AH or more specifically, to somatostatin, which is a constituent of the AH [17]. A fourth pathway that elicits the generation of T_{reg} cells occurs when novel antigens are expressed in the retina in response to transgenes driven by retina-specific promoters [18].

Regulatory T Cells Induced by Anterior Chamber-Associated Immune Deviation

The mechanisms and factors mentioned above act to either buffer or inhibit the expression of immune-mediated inflammation in an antigen-nonspecific manner. However, the eye has the capacity to promote the generation of T_{reg} cells that limit the expression of antigen-specific T cell-mediated inflammation. It has been recognized for almost 30 years that antigens introduced into the AC of the eye elicit an aberrant spectrum of systemic immune responses that are characterized by antigen-specific suppression of Th1 immune responses, such as DTH, while preserving antibody and CTL responses to many antigens (ACAID) [5]. Two categories of T_{reg} cells are generated in ACAID, CD4+ afferent-acting regulatory cells and CD8+ efferent-acting regulatory cells [2]. CD4+ T_{reg} cells inhibit the induction of DTH at the sensitization step and, thus, act at the afferent arm of the immune response [19, 20]. CD8+ T_{reg} cells are also induced by AC injection of antigen and act to prevent the expression of DTH by previously sensitized T cells and, therefore, function at the efferent arm of the immune response and are classified as efferent T_{reg} cells. The generation of these two T_{reg} cell populations is complex and involves the participation of several cell populations including: (a) F4/80+ antigen-presenting cells (APC) [21]; (b) B cells [22–24]; (c) γδ T cells [25, 26]; (d) NK1.1+ T cells [27–29], and (e) CD25+ CD4+ T cells [30].

ACAID CD4+ T_{reg} cells were first recognized for their capacity to inhibit T cell proliferative responses to antigens initially introduced into the AC [20]. Subsequent studies demonstrated that AC injection of antigen induced the development of CD4+ T cells that preferentially produced IL-10, but had diminished production of IFN-γ [31]. Kosiewicz and Streilein [32] also showed that CD8+ T_{reg} cells were produced by an MHC class II-restricted peptide, thereby suggesting an ancillary role for CD4+ T cells in the induction of ACAID. It is becoming increasingly clear that CD4+ T_{reg} cells play an important role in immune homeostasis [33]. In particular, naturally occurring CD4+ CD25+ T_{reg} cells constitute 5–10% of the CD4+ T cell population in mice and humans and play a critical role in controlling both the innate and adaptive immune responses [33–35]. Removal of CD4+ CD25+ T cells not only elicits autoimmunity, but also enhances immune responses to tissue grafts and tumors [36, 37]. CD4+ CD25+ T_{reg} cells are characterized by their preferential production of two anti-inflammatory cytokines, IL-10 and TGF-β [33]. It is noteworthy that CD4+ T cells isolated from ACAID spleens also express CD25, produce IL-10, and are required for the development of CD8+ efferent T_{reg} cells [30]. However, unlike conventional CD4+ CD25+ natural T_{reg} cells, the CD4+ afferent suppressor cells in ACAID do not require direct cell-cell contact to produce their regulatory effects [30]. There are conflicting reports as to whether the CD4+ T cells in ACAID are in fact CD4+ NK1.1+ T cells [30, 38]. Using an in vitro organ culture model of ACAID, Skelsey et al. [30] found that CD4+ T cell suspensions depleted of NK cells were able to induce the generation of CD8+ efferent ACAID T_{reg} cells. By contrast, Nakamura et al. [39] found compelling evidence indicating that CD4+ NKT cells, but not conventional CD4+ T cells, were necessary for the induction of ACAID. Among other things, these investigators found that ACAID could be induced in MHC class II−/− mice, which lack conventional CD4+ T cells, but still possess CD4+

NKT cells. However, both studies agree that production of IL-10 is a key function of the CD4+ T cells in the ACAID spleen. Neither study examined the CD4+ spleen cell populations for the expression of the Foxp3 transcription factor, which is specifically expressed on naturally occurring CD4+ CD25+ T_{reg} cells [40, 41].

The presence of CD8+ efferent T_{reg} cells has been demonstrated in all models of ACAID tested to date [2, 5]. The suppression produced by CD8+ efferent T_{reg} cells is antigen specific and inhibits the expression of DTH by previously sensitized T cells. Suppression can be produced by local adoptive transfer of CD8+ T_{reg} cells directly into the tissue site where antigen and DTH effector cells are deposited or by adoptive transfer via intraperitoneal or intravenous injection of CD8+ T_{reg} cells. The mechanism whereby CD8+ efferent T_{reg} cells exert their effects remains to be elucidated.

Pigment Epithelium-Induced Regulatory T Cells

The AH contains a potpourri of anti-inflammatory and immunosuppressive factors. Cells of the iris and ciliary body (I/CB) line the AC and are involved in the secretion of constituents of the AH. Earlier reports documented the immunomodulatory properties of I/CB cells [42–45]. Supernatants from cultures of I/CB tissue display immunosuppressive activity, largely due to the presence of TGF-β, although other immunomodulatory factors are also present [45]. However, the production of soluble factors alone does not explain the inhibitory effect of I/CB cells on T cell activity. Yoshida et al. [46] demonstrated that I/CB pigmented epithelial cells suppressed T cell proliferation and secretion of IFN-γ through a contact-dependent mechanism, which was not affected by neutralizing antibodies to TGF-β, IL-10 or TNF-α. In addition to exerting a direct immunosuppressive effect on T cells, I/CB cells induce the development of T_{reg} cells that inhibit anti-CD3-stimulated T cell proliferation and antigen-specific DTH [16]. The inhibitory effects of the I/CB-induced T_{reg} cells are mediated by the secretion of active and latent TGF-β. Thus, intraocular inflammation is controlled by multiple mechanisms. The myriad of immunosuppressive and anti-inflammatory molecules in the AH have an immediate impact on inflammatory cells that enter the eye. T cells that enter the eye via the I/CB route are directly inhibited by the contact-dependent immunosuppressive effects of I/CB cells, and the second wave of inflammatory T cells is extinguished by the inhibitory effects of the T_{reg} cells induced by I/CB cells.

Regulatory T Cells Induced by Aqueous Humor

One of the many immunosuppressive and anti-inflammatory constituents of the eye, α-melanocyte-stimulating hormone (α-MSH), suppresses IFN-γ production by activated T cells and enhances T cell production of anti-inflammatory cytokines, such as TGF-β_1 [47]. α-MSH also converts Th1 cells into CD4+ CD25+ T_{reg} cells that suppress antigen-specific DTH [48–50] and mitigate a Th1-mediated ocular inflammatory disease, experimental autoimmune uveoretinitis [48–50]. The induction of CD4+ CD25+ T_{reg} cells by α-MSH is mediated through the melanocortin 5 receptor that is expressed on primed CD4+ T cells [50]. In addition to α-MSH, vasoactive intestinal peptide and calcitonin gene-related peptide, another neuropeptide, somatostatin, is found in the AH [17]. Somatostatin not only suppresses IFN-γ production by activated T cells, but also induces the production of α-MSH, which is involved in the generation of CD4+ CD25+ T_{reg} cells [17]. Thus, the neuropeptides in the AH provide yet one more pathway for the generation of ocular T_{reg} cells.

Regulatory T Cells Induced by Endogenous Retinal Antigens

The induction of ACAID typically involves a single bolus injection of antigen delivered via glass needles or 30-gauge steel needles. Concerns have been raised about the physiological relevance of this technique. Such injections can produce significant leakage of the antigenic inocula and result in the deposition of antigens to the mucosal surface via drainage through the nasolacrimal duct, which conceivably might lead to the induction of mucosal tolerance. The mild trauma associated with using 30-gauge needles for AC injection provokes the local upregulation of TNF-α, which is required for the induction of ACAID [51]. This raises the question as to whether endogenous ocular antigens present in an intact, unmanipulated eye will elicit ACAID. With this in mind, Gregerson and Dou [18] produced transgenic mouse strains in which novel antigens were encoded by transgenes driven by retina-specific promoters. Endogenous retinal β-galactosidase expression led to depressed DTH responses to β-galactosidase and reduced lymphoproliferative responses to β-galactosidase-stimulated T cells, a phenotype that is reminiscent of ACAID [18]. The endogenous expression of self-retinal neoantigen (i.e. β-galactosidase) induced the development of T_{reg} cells that, when adoptively transferred, suppressed DTH responses to β-galactosidase in third-party, non-transgenic mice that had been previously immunized with β-galactosidase. However, the cytokine profile of the T_{reg} cells induced by endogenous retinal neoantigens departed from that found in ACAID T_{reg} cells and suggested that yet one more pathway was available for the generation of ocular T_{reg} cells.

Conclusions

There is remarkable redundancy in the mechanisms and factors that contribute to ocular immune privilege. Anatomical, physiological, and immunoregulatory features of the eye collectively reduce the induction, expression, and persistence of immune-mediated inflammation within the eye. The presence of at least four different pathways for the development of ocular T_{reg} cells indicates that in addition to redundancy, there is remarkable plasticity in the eye's capacity to sustain immune privilege. Gaining a better understanding of ocular T_{reg} cells will provide insights into how and why immune-mediated diseases circumvent immune privilege.

References

1 Niederkorn J: Immune privilege of the eye; in Chan LS (ed): Animal Models of Human Inflammatory Skin Diseases. New York, CRC Press, 2004, p 564.

2 Niederkorn JY: Immune privilege in the anterior chamber of the eye. Crit Rev Immunol 2002;22:13–46.

3 Niederkorn JY: Immunology and immunomodulation of corneal transplantation. Int Rev Immunol 2002;21:173–196.

4 Niederkorn JY: The immune privilege of corneal grafts. J Leukoc Biol 2003;74:167–171.

5 Streilein JW: Ocular immune privilege: therapeutic opportunities from an experiment of nature. Nat Rev Immunol 2003;3:879–889.

6 Streilein JW: Immune privilege as the result of local tissue barriers and immunosuppressive microenvironments. Curr Opin Immunol 1993;5:428–432.

7 Bora NS, Gobleman CL, Atkinson JP, Pepose JS, Kaplan HJ: Differential expression of the complement regulatory proteins in the human eye. Invest Ophthalmol Vis Sci 1993;34: 3579–3584.

8 Goslings WR, Prodeus AP, Streilein JW, et al: A small molecular weight factor in aqueous humor acts on C1q to prevent antibody-dependent complement activation. Invest Ophthalmol Vis Sci 1998;39:989–995.

9 Lass JH, Walter EI, Burris TE, et al: Expression of two molecular forms of the complement decay-accelerating factor in the eye and lacrimal gland. Invest Ophthalmol Vis Sci 1990;31: 1136–1148.

10 Griffith TS, Brunner T, Fletcher SM, Green DR, Ferguson TA: Fas ligand-induced apoptosis as a mechanism of immune privilege. Science 1995;270:1189–1192.

11 Ciccone E, Pende D, Vitale M, et al: Self class I molecules protect normal cells from lysis mediated by autologous natural killer cells. Eur J Immunol 1994;24:1003–1006.

12 Ljunggren HG, Karre K: In search of the 'missing self': MHC molecules and NK cell recognition. Immunol Today 1990;11:237–244.

13 Le Discorde M, Moreau P, Sabatier P, Legeais JM, Carosella ED: Expression of HLA-G in human cornea, an immune-privileged tissue. Hum Immunol 2003;64:1039–1044.

14 Niederkorn JY, Chiang EY, Ungchusri T, Stroynowski I: Expression of a nonclassical MHC class Ib molecule in the eye. Transplantation 1999;68:1790–1799.

15 Carosella ED, Moreau P, Aractingi S, Rouas-Freiss N: HLA-G: a shield against inflammatory aggression. Trends Immunol 2001;22:553–555.

16 Yoshida M, Kezuka T, Streilein JW: Participation of pigment epithelium of iris and ciliary body in ocular immune privilege. 2. Generation of TGF-beta-producing regulatory T cells. Invest Ophthalmol Vis Sci 2000;41:3862–3870.

17 Taylor AW, Yee DG: Somatostatin is an immunosuppressive factor in aqueous humor. Invest Ophthalmol Vis Sci 2003;44:2644–2649.

18 Gregerson DS, Dou C: Spontaneous induction of immunoregulation by an endogenous retinal antigen. Invest Ophthalmol Vis Sci 2002;43:2984–2991.

19 Kezuka T, Streilein JW: Analysis of in vivo regulatory properties of T cells activated in vitro by TGFβ2-treated antigen presenting cells. Invest Ophthalmol Vis Sci 2000;41:1410–1421.

20 Wilbanks GA, Streilein JW: Characterization of suppressor cells in anterior chamber-associated immune deviation (ACAID) induced by soluble antigen. Evidence of two functionally and phenotypically distinct T-suppressor cell populations. Immunology 1990;71:383–389.
21 Hara Y, Okamoto S, Rouse B, Streilein JW: Evidence that peritoneal exudate cells cultured with eye-derived fluids are the proximate antigen-presenting cells in immune deviation of the ocular type. J Immunol 1993;151:5162–5171.
22 D'Orazio TJ, Niederkorn JY: Splenic B cells are required for tolerogenic antigen presentation in the induction of anterior chamber-associated immune deviation (ACAID). Immunology 1998;95:47–55.
23 Niederkorn JY, Mayhew E: Role of splenic B cells in the immune privilege of the anterior chamber of the eye. Eur J Immunol 1995;25:2783–2787.
24 Skelsey ME, Mayhew E, Niederkorn JY: Splenic B cells act as antigen presenting cells for the induction of anterior chamber-associated immune deviation. Invest Ophthalmol Vis Sci 2003;44:5242–5251.
25 Skelsey ME, Mellon J, Niederkorn JY: Gamma delta T cells are needed for ocular immune privilege and corneal graft survival. J Immunol 2001;166:4327–4333.
26 Xu Y, Kapp JA: Gamma delta T cells are critical for the induction of anterior chamber-associated immune deviation. Immunology 2001;104:142–148.
27 Faunce DE, Stein-Streilein J: NKT cell-derived RANTES recruits APCs and CD8+ T cells to the spleen during the generation of regulatory T cells in tolerance. J Immunol 2002;169:31–38.
28 Sonoda KH, Exley M, Snapper S, Balk SP, Stein-Streilein J: CD1-reactive natural killer T cells are required for development of systemic tolerance through an immune-privileged site. J Exp Med 1999;190:1215–1226.
29 Wang Y, Goldschneider I, Foss D, et al: Direct thymic involvement in anterior chamber-associated immune deviation: evidence for a nondeletional mechanism of centrally induced tolerance to extrathymic antigens in adult mice. J Immunol 1997;158:2150–2155.
30 Skelsey ME, Mayhew E, Niederkorn JY: CD25+, interleukin-10-producing CD4+ T cells are required for suppressor cell production and immune privilege in the anterior chamber of the eye. Immunology 2003;110:18–29.
31 Li XY, D'Orazio LT, Niederkorn JY: Role of Th1 and Th2 cells in anterior chamber-associated immune deviation. Immunology 1996;89:34–40.
32 Kosiewicz MM, Streilein JW: Intraocular injection of class II-restricted peptide induces an unexpected population of CD8 regulatory cells. J Immunol 1996;157:1905–1912.
33 Shevach EM: CD4+ CD25+ suppressor T cells: more questions than answers. Nat Rev Immunol 2002;2:389–400.
34 Maloy KJ, Powrie F: Regulatory T cells in the control of immune pathology. Nat Immunol 2001;2:816–822.
35 Maloy KJ, Salaun L, Cahill R, et al: CD4+CD25+ T(R) cells suppress innate immune pathology through cytokine-dependent mechanisms. J Exp Med 2003;197:111–119.
36 Sakaguchi S, Sakaguchi N, Asano M, Itoh M, Toda M: Immunologic self-tolerance maintained by activated T cells expressing IL-2 receptor alpha-chains (CD25). Breakdown of a single mechanism of self-tolerance causes various autoimmune diseases. J Immunol 1995;155:1151–1164.
37 Yu P, Lee Y, Liu W, et al: Intratumor depletion of CD4+ cells unmasks tumor immunogenicity leading to the rejection of late-stage tumors. J Exp Med 2005;201:779–791.
38 Nakamura T, Sonoda KH, Faunce DE, et al: CD4+ NKT cells, but not conventional CD4+ T cells, are required to generate efferent CD8+ T regulatory cells following antigen inoculation in an immune-privileged site. J Immunol 2003;171:1266–1271.
39 Nakamura T, Terajewicz A, Stein-Streilein J: Mechanisms of peripheral tolerance following intracameral inoculation are independent of IL-13 or STAT6. J Immunol 2005;175:2643–2646.
40 Hori S, Nomura T, Sakaguchi S: Control of regulatory T cell development by the transcription factor Foxp3. Science 2003;299:1057–1061.
41 Hori S, Sakaguchi S: Foxp3: a critical regulator of the development and function of regulatory T cells. Microbes Infect 2004;6:745–751.

42 Helbig H, Gurley RC, Palestine AG, Nussenblatt RB, Caspi RR: Dual effect of ciliary body cells on T lymphocyte proliferation. Eur J Immunol 1990;20:2457–2463.
43 Hooper P, Bora NS, Kaplan HJ, Ferguson TA: Inhibition of lymphocyte proliferation by resident ocular cells. Curr Eye Res 1991;10:363–372.
44 Knisely TL, Bleicher PA, Vibbard CA, Granstein RD: Production of latent transforming growth factor-beta and other inhibitory factors by cultured murine iris and ciliary body cells. Curr Eye Res 1991;10:761–771.
45 Streilein JW, Bradley D: Analysis of immunosuppressive properties of iris and ciliary body cells and their secretory products. Invest Ophthalmol Vis Sci 1991;32:2700–2710.
46 Yoshida M, Takeuchi M, Streilein JW: Participation of pigment epithelium of iris and ciliary body in ocular immune privilege. 1. Inhibition of T-cell activation in vitro by direct cell-to-cell contact. Invest Ophthalmol Vis Sci 2000;41:811–821.
47 Taylor AW: Ocular immunosuppressive microenvironment; in Streilein JW (ed): Immune Response and the Eye. Chem Immunol. Basel, Karger, 1999, vol 73, pp 72–89.
48 Namba K, Kitaichi N, Nishida T, Taylor AW: Induction of regulatory T cells by the immunomodulating cytokines α-melanocyte-stimulating hormone and transforming growth factor-β2. J Leukoc Biol 2002;72:946–952.
49 Nishida T, Taylor AW: Specific aqueous humor factors induce activation of regulatory T cells. Invest Ophthalmol Vis Sci 1999;40:2268–2274.
50 Taylor A, Namba K: In vitro induction of CD25+ CD4+ regulatory T cells by the neuropeptide alpha-melanocyte stimulating hormone (α-MSH). Immunol Cell Biol 2001;79:358–367.
51 Ferguson TA, Herndon JM, Dube P: The immune response and the eye: a role for TNF alpha in anterior chamber-associated immune deviation. Invest Ophthalmol Vis Sci 1994;35:2643–2651.

Dr. Jerry Y. Niederkorn
Department of Ophthalmology, University of Texas Southwestern Medical Center
5323 Harry Hines Boulevard
Dallas, TX 75390–9057 (USA)
Tel. +1 214 648 3829, Fax +1 214 648 9061, E-Mail jerry.niederkorn@utsouthwestern.edu

Niederkorn JY, Kaplan HJ (eds): Immune Response and the Eye.
Chem Immunol Allergy. Basel, Karger, 2007, vol 92, pp 140–154

The Role of Fas Ligand and TNF-Related Apoptosis-Inducing Ligand (TRAIL) in the Ocular Immune Response

Thomas A. Ferguson[a], *Thomas S. Griffith*[b]

[a]Department of Ophthalmology and Visual Sciences, Washington University School of Medicine, St. Louis, Mo., [b]Department of Urology, University of Iowa, Iowa City, Iowa, USA

Abstract

The host response to pathogenic insults involves complex inflammatory responses and cellular immune reactions. While these are central to host defense and vital to clearing dangerous invaders, they are often associated with nonspecific injury to nearby tissue. These localized reactions function to successfully deal with pathogens before they spread to other areas. They are generally effective since most organ systems can tolerate these responses without permanent consequences. There are sites, however, that prohibit the spread of inflammation because these episodes can threaten organ integrity and function. The most prominent examples of these are the eye, brain, and reproductive organs (testis and ovary) where even minor bouts of inflammation can have long-term consequences on the survival of the organism. In these areas, immune responses either do not proceed, or proceed in a manner different from other areas; thus, they are called 'immunologically privileged'. Studies by a number of laboratories have determined that there are a number of mediators of ocular immune privilege. These include locally produced immunosuppressive cytokines, neuropeptides, limited expression of major histocompatibility complex class I and class II, complement-regulatory proteins, immune deviation, natural killer cell inhibitors, and the expression of the death-inducing ligands Fas ligand (FasL) and tumor necrosis factor (TNF)-related apoptosis-inducing ligand (TRAIL). The death-inducing molecules are poised to effectively deal with inflammatory cells once they pass the natural barriers of the eye, and effectively limit the spread of inflammatory cells and tumor cells within the confines of the eye by inducing apoptosis. The function of FasL and TRAIL will be the subject of this chapter.

Get your facts first, and then you can distort them as much as you please

Mark Twain

The mechanisms traditionally assigned to immune-privileged sites receive emphasis depending on the investigators and their area of expertise. However, there are several points that need to be made when considering the mediators of immune privilege. First, no single mechanism truly defines immune privilege. Privilege is no more 'just' anterior chamber (AC)-associated immune deviation (ACAID), than it is 'just' Fas ligand (FasL). Actually, the original definition was established based on the success of allografts when these sites were compared to conventional sites (e.g. the skin). Second, none of the mechanisms of immune privilege are unique to the eye. All assigned mediators (e.g. FasL, TGF-β, or immune deviation) are found (or happen) elsewhere. What is unique for the eye is that these processes have all come together in one site to provide a unique immunosuppressive microenvironment. Third, the loss of any single mechanism does not lead to spontaneous inflammation in the eye. Only the loss of FasL or tumor necrosis factor (TNF)-related apoptosis-inducing ligand (TRAIL) has been shown to have consequences [1–3], and this was not revealed until serious insult to the eye, such as infection or physical trauma, occurred. Consequently, considering immune privilege from the perspective of one or two mediators does not give the entire picture. However, this chapter was commissioned to deal with death-inducing ligands and we will restrict our discussion to these molecules, keeping in mind that the two molecules reviewed (FasL and TRAIL) are only part of the picture. A more thorough analysis of all proposed mediators of immune privilege can be found in any number of recent reviews [4–6].

Death Receptors and the Eye

Dyin' ain't no way to make a livin'

Outlaw *Josey Wales*

Fas Ligand

Overview

In the immune response, apoptosis plays a role in thymic deletion, control of clonal expansion, and cytotoxic T lymphocyte activity (CTL) activity. This type of cell death also plays an important regulatory role for the immune response. One hallmark of death by apoptosis is that any immune response that might develop against the dead cells, or as a result of the release of cell components, is minimized. This is because apoptotic cells can be recognized and removed without the induction of an inflammatory or immune reaction. It turns out that apoptotic cells not only inhibit immunity, they also induce immune tolerance (see below). Apoptosis is an indispensable part of adaptive immunity, as the immune system must not only deal with pathogens, it must deal with its own potentially damaging cells to prevent the formation of self-reactive responses that could lead to autoimmunity. Many aspects of apoptosis in the immune system rely on the Fas/FasL system, where peripheral deletion and control of clonal expansion are regulated by the Fas antigen (CD95) and its ligand, FasL (CD178) [7, 8].

FasL is a type II membrane protein belonging to the TNF family. FasL is expressed primarily on activated T cells, some tumor cells, and immune-privileged sites such as the eye and the testis [9]. FasL induces apoptosis in cells expressing the Fas receptor. Fas is a type I membrane protein of the TNF receptor family that was discovered due to the ability of specific antibodies to induce apoptosis in lymphoid tumor lines expressing the molecule. Two naturally occurring mutations in mice have emphasized the importance of Fas and FasL in the control of autoimmunity, the *lpr* and *gld* mutations, respectively. These mice display increased autoimmunity, which is characterized by a generalized and progressive lymphoproliferation resembling systemic lupus erythematosus. They suffer from a large accumulation of CD4− CD8− T cells in the spleen and lymph nodes. Genetic analysis has determined that a retroviral insertion into the *Fas* gene causes premature interruption of transcription in *lpr* mice. A point mutation in the *FasL* gene disrupts FasL function, resulting in the autoimmune syndrome in *gld* mice [10]. Recently, it was shown that these mutations, although they result in autoimmunity, did not result in complete loss of function. The targeted deletion of either *Fas* [11] or *FasL* [12] resulted in more severe pathology in these strains. Whether this means that data using *lpr* and *gld* mice must be reinterpreted is currently unknown.

The Discovery

The initial demonstration of a role for FasL in ocular immune privilege was based on two sets of observations: (a) functional FasL is expressed in the eye, and (b) loss of functional FasL expression exacerbates damage during immune responses [2]. Constitutive expression of functional FasL in the eye was shown by culturing murine or human corneas with target cells, which were then assessed for apoptosis [13]. Fas+ but not Fas− target cells underwent apoptosis, and in Fas+ cells, apoptosis was blocked by soluble Fas (sFasL). Furthermore, Fas+ T cells, but not those from *lpr* mice, underwent apoptosis upon injection into the eyes of wild-type, but not *gld* mice. These data clearly showed that functional FasL is present in the eye. Subsequently, studies showed that human retinal pigment epithelial cells induce apoptosis of activated T cells and the Fas+ Jurkat T cell line [14]. A cis-acting element in the FasL promoter was identified as being responsible for constitutive FasL expression in corneal endothelial cells [15]. These cells are responsible for the FasL-mediated protection of the cornea following grafting.

Studies have also shown that introduction of herpes simplex virus into the eyes of wild-type mice produced a transient inflammation wherein the infiltrating cells underwent apoptosis [2]. In *gld* mice, the lack of FasL-induced apoptosis in these inflammatory cells resulted in massive inflammatory damage. Experiments with bone marrow chimeras demonstrated that FasL expression in parenchymal (not bone marrow-derived) tissues was required for this protection. In subsequent studies, this effect was not restricted to viral infection as introduction of *Toxoplasma* similarly resulted in a transient inflammatory response. In animals lacking functional FasL, this erupted into immunological damage [16].

Localization

FasL is displayed abundantly in a number of strategic locations throughout the eye, including the cornea, retina, iris, and ciliary body. It is placed at or near areas that comprise the blood-ocular barrier, as well as in locations where there is an opportunity for interaction between ocular tissue and inflammatory cells. In the cornea, FasL is expressed on the endothelium and epithelium, suggesting its importance in controlling inflammatory cells that would enter from the conjunctiva or AC, respectively. In vitro studies with the cornea have revealed that FasL is readily available to kill cells in the normal eye. Accessible FasL on the cornea suggests that it is probably fully functional on other ocular structures within this organ. FasL is expressed on the iris and ciliary body where it can contact and kill cells entering from the vessels prominent in this tissue [2]. sFasL can be detected in serum [17] and the aqueous humor of uveitis patients [18]. In addition, sFasL has been shown to be chemotactic for neutrophils and is inhibitory to the apoptotic functions of FasL, but it remains to be shown if sFasL has relevance to ocular disease.

In the retina, FasL is expressed on the retinal pigment epithelial (RPE) cells, which comprise the outermost retinal layer, where it seems to have set up a barrier to the outside. Interestingly, it is prominently expressed on the photoreceptors (rods and cones) and throughout the neurosensory retina, where it may play a vital protective role to these cells important to visual transduction. It is not known if a compromise in FasL expression might lead to severe and sight-threatening episodes of inflammation [2]. However, FasL on RPE cells has been shown to be important in laser-induced choroidal neovascularization (see below).

Corneal Transplantation

FasL expression in the eye is important for the success of corneal transplants [13]. The cornea is the second most common tissue for transplantation in humans, and success rates of 80–90% are achieved without the use of systemic immunosuppressive therapy (or even tissue matching). In a mouse model, FasL+ corneas grafted across a fully allogeneic barrier typically result in a 60–70% acceptance rate. However, when allogeneic corneas from FasL-defective *gld* mice were transplanted, graft failure was near 100%. It was also demonstrated that cells entering the FasL+ grafts underwent apoptosis, while cells infiltrating the FasL− grafts did not. The role of FasL in human corneal transplantation was implicated when it was shown that humans express functional FasL on the endothelial and epithelial layers of the cornea.

The importance of FasL to corneal integrity and protection from the immune response was further supported in a system using heterotopic corneal transplantation [19]. In these studies, fully allogeneic corneas were placed beneath the kidney capsule. FasL+ corneas maintained clarity for several weeks while FasL− corneas from *gld* animals were rapidly rejected. As in the orthotopic graft model, the integrity of the allogeneic cornea was maintained by FasL expression on the corneal endothelium. Thus, FasL expression on the cornea is vital to the survival of allogeneic corneal grafts.

Immune Tolerance

Apoptosis (by Fas/FasL and other means) is an important component in several tolerance pathways [2, 20, 21]. In these systems, apoptotic cells are thought to enter the cross priming pathway and promote immune tolerance. Necrotic cells do not have this capacity and can release pro-inflammatory mediators. This difference accounts for the differing ways in which the immune system handles necrosis and apoptosis [for discussion, see ref. 6].

The first in vivo demonstration that apoptotic cells were, in fact, tolerogenic, was done using the HSV-1 ACAID model [22]. When virus was injected into the AC of the eye in wild-type mice, infiltrating inflammatory cells underwent apoptosis within 48 h, and tolerance (as measured by systemic delayed-type hypersensitivity, DTH) developed to the viral antigens. When the same experiments were done with *gld* and *lpr* mice, where HSV-1 infection does not result in death of inflammatory cells, DTH tolerance did not occur. Tolerance could be reestablished in *lpr* mice if cell death was restored by replacing the *lpr* lymphoid system with wild-type lymphoid cells, as in wild-type → *lpr* radiation bone marrow chimeras. Furthermore, if the eye (containing the dead cells) of normal mice is removed within the first 3 days of viral injection, tolerance is not established. These enucleated mice actually become immune by displaying a normal DTH response to the virus, suggesting that sufficient virus can leave the eye to induce immunity, but the eye must remain intact for a time so tolerance can be established. We believe this allows the dead cells within the eye to initiate the systemic tolerance response.

Using the experimental system where trinitrophenyl (TNP)-coupled spleen cells are injected into the eye, it became clear that cell death had a significant role in tolerance induction. In this situation where the type of cell injected and the recipient can be easily controlled, it became evident that the presence of Fas on the injected cells and FasL on the eye were essential for tolerance to follow. When either molecule was defective, immune tolerance was not established. A surprising and interesting finding was that while it was FasL-induced death in the eye that led to tolerance, it was the process of apoptotic cell death that was the critical factor. This was readily shown using *lpr* TNP-coupled spleen cells, which did not undergo apoptosis or induce tolerance when injected into the AC of wild-type mice. If apoptotic cell death is initiated in these cells by lethal irradiation or heat shock prior to injection, tolerance develops. Death of these cells by necrotic means, such as freeze-thaw cycles, does not work, nor is tolerance established if apoptosis is prevented by rapid fixation or overexpression of Bcl-X_L. The implication from these studies with virus or TNP-coupled spleen cells was that the FasL-induced dead cells actually performed a function in the tolerance scheme, overriding (or regulating) the induction of immunity. Furthermore, the results implied that the presence of an anti-inflammatory component within the apoptotic event in the eye was manifested through the inhibition of systemic immune responses [9].

Neovascularization

Angiogenesis is a fundamental process during development and wound healing. New vessel growth, however, can be detrimental in pathologic conditions such as retinopathy, inflammatory diseases, and tumor progression. In diabetic retinopathy, retinopathy of prematurity, and age-related macular degeneration, vessel growth itself causes retinal detachment and loss of vision. In a mouse model of age-related macular degeneration (laser-induced choroidal neovascularization), Kaplan et al. [23] showed that vessel growth beneath the retina was exacerbated in *gld* mice compared to wild-type mice. It was further demonstrated that it was FasL on retinal pigment epithelium that regulated the spread of the new vessels induced by laser damage. Similarly, in the mouse model of retinopathy of prematurity, exposure to oxygen induces more severe neovascularization in *gld* compared to wild-type mice [24]. Finally, corneal neovascularization, an important component of graft rejection and corneal disease, is also regulated by FasL expression [25]. Thus, FasL not only controls invasion of the eye by lymphocytes, it blocks the growth of blood vessels that can damage the eye and impair vision. Clearly, the exclusion of a sight-threatening process such as blood vessel growth shows that the principles of 'privilege' extend to other physiological processes.

It is interesting that *gld* and *lpr* mice have eyes that appear normal [23, 24]. There are no natural abnormalities in these eyes and we have not found evidence for increased lymphocytic infiltration in these mice. Thus, Fas and FasL play no role in vascular development in the eye.

The Microenvironment

One important (and often overlooked) component of FasL-mediated effects in immune-privileged sites is the site itself. In other words, the microenvironment for the Fas-FasL interaction influences the outcome. In the eye, for example, Fas and FasL interact in the presence of other immunosuppressive factors, which can contribute to the function of FasL. Complementary mechanisms known to be operative in the eye involve the constitutive expression of immunosuppressive cytokines, e.g. transforming growth factor (TGF)-β and vasoactive intestinal peptide. The importance of cofactors in FasL-mediated protection of immune-privileged sites was demonstrated by Chen et al. [26]. These authors examined the role of TGF-β in FasL mediated tumor surveillance. They observed that forced expression of FasL in a colon carcinoma resulted in granulocytic infiltration when the tumor was transplanted subcutaneously. When the tumors were placed in the eye (where TGF-β and immune-privileged mediators are abundant), granulocyte infiltration was absent and the tumors grew. Co-expression of TGF-β and FasL conferred protection on this allograft when transplanted to the skin. These authors further showed that TGF-β inhibited neutrophil activation. Thus, the microenvironment consisting of FasL and TGF-β promoted immune tolerance and graft protection [9].

It was also found that cells resistant to death induced by ocular FasL were sensitized for Fas-mediated apoptosis by the pro-inflammatory cytokine TNF [27]. This effect was mediated by the TNF receptor 2, not the conventional apoptosis-inducing TNF receptor 1. The mechanism for this was downmodulation of anti-apoptotic proteins within the cell, which sensitized the cells for death. Thus, complicity between FasL and elements of the inflammatory response exists to control inflammation.

Inducible (Induced?) Immune Privilege

While there are clearly constitutive immune-privileged sites that are protected because of their importance to survival, this status is extended to other organs that are just as vital. These sites may want to limit the spread of inflammation, but they would not want to completely prohibit the expression of immunity. The anti-inflammatory effects of constitutive immune privilege might actually be dangerous to systemic immunity because they are areas of high lymphoid traffic. Organs such as the liver, lung, skin, and small intestine would fall into this category. These organs employ a strategy we call 'inducible immune privilege'. Here immunity is vital, lymphoid traffic is high, but out-of-control immunity could compromise their important physiological functions.

Induced immune privilege was first observed with superantigen deletion where FasL expression was increased in response to T cell activation. In this system, systemic injection of the superantigen (staphylococcal enterotoxin B) results in rapid T cell expansion followed by deletion of the reactive cells. Deletion is defective in *lpr* and *gld* mice, and therefore, the Fas-FasL interaction participates in the removal of these cells [28]. It was assumed that deletion was suicide (or at least fratricide) of responding Vβ8+ cells. However, when radiation bone marrow chimeras were made between *gld* and wild-type mice, it was discovered that T cells from *gld* mice were deleted when they were present in normal mice (ruling out fratricide/suicide). In contrast, wild-type T cells could not be deleted in *gld* mice, suggesting that non-lymphoid FasL was responsible for removing Fas+ T cells. This study also showed that immunization induced an upregulation of functional FasL in the liver and small intestine, and that this required the presence of activated T cells. This concept was recently extended to TCR transgenic T cells responding to peptide antigens [29]. Therefore, such inducible, peripheral, non-lymphoid FasL may be involved in the phenomenon of peripheral deletion.

The skin also uses immune privilege to protect itself from damage. In one elegant study, FasL induction following UV irradiation of the skin prevented the accumulation of p53 mutations in the epidermis. This effect was absent in *gld* and *lpr* mice [30]. UV irradiation of the skin also causes an increased FasL expression in keratinocytes leading to the elimination of T cells in psoriasis [31]. In these examples, organs use 'immune privilege' (and FasL) as a protective mechanism, but expression is induced, not constitutive.

Pro-Inflammatory Properties

> A scientist will never show any kindness for a theory which he did not start himself
>
> *Mark Twain*

The discussion thus far has focused on the anti-inflammatory properties of FasL and its ability to induce apoptotic cell death in cells invading the eye. There are, however, situations where FasL expression in the eye appears to have a pro-inflammatory component. Recently, tumor cells overexpressing wild-type FasL, membrane-bound FasL, or sFasL were injected into the eyes of mice [32]. Tumors expressing only wild-type FasL or sFasL failed to trigger inflammation and grew progressively. Tumors expressing only membrane-bound FasL induced neutrophil-mediated inflammation and were rejected. Under these circumstances, the authors concluded that membrane-bound FasL terminates immune privilege and activates innate immunity. Whether this suggests that the original function of FasL in the eye should be reevaluated or whether these data emphasize the problems with enforced overexpression of FasL is not clear. Of note, wild-type FasL did not terminate immune privilege or activate innate immunity. Since in the presence of wild-type FasL there is both sFasL and membrane-bound FasL, this balance may block the pro-inflammatory aspect of this protein and promote the anti-inflammatory component. Maybe this is why the eye expresses a form of FasL that can be soluble and membrane bound.

Whether the results with tumor cells are physiologically relevant or yet another example of an overexpression artifact is not clear. However, a recent study of bacterial endophthalmitis suggests that there may indeed be a pro-inflammatory role for FasL in bacterial infections of the eye [33]. These authors observed that mice defective in FasL had difficulty in clearing an intraocular infection with *Staphylococcus aureus*. They also observed, in contrast to observations with viral infection, that a significantly greater number of phagocytes were recruited to the intraocular infection site in mice expressing FasL compared with either *gld* or *lpr* mice. Thus, it was hypothesized that FasL activates cells, either resident cells or possibly infiltrating neutrophils, to release factors that attract granulocytes. These results are quite interesting and point to the complexity of constitutive death ligand expression. Perhaps cells entering in response to bacterial infections rapidly become resistant to Fas-mediated death. It is even likely that important cofactors (TGF-β or TNF-α) are regulated differently during bacterial infection. Whatever the reason, these interesting observations certainly do not suffer from the overexpression 'problem' from which many studies of FasL suffer. Elucidation of this mechanism will give important insights into the function of FasL in the eye.

TNF-Related Apoptosis-Inducing Ligand/Apo-2L

> I cannot give any scientist of any age better advice than this: the intensity of a conviction that a hypothesis is true has no bearing over whether it is true or not
>
> *Peter Medawar*

Expression and Receptors

The TNF family of cytokines influences a variety of immunological functions, such as cell activation and death. Programmed cell death, or apoptosis, is a vital process in the life of complex organisms, and this death is regulated in situ by many intracellular and extracellular signals. For example, CD40 ligand (CD40L; CD154) inhibits apoptotic cell death, whereas TNF and FasL function as inducers of apoptosis in many physiological events, such as autoimmunity, activation-induced cell death, immune privilege, and evasion of tumors from the immune system. TRAIL (Apo-2L) is another family member capable of inducing apoptosis and has recently received great attention because of its therapeutic potential as a tumoricidal agent.

Early studies identified two unique characteristics of TRAIL. First, TRAIL-induced apoptosis occurs only in tumor cells or transformed cells and not normal cells [34]. Analogous to the other death-inducing members of the TNF family (i.e. FasL and TNF), cells undergoing TRAIL-induced death exhibited many of the hallmarks of apoptosis, including DNA fragmentation, expression of prophagocytic signals (i.e. phosphatidylserine) on the cell membrane, and cleavage of multiple intracellular proteins by caspases [34–37]. Soluble TRAIL was tumoricidal for over 75% of the more than sixty hematopoietic and non-hematopoietic tumor cell lines tested in vitro, suggesting that TRAIL could be used as a broad-spectrum, anti-tumor molecule in vivo [34, 35, 38, 39]. TRAIL may be important in activation-induced cell death of T cells during HIV infection [40]. In humans, peripheral blood T cells express TRAIL after CD3 crosslinking and type I interferon stimulation, perhaps also contributing to the activation-induced cell death of T cells in the natural setting [41].

Second, human natural killer cells, monocytes, and dendritic cells express TRAIL following cytokine stimulation, transforming them into potent killers of tumor cells [42–44]. Recent work has revealed that CpG-containing oligonucleotides are also potent inducers of TRAIL on human peripheral blood mononuclear cells (especially monocytes and B cells) via an interferon-α-dependent mechanism [45]. In contrast to other TNF family members whose expression is tightly regulated and often transiently expressed, mRNA for TRAIL is detected in a wide range of tissues, including peripheral blood lymphocytes, spleen, thymus, prostate, ovary, small intestine, colon and placenta [34].

Unlike FasL and TNF, which interact with a single or pair of receptors, respectively, TRAIL specifically binds to five distinct receptors: DR4 [46], DR5/TRAIL-R2 [47–49], TRID/DcR1/TRAIL-R3 [47, 48, 50], TRAIL-R4/DcR2 [38, 51] (hereafter referred to as TRAIL-R1, -R2, -R3, and -R4, respectively), and osteoprotegerin (OPG) [52]. Both TRAIL-R1 and TRAIL-R2 contain a cytoplasmic death domain, and crosslinking by TRAIL or receptor-specific monoclonal antibodies activates the apoptosis signaling pathway in sensitive cells [37, 46–49]. In contrast, neither TRAIL-R3 (which is glycosyl-phosphatidyl inositol linked) nor TRAIL-R4 (which is a type I membrane protein) contains a complete cytoplasmic death domain, and neither can mediate apoptosis upon ligation [38, 47, 48, 50, 51]. OPG is a soluble receptor capable of binding to TRAIL in vitro and blocking TRAIL-induced apoptosis [52]. Because TRAIL-R3, TRAIL-R4, and OPG bind to TRAIL without directly signaling for cell death, it was initially proposed that these receptors inhibit TRAIL-induced apoptosis by acting either as membrane-bound or soluble antagonistic receptors [47, 48, 50, 52] or via transduction of an anti-apoptotic signal [38]. Therefore, the presence or absence of TRAIL-R3, TRAIL-R4, and/or OPG was thought to determine whether a cell is resistant or sensitive, respectively, to TRAIL-induced apoptosis [47, 48, 51, 52]. Further investigation of many tumor cell lines, however, disproved this theory as the sole mechanism regulating TRAIL sensitivity and resistance [36, 44].

Immune Privilege

An animal's eyes have the power to speak a great language
Martin Buber

The importance for FasL in maintaining immune privilege was highlighted by studies in the eye, testis, and placenta [2, 22, 53, 54]. Because of its ability to kill activated lymphocytes and having the highest homology with FasL, investigation into the potential of the TRAIL-TRAIL receptor system to protect these same sites from immune attack was also explored. Indeed, TRAIL performs many of the same functions within the eye and placenta. Within the eye, TRAIL is constitutively expressed on numerous ocular structures, including the cornea and retina [3], suggesting a role for TRAIL in tumor surveillance within the eye. Ocular expression of TRAIL may also explain the paucity of clinical cases of ocular tumors; however, it is unknown whether TRAIL plays any role in the success of corneal transplants. Studies investigating the expression of TRAIL in first trimester placentas found prominent expression in syncytiotrophoblasts, where it was localized primarily to the apical brush border [55]. In addition, TRAIL was present on villous stroma and stromal cells, particularly the Hofbauer cells (placental macrophages), amnion epithelial cells, and maternal decidual cells. Expression was low to absent in fibroblastic mesenchymal cells and endothelial cells. In addition to the high level of TRAIL expression, trophoblasts also expressed significant levels of the nonsignaling TRAIL receptor, TRAIL-R3. Based on the expression of these two molecules, it was concluded that TRAIL may be an important contributor to immune tolerance during pregnancy.

Examination of TRAIL in the mouse eye reveals several findings relevant to immune privilege. It was found that TRAIL mRNA and protein are constitutively expressed on numerous ocular structures, including the cornea and retina [3]. The pattern of expression for TRAIL in the eye is remarkably similar to that of FasL, where these ligands are positioned at sites of interaction between the internal structures of the eye and the 'outside' world. FasL/TRAIL expression on the corneal epithelium can prevent cells from entering from the conjunctiva, while expression in vascularized iris can prevent entry of cells via iris blood vessels, whereas expression on the corneal endothelium protects this very important single layer of non-regenerating cells essential to the maintenance of corneal integrity and clarity. Expression on the RPE cell forms a barrier between the photoreceptors and the vascularized choroid. It is interesting to note that most ocular tumors take up residence in the choroid, just outside the barrier formed by TRAIL and FasL. Recently, TRAIL receptor was documented on ocular melanomas, suggesting that TRAIL may be a potential target for these tumors. However, these data were derived from analysis of long-term cultured cell lines. Thus, the importance of the TRAIL/TRAIL-R system to primary ocular melanomas is uncertain.

Most importantly, ocular tissue displays functional TRAIL as determined by in vitro killing of TRAIL-sensitive tumor cell lines. When TRAIL-sensitive tumors (that were not FasL sensitive) were injected into the AC of the eye, the growth of these cells was significantly inhibited compared to TRAIL-insensitive cells [3]. The relative contribution of TRAIL and FasL for tumor cell killing in the eye was also examined. It was found that ocular tissue can kill cells via either ligand. This suggests that a compensatory mechanism between TRAIL and FasL might exist. This may help explain why FasL-defective *gld* mice or TRAIL−/− mice do not show spontaneous inflammation. When *gld* × TRAIL−/− mice are generated, this question can be more directly addressed. Whether TRAIL serves any function in corneal transplantation, the induction of systemic tolerance, or the regulation of herpes simplex virus replication is currently unknown. However, there is good physiological evidence for ocular TRAIL expression, and a role for this molecule in tumor surveillance in an immune privileged site.

Conclusions

A conclusion is the place where you got tired thinking
Martin Henry Fischer

The protection of the visual axis by inhibitors of inflammation is well documented. It is clear that the constitutive expression of inhibitory cytokines, inhibitory neuropeptides, the blood-ocular barrier, FasL, and TRAIL provide a basis for immune privilege. Studies examining how these mediators collaborate to ensure immune privilege is the challenge for the future.

Acknowledgment

This work was supported by National Institutes of Health grants EY06765 (T.A.F.) and CA109446 (T.S.G.), and the Department of Ophthalmology and Visual Sciences core grant (EY08972). Support was also received from the Foundation for Fighting Blindness (Owings Mills, Md., USA) and from Research to Prevent Blindness (New York, N.Y., USA).

References

1 Ferguson TA, Griffith TS: A vision of cell death: insights into immune privilege. Immunol Rev 1997;156:167–184.

2 Griffith TS, Brunner T, Fletcher SM, Green DR, Ferguson TA: Fas ligand-induced apoptosis as a mechanism of immune privilege. Science 1995;270:1189–1192.

3 Lee HO, Herndon JM, Barreiro R, Griffith TS, Ferguson TA: TRAIL: a mechanism of tumor surveillance in an immune privileged site. J Immunol 2002;169:4739–4744.
4 Streilein JW: Ocular immune privilege: the eye takes a dim but practical view of immunity and inflammation. J Leukoc Biol 2003;74:179–185.
5 Niederkorn JY: The immune privilege of corneal grafts. J Leukoc Biol 2003;74:167–171.
6 Ferguson TA, Stuart PM, Herndon JM, Griffith TS: Apoptosis, tolerance, and regulatory T cells – old wine, new wineskins. Immunol Rev 2003;193:111–123.
7 Abbas AK: Die and let live: eliminating dangerous lymphocytes. Cell 1996;84:655–657.
8 Abbas AK, Lohr J, Knoechel B, Nagabhushanam V: T cell tolerance and autoimmunity. Autoimmun Rev 2004;3:471–475.
9 Ferguson TA, Green DR: Fas-ligand and immune privilege: the eyes have it. Cell Death Differ 2001;8:771–772.
10 Nagata S, Suda T: Fas and Fas ligand: lpr and gld mutations. Immunol Today 1995;16:39–43.
11 Adachi M, Suematsu S, Suda T, et al: Enhanced and accelerated lymphoproliferation in Fas-null mice. Proc Natl Acad Sci USA 1996;93:2131–2136.
12 Karray S, Kress C, Cuvellier S, et al: Complete loss of Fas ligand gene causes massive lymphoproliferation and early death, indicating a residual activity of gld allele. J Immunol 2004;172: 2118–2125.
13 Stuart PM, Griffith TS, Usui N, Pepose J, Yu X, Ferguson TA: CD95 ligand (FasL)-induced apoptosis is necessary for corneal allograft survival. J Clin Invest 1997;99:396–402.
14 Jorgensen A, Wiencke AK, la Cour M, et al: Human retinal pigment epithelial cell-induced apoptosis in activated T cells. Invest Ophthalmol Vis Sci 1998;39:1590–1599.
15 Zhang J, Ma B, Marshak-Rothstein A, Fine A: Characterization of a novel cis-element that regulates Fas ligand expression in corneal endothelial cells. J Biol Chem 1999;274:26537–26542.
16 Hu MS, Schwartzman JD, Yeaman GR, et al: Fas-FasL interaction involved in pathogenesis of ocular toxoplasmosis in mice. Infect Immun 1999;67:928–935.
17 Tanaka M, Suda T, Haze K, et al: Fas ligand in human serum. Nat Med 1996;2:317–322.
18 Sotozono C, Sano Y, Suzuki T, et al: Soluble Fas ligand expression in the ocular fluids of uveitis patients. Curr Eye Res 2000;20:54–57.
19 Hori J, Joyce N, Streilein JW: Epithelium-deficient corneal allografts display immune privilege beneath the kidney capsule. Invest Ophthalmol Vis Sci 2000;41:443–452.
20 Ferguson TA, Herndon J, Elzey B, Griffith TS, Schoenberger S, Green DR: Uptake of apoptotic antigen-coupled cells by lymphoid dendritic cells and cross-priming of $CD8^+$ T cells produce active immune unresponsiveness. J Immunol 2002;168:5589–5595.
21 Hill LL, Shreedhar VK, Kripke ML, Owen-Schaub LB: A critical role for Fas ligand in the active suppression of systemic immune responses by ultraviolet radiation. J Exp Med 1999;189: 1285–1294.
22 Griffith TS, Yu X, Herndon JM, Green DR, Ferguson TA: CD95-induced apoptosis of lymphocytes in an immune privileged site induces immunological tolerance. Immunity 1996;5:7–16.
23 Kaplan HJ, Leibole MA, Tezel T, Ferguson TA: Fas ligand (CD95 ligand) controls angiogenesis beneath the retina. Nat Med 1999;5:292–297.
24 Barreiro R, Schadlu R, Herndon J, Kaplan HJ, Ferguson TA: The role of Fas-FasL in the development and treatment of ischemic retinopathy. Invest Ophthalmol Vis Sci 2003;44:1282–1286.
25 Stuart PM, Pan F, Plambeck S, Ferguson TA: FasL-Fas interactions regulate neovascularization in the cornea. Invest Ophthalmol Vis Sci 2003;44:93–98.
26 Chen JJ, Sun Y, Nabel GJ: Regulation of the proinflammatory effects of Fas ligand (CD95L). Science 1998;282:1714–1717.
27 Elzey BD, Griffith TS, Herndon JM, Barreiro R, Tschopp J, Ferguson TA: Regulation of Fas ligand-induced apoptosis by TNF. J Immunol 2001;167:3049–3056.
28 Bonfoco E, Stuart PM, Brunner T, et al: Inducible nonlymphoid expression of Fas ligand is responsible for superantigen-induced peripheral deletion of T cells. Immunity 1998;9:711–720.
29 Pinkoski MJ, Droin NM, Lin T, Genestier L, Ferguson TA, Green DR: Nonlymphoid Fas ligand in peptide-induced peripheral lymphocyte deletion. Proc Natl Acad Sci USA 2002;99:16174–16179.
30 Hill LL, Ouhtit A, Loughlin SM, Kripke ML, Ananthaswamy HN, Owen-Schaub LB: Fas ligand: a sensor for DNA damage critical in skin cancer etiology. Science 1999;285:898–900.

31 Gutierrez-Steil C, Wrone-Smith T, Sun X, Krueger JG, Coven T, Nickoloff BJ: Sunlight-induced basal cell carcinoma tumor cells and ultraviolet-B-irradiated psoriatic plaques express Fas ligand (CD95L). J Clin Invest 1998;101:33–39.
32 Gregory MS, Repp AC, Holhbaum AM, Saff RR, Marshak-Rothstein A, Ksander BR: Membrane Fas ligand activates innate immunity and terminates ocular immune privilege. J Immunol 2002;169:2727–2735.
33 Engelbert M, Gilmore MS: Fas ligand but not complement is critical for control of experimental *Staphylococcus aureus* endophthalmitis. Invest Ophthalmol Vis Sci 2005;46:2479–2486.
34 Wiley SR, Schooley K, Smolak PJ, et al: Identification and characterization of a new member of the TNF family that induces apoptosis. Immunity 1995;3:673–682.
35 Pitti RM, Marsters SA, Ruppert S, Donahue CJ, Moore A, Ashkenazi A: Induction of apoptosis by Apo-2 ligand, a new member of the tumor necrosis factor cytokine family. J Biol Chem 1996;271:12687–12690.
36 Griffith TS, Chin WA, Jackson GC, Lynch DH, Kubin MZ: Intracellular regulation of TRAIL-induced apoptosis in human melanoma cells. J Immunol 1998;161:2833–2840.
37 Griffith TS, Rauch CT, Smolak PJ, et al: Functional analysis of TRAIL receptors using monoclonal antibodies. J Immunol 1999;162:2597–2605.
38 Degli-Esposti MA, Dougall WC, Smolak PJ, Waugh JY, Smith CA, Goodwin RG: The novel receptor TRAIL-R4 induces NF-κB and protects against TRAIL-mediated apoptosis, yet retains an incomplete death domain. Immunity 1997;7:813–820.
39 Griffith TS, Lynch DH: TRAIL: a molecule with multiple receptors and control mechanisms. Curr Opin Immunol 1998;10:559–563.
40 Katsikis PD, Garcia-Ojeda ME, Torres-Roca JF, et al: Interleukin-1β converting enzyme-like protease involvement in Fas-induced and activation-induced peripheral blood T cell apoptosis in HIV infection. TNF-related apoptosis-inducing ligand can mediate activation-induced T cell death in HIV infection. J Exp Med 1997;186:1365–1372.
41 Kayagaki N, Yamaguchi N, Nakayama M, Eto H, Okumura K, Yagita H: Type I interferons (IFNs) regulate tumor necrosis factor-related apoptosis-inducing ligand (TRAIL) expression on human T cells: a novel mechanism for the antitumor effects of type I IFNs. J Exp Med 1999;189:1451–1460.
42 Zamai L, Ahmad M, Bennett IM, Azzoni L, Alnemri ES, Perussia B: Natural killer (NK) cell-mediated cytotoxicity: differential use of TRAIL and Fas ligand by immature and mature primary human NK cells. J Exp Med 1998;88:2375–2380.
43 Griffith TS, Wiley SR, Kubin MZ, Sedger LM, Maliszewski CR, Fanger NA: Monocyte-mediated tumoricidal activity via the tumor necrosis factor-related cytokine, TRAIL. J Exp Med 1999;189:1343–1354.
44 Fanger NA, Maliszewski CR, Schooley K, Griffith TS: Human dendritic cells mediate cellular apoptosis via tumor necrosis factor-related apoptosis-inducing ligand (TRAIL). J Exp Med 1999;190:1155–1164.
45 Kemp TJ, Elzey BD, Griffith TS: Plasmacytoid dendritic cell-derived IFN-α induces TNF-related apoptosis-inducing ligand/Apo-2L-mediated antitumor activity by human monocytes following CpG oligodeoxynucleotide stimulation. J Immunol 2003;171:212–218.
46 Pan G, O'Rourke K, Chinnaiyan AM, et al: The receptor for the cytotoxic ligand TRAIL. Science 1997;276:111–113.
47 Pan G, Ni J, Wei YF, Yu G, Gentz R, Dixit VM: An antagonist decoy receptor and a death domain-containing receptor for TRAIL. Science 1997;277:815–818.
48 Sheridan JP, Marsters SA, Pitti RM, et al: Control of TRAIL-induced apoptosis by a family of signaling and decoy receptors. Science 1997;277:818–821.
49 Walczak H, Degli-Esposti MA, Johnson RS, et al: TRAIL-R2: a novel apoptosis-mediating receptor for TRAIL. EMBO J 1997;16:5386–5397.
50 Degli-Esposti MA, Smolak PJ, Walczak H, et al: Cloning and characterization of TRAIL-R3, a novel member of the emerging TRAIL receptor family. J Exp Med 1997;186:1165–1170.
51 Marsters SA, Sheridan JP, Pitti RM, et al: A novel receptor for Apo2L/TRAIL contains a truncated death domain. Curr Biol 1997;7:1003–1006.
52 Emery JG, McDonnell P, Burke MB, et al: Osteoprotegerin is a receptor for the cytotoxic ligand TRAIL. J Biol Chem 1998;273:14363–14367.

53 Bellgrau D, Gold D, Selawry H, Moore J, Franzusoff A, Duke RC: A role for CD95 ligand in preventing graft rejection. Nature 1995;377:630–632.
54 Hunt JS, Vassmer D, Ferguson TA, Miller L: Fas ligand is positioned in mouse uterus and placenta to prevent trafficking of activated leukocytes between the mother and the conceptus. J Immunol 1997;158:4122–4128.
55 Phillips TA, Ni J, Pan G, et al: TRAIL (Apo-2L) and TRAIL receptors in human placentas: implications for immune privilege. J Immunol 1999;162:6053–6059.

Dr. Thomas A. Ferguson
Department of Ophthalmology and Visual Sciences, Washington University School of Medicine
660 South Euclid, Box 8096
St. Louis, MO 63110 (USA)
Tel. +1 314 362 3745, Fax +1 314 747 4238, E-Mail Ferguson@vision.wustl.edu

Niederkorn JY, Kaplan HJ (eds): Immune Response and the Eye.
Chem Immunol Allergy. Basel, Karger, 2007, vol 92, pp 155–165

Impact of Inflammation on Ocular Immune Privilege

Jun-Song Mo[a,b], *Wei Wang*[a,b], *Henry J. Kaplan*[a]

Departments of [a]Ophthalmology and Visual Sciences, and [b]Microbiology and Immunology, University of Louisville School of Medicine, Louisville, Ky., USA

Abstract

The immune-privileged status of the anterior chamber of the eye is altered in experimentally induced intraocular inflammation and in the pigment dispersion syndrome of DBA/2J mice. However, the eye has developed multiple mechanisms to maintain ocular immune privilege even in the presence of intraocular inflammation.

Ocular immune privilege depends upon the integrity of the anatomical and biochemical structures of the eye and is important in preventing the loss of vision from the innate and adaptive immune responses to potential ocular pathogens [1]. It was assumed that ocular immune privilege and inflammation could not coexist and that intraocular inflammation would damage and eliminate immune privilege. In the past 6 years, we have tested this assumption and systemically analyzed how intraocular inflammation can alter ocular immune privilege. Our results indicate that the eye has developed multiple mechanisms to maintain ocular immune privilege with a new mechanism used to establish immune privilege when the old mechanism is destroyed.

Indicators of Ocular Immune Privilege

There are at least four signs that ocular immune privilege may exist in the anterior chamber (AC) of the eye: (1) integrity of the blood-aqueous humor (AH) barrier [2]; (2) the immunosuppressive microenvironment of the eye; (3) the capacity of the eye to support AC-associated immune deviation (ACAID)

[6, 7], and (4) survival of a foreign tissue graft in the AC. (1) The tight epithelial junctions of the iris and ciliary body prevent the leakage of plasma proteins and the infiltration of leukocytes from the circulation into the eye. (2) AH has the capacity to suppress the function of both innate immunity (e.g. macrophages) and adaptive immunity (e.g. T cells) [3]. The ocular immunosuppressive microenvironment can be analyzed in vitro by studying the capacity of AH to suppress T cell proliferation stimulated by anti-CD3 monoclonal antibody (2C11) [4]. Small neuropeptides and latent transforming growth factor (TGF)-β are present in native AH. Since most of the TGF-β is in its latent form and must be activated to have biological effects, it is believed that small neuropeptides are the major source of immunosuppression in native AH [5]. (4) Survival of a foreign tissue graft in the AC is direct evidence of immune privilege [8]. A conventional measurement is the survival of DBA/2-derived mastocytoma P815 tumor cells in the AC of BALB/c mice. DBA/2 and BALB/c mice share the same major histocompatibility complex but differ in minor histocompatibility antigens. P815 tumor cells are rejected and never form a tumor if they are placed in a conventional immunological site, such as the subcutaneous space, in BALB/c mice. However, P815 cells survive and form tumors if they are placed in the AC of BALB/c mouse eyes. Survival of P815 tumor in the BALB/c mouse eye is a direct indicator of ocular immune privilege. Similarly, survival of the BALB/c-derived, chemically induced colon carcinoma cell line CT26.WT [9] in the AC of DBA/2J mice is direct evidence of ocular immune privilege.

Animal Models of Intraocular Inflammation

The immune-privileged status of the eye has been analyzed in the following models of intraocular inflammation.

Experimental autoimmune uveitis (EAU) [10, 11] was induced by immunizing subcutaneously B10.A mice with the ocular autoantigen interphotoreceptor binding protein in complete Freund's adjuvant (CFA). This form of intraocular inflammation is a Th1-mediated disease that persisted for more than 28 days. AH protein levels increased and peaked at 11 days (4–5 mg/ml) and then decreased at 28 days. Leukocytes began to appear in the AH at 11 days and continued to increase so that on day 28, the AH leukocyte count reached 140/μl.

Endotoxin-induced uveitis (EIU) was induced by systemically administering a large amount (200 μg) of lipopolysaccharide (LPS; systemic EIU) [11, 12] in C3H/HeN mice. Systemic EIU lasted for 2 days after LPS administration. The intraocular inflammation reached a peak at 12 h with AH protein levels at 6 mg/ml and leukocyte counts at 70/μl. The presence of ACAID was not tested in these animals because the large amount of LPS received by these mice prevented the development of delayed-type hypersensitivity (DTH).

EIU was also induced by intravitreal injection of a tiny amount (1 ng) of LPS (local EIU) [4]. In order to produce an intense intraocular inflammation in BALB/c mice without influencing the systemic immune system, one ng of LPS was injected into the vitreous cavity of the BALB/c mouse. This intravitreal LPS-induced uveitis lasted 48 h. AH protein levels reached a peak at 6 h (35 mg/ml) and AH leukocyte counts peaked at 9 h (3500/μl) after injection. P815 tumor cells inoculated into the AC demonstrated the existence of ocular immune privilege since uveitis was induced in BALB/c mice.

Mycobacterium tuberculosis (MT) *adjuvant-induced uveitis* (MTU) [13]: intravitreal injection of 15 μg of MT adjuvant induced severe inflammation in BALB/c mouse eyes. The uveitis lasted for 8 days after injection. AH protein levels peaked after 9–24 h (18–23 mg/ml) and AH leukocyte counts peaked at 12 h (6,830/μl).

Pigment dispersion syndrome (PDS) [14]: DBA/2J mice spontaneously developed PDS and intraocular inflammation as they aged. The inflammation lasted more than 6 months. The blood-aqueous barrier was compromised when the mice were 4 months old and AH protein levels continued to increase through 10 months. Leukocytes began to appear in the AC after 6 months, reached a peak at 7 months, and then decreased by 10 months [15].

Influence of Inflammation on the Ocular Immunosuppressive Microenvironment

AH humor harvested from eyes with EAU [11] and systemic EIU [16, 17] transiently lost their capacity to suppress T cell proliferation. The AH contained IL-6, which is mitogenic to T cells, and the loss of the AH capacity to suppress T cell activation correlated with the production of IL-6. Furthermore, blocking IL-6 activity in the AH with neutralizing antibodies enabled the AH to re-acquire its capacity to suppress T cell activation. TGF-β was activated in the AH from eyes with EAU and systemic EIU, and was responsible for the return of the capacity of the AH to suppress T cell activation after IL-6 activity was neutralized. The capacity of the AH to suppress T cell activation in EAU eyes on days 17 and 28, when IL-6 was no longer detectable, was also dependent on active TGF-β. Although normal AH inhibits T cell activation, it is the small neuropeptides, such as vasoactive intestinal polypeptide, which are responsible for T cell suppression since most of the TGF-β in the AH is in its latent form. Therefore, a secondary immunosuppressive microenvironment was reestablished in these inflamed eyes by transforming latent TGF-β to its active form.

The reappearance of T cell suppression activity in the AH preceded resolution of EAU, a self-limited, autoimmune intraocular inflammatory disease.

AH collected from eyes with local EIU and MTU never lost its capacity to suppress T cell activation even though the AH also contained IL-6 [4, 13]. The injection of LPS or MT adjuvant directly into the eye induced a large increase in AH protein levels, which was able to neutralize the mitogenic activity of IL-6.

Of particular interest is the failure of AH from DBA/2J mice with PDS to suppress T cell activation [15]. In DBA/2J mouse AH, the capacity to suppress T cell activation was lost already at 2 months of age when there were no clinical signs of intraocular inflammation or pigment dispersion. The T cell-suppressive capacity of the AH never appeared in DBA/2J mice, even though intraocular inflammation and pigment dispersion from the iris and ciliary body continued to progress, leading to the destruction of ocular tissues, the blockage of AH outflow drainage pathway, an increase in intraocular pressure, and the development of glaucomatous optic neuropathy. It seems that eyes that experience a self-limited, autoimmune disease, such as EIU, and eyes that have progressive destruction from inflammation, such as PDS, differ in their capacity to reestablish an intraocular immunosuppressive microenvironment.

Influence of Inflammation on the Induction of ACAID

Soluble ovalbumin (OVA) was injected into the inflamed AC of the mouse eye to study the capacity of an inflamed eye to support ACAID induction. One week later, the mouse was immunized subcutaneously with OVA plus CFA, then after another week, OVA was injected into the ear dermis and DTH (ear thickness) was measured at 24 h. Injection of OVA into the AC of the EAU eye [11] on day 17 after immunization with interphotoreceptor binding protein failed to suppress DTH, indicating loss of the capacity to induce ACAID by the EAU eye. In contrast, injection of OVA into the local EIU [4] eye induced ACAID even though the eye was experiencing a much more intense intraocular inflammation, as documented by the amount of total protein and number of leukocytes in the AH. These results suggest that ACAID can be induced in an eye with a severely compromised blood-aqueous barrier and intense intraocular inflammation. Furthermore, the type of intraocular inflammation and not the intensity of inflammation is the determining factor.

EAU is mediated by Th1 effector cells which produce IFN-γ. It has been reported that the local intraocular production of IFN-γ by transgenic mice also failed to support ACAID induction [18]. It is possible that only the eye with a Th1 immune response cannot induce ACAID. To test this hypothesis, we used the model of MTU. MT organisms in CFA induce T cells to differentiate down the Th1 pathway. Injection of CFA into the vitreous cavity of BALB/c mouse eyes induced the production of IL-12 [13]. Injection of OVA into the AC of these eyes, 3 h after intravitreal adjuvant, failed to induce ACAID and correlated with the production of intraocular IL-12. Furthermore, MTU eyes recovered their capacity to induce ACAID when OVA was injected on day 8 when there was no IL-12 in the AH. Whether intraocular IL-12 is responsible for the failure of MTU eyes to support ACAID induction will require further study using neutralizing antibodies.

Pigment continues to be released from the iris and ciliary epithelium as DBA/2J mice age. These melanin particles float in the AH, and adhere to the surface of the lens, iris, and cornea [14]. Melanin particles are known to have adjuvant activities that enhance Th1-mediated DTH. IL-18, also known as IFN-γ-inducing factor, is a major stimulant of Th1 differentiation. A significant increase in IL-18 gene expression and IL-18 protein production were detected in the iris, ciliary body, and AH of DBA/2J mouse eyes as they aged, suggesting the existence of Th1 immunity in these eyes. Injection of OVA into the AC of 2-month-old DBA/2J mice marginally suppressed DTH. However, the injection of OVA into 4- and 6-month-old DBA/2J mouse eyes failed to induce ACAID. These results strongly support the hypothesis that ACAID cannot be induced in eyes with Th1 type immunity (IL-12, IL-18, and IFN-γ) – i.e. Th1 immunity-destroyed ACAID induction.

Surprisingly, the injection of OVA into 7-month-old DBA/2J mouse eyes induced ACAID (fig. 1) even though Th1 intraocular inflammation was ongoing. It is possible that the aged DBA/2J mice might have developed an alternative mechanism to regain the ability to induce ACAID in the presence of a Th1 immune response. Interestingly, it was reported that the density of nerve terminals in the iris and ciliary body, containing calcitonin gene-related peptide, increased as the mice aged and that these nerve terminals surrounded the F4/80+ antigen-presenting cells within the eye [19]. Subcutaneous injection of calcitonin gene-related peptide was observed to overcome Th1-mediated skin DTH [20], possibly through an IL-10-dependent mechanism [21], or through the secretion of Th2 cytokines, such as IL-4 [22]. Whether 7-month-old DBA/2J mouse eyes used calcitonin gene-related peptide or other neuropeptides as an alternative mechanism to re-establish ACAID requires further study.

Influence of Inflammation on Ocular Immune Privilege

Immune privilege can be assessed directly by observing the survival of minor histocompatibility-incompatible tumor cells in the AC of mouse eyes. Despite the intense intraocular inflammations of local EIU and MTU in

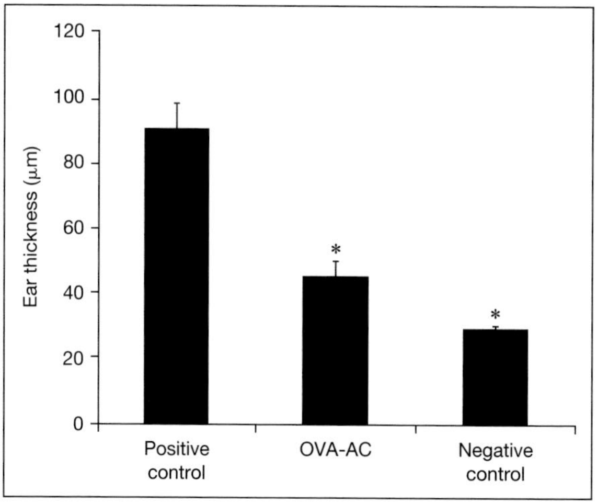

Fig. 1. Induction of OVA-specific ACAID in 7-month-old DBA/2J mice. OVA was injected (50 μg in 2 μl HBSS) into the AC of one eye of 7-month-old DBA/2J mice; 7 days later, these mice were immunized with 100 μg s.c. OVA emulsified 1:1 in CFA (total volume 100 μl). Positive control mice received subcutaneous immunization without any previous exposure to OVA. After another 7 days, 200 μg/10 μl OVA were injected intradermally into one ear pinna, and swelling of the injected ear was assessed 24 h later using an engineer's micrometer (Mitutoyo 227-101). Negative controls received only intrapinna injections of OVA. Ear swelling is expressed as: 24-hour measurement of the ear – 0-hour measurement of the ear. *$p < 0.01$ vs. positive control.

BALB/c mouse eyes, DBA/2-derived mastocytoma P815 tumor cells survived and formed tumors in those inflamed eyes, and the growth of P815 tumor in these inflamed eyes was comparable to that in normal, uninflamed BALB/c eyes. Thus, it appeared that immune privilege was not lost in eyes with local EIU or MTU [4, 13]. The results suggested that multiple mechanisms are developed by the eye to maintain immune privilege, and that an intact, anatomical blood-aqueous barrier is not required for immune privilege.

In 7-month-old DBA/2J mouse eyes, the blood-aqueous barrier was breached, the AH humor failed to suppress T cell activation [15], and ACAID induction was only recently restored (fig. 1). BALB/c-derived CT26.WT tumor cells were injected into the AC of 7-month-old DBA/2J eyes to test immune privilege. The transplanted CT26.WT cells survived although tumor growth was delayed compared to 2-month-old DBA/2J mice, implying a compromised immune privilege in these eyes. However, these tumors continued to grow, and eventually completely filled the AC, indicating that immune privilege was only temporarily compromised. Thus, a disrupted blood-aqueous barrier did not interfere with either the ability to maintain an immunosuppressive microenvironment (i.e. induce ACAID) or immune privilege in the 7-month-old DBA/2J mouse eye.

Neural Control of Ocular Immune Privilege and Inflammation

The eye is extensively innervated by sensory and autonomic nerves, including sympathetic and parasympathetic nerves [23]. These nerve terminals contain neuropeptides that have immune-modulating capability. The corneal surface is innervated by the trigeminal nerve entering from the limbus and extending toward the central cornea [24]. Stimulation of the corneal surface elicits a local ocular stress response in which the blood-aqueous barrier breaks down [25] and plasma proteins, including inactive proenzyme proteins such as plasminogen, leak into the AH, and intraocular pressure increases. Corneal stimulation also induces a systemic stress response through the trigeminal pathway, activating the sympathetic nervous system, leading to an increase in heart rate, arterial pressure, and plasma concentrations of adrenocorticotropin, epinephrine, and norepinephrine [26].

Ocular sympathetic innervation appears to regulate ocular immune privilege. Although most of the TGF-β in normal AH is in a latent form, a small amount of active TGF-β is still detectable indicating an ongoing mechanism that continuously transforms latent TGF-β into its active form. Superior cervical ganglionectomy of mice effectively eliminated sympathetic innervation of the eye, significantly lowered the amount of active TGF-β in the AH [27], and abrogated immune privilege for P815 tumor cells. Apparently, the sympathetic nervous system contributes to the maintenance of intraocular immune homeostasis by activating a small amount of TGF-β and is essential for the support of ocular immune privilege.

Corneal innervation also contributes to the existence of ACAID within the eye. A circumferential, non-penetrating cut of the cornea eliminated nerve axons on the corneal surface and stroma extending from the limbus [28]. These eyes lost their capacity to support ACAID when an antigen was injected into the AC, suggesting that afferent neural stimuli from the cornea were important for this phenomenon. Since introduction of antigen into the AC is accompanied by penetrating trauma to the cornea, we analyzed the effect of a simple corneal injury on ACAID. Scratching of the central cornea, using the tip of a 30-gauge syringe needle, induced an immediate disruption of the blood-aqueous barrier, causing plasma proteins to enter the AC (fig. 2). Accordingly, the amount of active TGF-β in the AH rapidly increased and reached a peak in 30 min. It

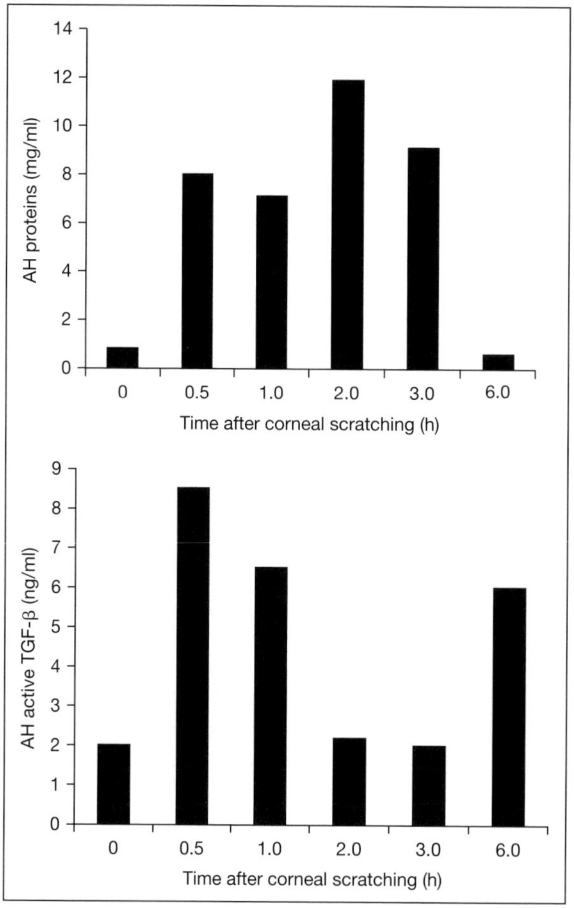

Fig. 2. Total proteins and active TGF-β activity in AH after corneal injury. A scratch was placed on the central cornea with the tip of a 30-gauge syringe needle of 2-month-old BALB/c mice under systemic anesthesia. AH was collected and pooled from eyes at different times after the scratching. Total protein content in the AH was analyzed using the BCA protein assay kit. TGF-β activity in the AH was analyzed by a bioassay using mink lung cells.

seems that the eye responds to corneal trauma by immersing ocular tissues with active TGF-β that establishes a new immunosuppressive microenvironment.

The mechanism by which the latent form of TGF-β in the AH was activated is not known. It has been established that neurons in the iris and ciliary body contain large amounts of tissue plasminogen activator [29]. Since tissue plasminogen activator was released into the AH upon sympathetic stimulation

[30], it is reasonable to postulate that activated plasminogen within the traumatized eye formed plasmin, and that plasmin split products converted the latent TGF-β into its active form [31]. Consistent with this mechanism is our recent observation that after the injection of OVA into the AC, active TGF-β can be found in the AH [32]. In vitro experiments have shown that active TGF-β can transform macrophages into ACAID-inducing antigen-presenting cells [33]. The induction of ACAID after the injection of antigens into the AC may be a secondary ocular stress response to the trauma involving the activation of TGF-β.

In summary, it appears that there are multiple mechanistic layers to the preservation of immune privilege in the eye. The first layer involves an intact anatomical blood-ocular barrier and immunosuppressive neuropeptides in native AH. The second layer relies on the ability of the eye to re-establish an immunosuppressive microenvironment by activating latent TGF-β and reestablishing ACAID. The third layer involves a mechanism that is not yet identified, but that has the ability to overcome a Th1 intraocular immune response and to reestablish ACAID, as shown in 7-month-old DBA/2J mice. Understanding these mechanisms should help us to develop new treatments to prevent damage to the eye from inflammation that is a protective response against pathogens that present a danger to the integrity of the eye.

Acknowledgments

This work was supported by NIH grant R03EY014578 (J.S.M.). Seven-month-old DBA/2J mice were provided by Dr. Simon John of the Jackson Laboratory when J.S.M. was working with Dr. J. Wayne Streilein in Boston.

References

1 Streilein JW: Ocular immune privilege and the Faustian dilemma. The Proctor lecture. Invest Ophthalmol Vis Sci 1996;37:1940–1950.
2 Freddo TF: Shifting the paradigm of the blood-aqueous barrier. Exp Eye Res 2001;73:581–592.
3 Taylor AW, Streilein JW, Cousins SW: Immunoreactive vasoactive intestinal peptide contributes to the immunosuppressive activity of normal aqueous humor. J Immunol 1994;153:1080–1086.
4 Mo JS, Streilein JW: Immune privilege persists in eyes with extreme inflammation induced by intravitreal LPS. Eur J Immunol 2001;31:3806–3815.
5 Taylor JW: Ocular immunosuppressive microenvironment; in Streilein JW (ed): Immune Response and the Eye. Chem Immunol. Basel, Karger, 1999, vol 73, pp 72–89.
6 Kaplan HJ, Streilein JW: Immune response to immunization via the anterior chamber of the eye. I. F1-lymphocyte-induced immune deviation. J Immunol 1977;118:809–814.
7 Streilein JW, Niederkorn JY: Induction of anterior chamber-associated immune deviation requires an intact, functional spleen. J Exp Med 1981;153:1058–1067.
8 Streilein JW, Niederkorn JY: Characterization of the suppressor cell(s) responsible for anterior chamber-associated immune deviation (ACAID) induced in BALB/c mice by P815 cells. J Immunol 1985;134:1381–1387.

9 Wang M, Bronte V, Chen PW, Gritz L, Panicali D, Rosenberg SA, Restifo NP: Active immunotherapy of cancer with a nonreplicating recombinant fowlpox virus encoding a model tumor-associated antigen. J Immunol 1995;154:4685–4692.
10 Silver PB, Chan CC, Wiggert B, Caspi RR: The requirement for pertussis to induce EAU is strain-dependent: B10.RIII, but not B10.A mice, develop EAU and Th1 responses to IRBP without pertussis treatment. Invest Ophthalmol Vis Sci 1999;40:2898–2905.
11 Ohta K, Wiggert B, Taylor AW, Streilein JW: Effects of experimental ocular inflammation on ocular immune privilege. Invest Ophthalmol Vis Sci 1999;40:2010–2018.
12 Kasner L, Chan CC, Whitcup SM, Gery I: The paradoxical effect of tumor necrosis factor alpha (TNF-alpha) in endotoxin-induced uveitis. Invest Ophthalmol Vis Sci 1993;34:2911–2917.
13 Mo JS, Streilein JW: Analysis of immune privilege in eyes with Mycobacteria tuberculosa adjuvant-induced uveitis. Ocul Immunol Inflamm 2005;13:139–147.
14 John SW, Smith RS, Savinova OV, Hawes NL, Chang B, Turnbull D, Davisson M, Roderick TH, Heckenlively JR: Essential iris atrophy, pigment dispersion, and glaucoma in DBA/2J mice. Invest Ophthalmol Vis Sci 1998;39:951–962.
15 Mo JS, Anderson MG, Gregory M, Smith RS, Savinova OV, Serreze DV, Ksander BR, Streilein JW, John SW: By altering ocular immune privilege, bone marrow-derived cells pathogenically contribute to DBA/2J pigmentary glaucoma. J Exp Med 2003;197:1335–1344.
16 Ohta K, Yamagami S, Taylor AW, Streilein JW: IL-6 antagonizes TGF-beta and abolishes immune privilege in eyes with endotoxin-induced uveitis. Invest Ophthalmol Vis Sci 2000;41:2591–2599.
17 Ohta K, Wiggert B, Yamagami S, Taylor AW, Streilein JW: Analysis of immunomodulatory activities of aqueous humor from eyes of mice with experimental autoimmune uveitis. J Immunol 2000;164:1185–1192.
18 Geiger K, Sarvetnick N: Local production of IFN-gamma abrogates the intraocular immune privilege in transgenic mice and prevents the induction of ACAID. J Immunol 1994;153:5239–5246.
19 Adamek-Kotowicz E, Lutjen-Drecoll E: Development of F4/80 positive cells and CGRP nerve terminals in the mouse uvea (abstract). Invest Ophthalmol Vis Sci 2003;44:744.
20 Kitazawa T, Streilein JW: Hapten-specific tolerance promoted by calcitonin gene-related peptide. J Invest Dermatol 2000;115:942–948.
21 Streilein JW, Alard P, Niizeki H: Neural influences on induction of contact hypersensitivity. Ann NY Acad Sci 1999;885:196–208.
22 Levite M: Nerve-driven immunity. The direct effects of neurotransmitters on T-cell function. Ann NY Acad Sci 2000;917:307–321.
23 ten Tusscher MP, Beckers HJ, Vrensen GF, Klooster J: Peripheral neural circuits regulating IOP? A review of its anatomical backbone. Doc Ophthalmol 1994;87:291–313.
24 Rozsa AJ, Beuerman RW: Density and organization of free nerve endings in the corneal epithelium of the rabbit. Pain 1982;14:105–120.
25 Unger WG: Review: mediation of the ocular response to injury. J Ocul Pharmacol 1990;6:337–353.
26 Bereiter DA, Bereiter DF, Hathaway CB: The NMDA receptor antagonist MK-801 reduces Fos-like immunoreactivity in central trigeminal neurons and blocks select endocrine and autonomic responses to corneal stimulation in the rat. Pain 1996;64:179–189.
27 Vega J, Keino H, Streilein JW: Immune privilege in the anterior chamber of the eye is disrupted by removal of the superior cervical ganglion. Fort Lauderdale, American Uveitis Society Meeting, April 24, 2004; www.uveitissociety.org
28 Streilein JW, Bradley D, Sano Y, Sonoda Y: Immunosuppressive properties of tissues obtained from eyes with experimentally manipulated corneas. Invest Ophthalmol Vis Sci 1996;37:413–424.
29 Wang Y, Hand AR, Gillies C, Grunnet ML, Cone RE, O'Rourke J: Morphologic evidence for a preferential storage of tissue plasminogen activator (t-PA) in perivascular axons of the rat uvea. Exp Eye Res 1997;65:105–116.
30 Peng T, Jiang X, Wang Y, Hand A, Gillies C, Cone RE, O'Rourke J: Sympathectomy decreases and adrenergic stimulation increases the release of tissue plasminogen activator (t-PA) from blood vessels: functional evidence for a neurologic regulation of plasmin production within vessel walls and other tissue matrices. J Neurosci Res 1999;57:680–692.
31 Yehualaeshet T, O'Connor R, Green-Johnson J, Mai S, Silverstein R, Murphy-Ullrich JE, Khalil N: Activation of rat alveolar macrophage-derived latent transforming growth factor beta-1 by

plasmin requires interaction with thrombospondin-1 and its cell surface receptor, CD36. Am J Pathol 1999;155:841–851.
32 Mo JS, Streilein JW: Ocular trauma induced a secondary immunosuppressive microenvironment containing active TGF-beta (abstract). Invest Ophthalmol Vis Sci 2005;46:5044.
33 D'Orazio TJ, Niederkorn JY: A novel role for TGF-beta and IL-10 in the induction of immune privilege. J Immunol 1998;160:2089–2098.

Dr. Jun-Song Mo
Department of Ophthalmology and Visual Sciences
University of Louisville School of Medicine
301 East Muhammad Ali Boulevard, Room 3318
Louisville, KY 40202 (USA)
Tel. +1 502 852 0733, Fax +1 502 852 7311, E-Mail jun.mo@louisville.edu

Niederkorn JY, Kaplan HJ (eds): Immune Response and the Eye.
Chem Immunol Allergy. Basel, Karger, 2007, vol 92, pp 166–175

Allergy and Contact Lenses

Mohammad Siddique, Bita Manzouri, Tom H. Flynn, Santa J. Ono

Department of Ocular Immunology, Institute of Ophthalmology and Moorfields Eye Hospital, University College London, London, UK

Abstract

Allergic conjunctivitis is a response to environmental allergens, as well as a genetic predisposition of the patient. It is classified as either acute (seasonal allergic conjunctivitis) or chronic (perennial allergic conjunctivitis, vernal keratoconjunctivitis, atopic keratoconjunctivitis and giant papillary conjunctivitis). The immune mechanism of these diseases will be discussed, as well as the allergic response to contact lens wear.

Typical eye allergy develops when pollen and dust come into contact with the eye and activate mast cells in the conjunctiva leading to mast cell degranulation and, thus, the release of histamine, prostanoids, kinins, proteases and other pro-inflammatory mediators. Acute allergic conjunctivitis is a type I IgE-mediated response while chronic conjunctivitis is a mixed cell response, mainly consisting of eosinophils and basophils [1, 2]. The main symptoms of allergic conjunctivitis are burning, itching, and a watery and ropy discharge; the main signs are redness, chemosis of the conjunctiva, and edema of the lids. Due to the chronic nature of atopic and vernal keratoconjunctivitis, there is frequently vision loss due to corneal involvement [3].

Mechanism of Ocular Allergy

In all forms of allergic eye disease, the clinical response is due to mast cell activation either directly via antigen-mast cell linkage, or by T cell activation of mast cells, resulting in mast cell release of inflammatory factors and cytokines. In the milder forms of allergic eye disease, such as seasonal allergic conjunctivitis (SAC) and perennial allergic conjunctivitis (PAC), mast cell numbers alone are increased, while in vernal keratoconjunctivitis (VKC) and atopic keratoconjunctivitis (AKC), mast cell and T cell numbers are increased [4, 5]. In the normal subject, there are few conjunctival T cells, and those that are present are naïve; in chronic allergic conditions, i.e. AKC, VKC and giant papillary conjunctivitis (GPC), there is an increase in CD4 memory T cells. In VKC and GPC, 50% of T cells co-express CD45RO and CD45RA suggesting that T cells may be produced locally. In contrast, these cell surface markers are rare in AKC, a disease associated with systemic atopy, suggesting that these T cells are recruited from circulating memory T cells [6, 7].

Conjunctival mast cells exist in two forms, characterized by their staining pattern to the proteases tryptase and chymase. The MC_{TC} form (found in the skin) contains both tryptase and chymase, and the MC_T form (found in mucus membranes and increased in aero-allergen-driven disease) contains tryptase only [8]. The latter is increased in allergic eye disease.

The Role of Mast Cells

Mast cell activation results from a multivalent allergen cross-linking cell surface IgE with high affinity FcεRI mast cell receptors [9]. Conjunctival mast cell activation leads to the release of histamine and locally synthesized mediators, e.g. prostaglandin D_2, leukotriene C_4, tryptase, chymase, carboxypeptidase A, cathepsin G, and platelet-activating factor, a powerful eosinophil chemotactic agent and other eosinophil and neutrophil chemoattractants. Allergen challenge in atopic patients leads to an early phase response, which is maximal at 20 min, with increased tear levels of histamine, the mast cell protease tryptase, leukotrienes and eosinophils [10].

At 6 h there is a dose-dependent late phase response, with a second peak in tear concentrations of histamine and eosinophil cationic protein levels. Tryptase is not increased, suggesting that either mast cells are still degranulated, or that other cells such as basophils, whose conjunctival numbers are increased at this stage, are involved. The tissue adhesion molecules E-selectin and ICAM-1, but not VCAM-1, are increased at 6 h consistent with the increased conjunctival levels of granulocytes and eosinophils [11]. IgE is produced in the conjunctiva, under mast cell control, and most patients with allergic eye disease have a positive family history of atopy with raised serum and tear levels of allergen-specific IgE. Mast cells induce B cell IgE production independently of T cells, suggesting that mast cells may be involved in the autoregulation of IgE production through the CD40/CD40 ligand [12].

The clinical effectiveness of the histamine H_1 receptor antagonist emedastine supports the involvement of mast cells in allergic eye responses; emedastine potently inhibited histamine-induced secretion of interleukin (IL)-6, IL-8 and granulocyte-macrophage colony-stimulating factor, as well as the topical mast cell stabilizers, e.g. sodium cromoglycate, lodoxamide [13, 14] and nedocromil [15], which reduce tear concentrations of tryptase. Topically applied antihistamines (e.g. levocabastine [16]) and systemic histamine H_1 receptor antagonists (e.g. astemizole, terfenadine and loratadine) are also effective in the treatment of SAC and PAC [17].

Mast cell release of histamine and leukotrienes contributes to the inflammatory response by the recruitment of eosinophils and neutrophils. Eosinophil numbers are also increased in the chronic forms of allergic eye disease [18]. In AKC and VKC, they are not only increased in the deep layers of the conjunctiva (lamina propria) but also migrate into the epithelium [19]. In VKC, there are increased tear levels of eosinophil cationic protein, eosinophil granule major basic protein and Charcot-Leyden crystal protein. Eosinophil granule-derived proteins have been localized to the base of vernal ulcers [20]. Neutrophil numbers are also increased in the conjunctiva of atopic subjects after allergen challenge [17]. Histamine, through H_1 receptors in the conjunctiva, appears to couple to inositol phosphate, increasing intracellular calcium, and results in the development of pruritus. Histamine stimulation of H_2 receptors on the ocular surface causes vasodilation [11].

Cytokine Responses

How does the mast cell influence the conjunctival allergic response apart from the release of inflammatory factors? The mast cell has been shown to store, release and synthesize the cytokines IL-4, IL-5, IL-6, IL-8, IL-13 and tumor necrosis factor (TNF)-α [21]. Recent work has shown that the two types of conjunctival mast cells are heterogeneous with respect to cytokine storage [22]. In SAC, IL-4 and IL-13 are predominately localized to MC_{TC} cells while IL-5 and IL-6 are localized to MC_T cells. IL-4 promotes T cell growth, induces the switching of B cells from IgM to IgE production and directs Th2 differentiation. In the mast cell, there are two types of IL-4. One form is contained in granules throughout the cytoplasm (i.e. the stored form) and found in inactive SAC, and the other is found in increased amounts only in the cell membrane in active SAC [23].

In situ hybridization techniques using riboprobes to IL-4 mRNA have demonstrated the production of IL-4 within the mast cell [24]. The adhesion molecule VCAM-1 is under the regulatory influence of IL-4 and is strongly expressed in VKC but not in SAC [25]. It has been shown that there is a correlation between the level of adhesion molecule expression, the activity of the allergic eye disease and the different types of inflammatory cell infiltrates encountered [26]. There is a positive correlation between ICAM-1 and E-selectin levels with granulocyte and lymphocyte infiltration, and VCAM-1 expression with eosinophil infiltration [27]. Thus, VCAM-1 levels are higher in VKC than in SAC, and the conjunctival levels of CD4+ T cells and eosinophils are increased in VKC but not SAC.

Stem Cell Factor and TNF-α

Stem cell factor (SCF) is an essential growth factor for mast cells, and enhances IgE-dependent mast cell mediator release, as well as cytokine generation and release, and is a chemoattractant for mast cells [28]. It has recently been shown that the mast cell not only stores but also manufactures SCF, and there is a fourfold increase in SCF in SAC giving the mast cell the potential for its own autoregulation [11].

TNF-α is an early mediator of the conjunctival allergic response. The mast cell may be a source of TNF-α with its release following the activation of IgE [29]. It is also produced by lymphocytes, neutrophils and eosinophils and upregulates endothelial cell adhesion molecules leading to the recruitment of inflammatory cells. Conjunctival tissue levels of TNF-α have not been found to be significantly increased in SAC.

Seasonal and Perennial Allergic Conjunctivitis

The symptoms and signs of SAC and PAC include burning, itching, watery discharge, conjunctival redness, chemosis and fine follicles. The follicles result from the release of mediators such as histamine, leukotrienes and prostaglandins. This early phase reaction is followed by a late phase reaction in which eosinophils and T lymphocytes are the predominant cells.

Mast cells have been discovered as a source of Th2-type helper cytokines, IL-4, IL-5, IL-6 and IL-13 [12]. MC_{TC} secrete IL-4 and IL-13 while MC_{T} release IL-5 and IL-6 [30]. The latter is the predominant type in ocular allergy. The release of such cytokine mediators from mast cells helps in eosinophil recruitment, activation and inflammatory cell mediator release [30]. High levels of TNF-α upregulate intracellular adhesion molecules on conjunctival epithelial cells, which in turn mediate the epithelial leukocyte interaction with an increase in IL-5. There is also a decrease in IL-10, which has anti-inflammatory properties [27].

Using the presence of the neutral protease tryptase as an immunohistochemical marker, mast cell numbers have been found to be raised in SAC and PAC. IgE is the activator of mast cells and is bound to high affinity receptors FcεRI on the cell surface. There are raised levels of allergen-specific IgE in patients with a history of atopy [29, 31]. The symptomatology of SAC and PAC relates to the number of mast cells present in the conjunctiva. SCF regulates mast cell growth and maturation. It is a chemoattractant for mast cells and enhances IgE-dependent mast cell mediator release and cytokine generation. Pro-inflammatory cytokines IL-4 and IL-5 are stored in the eosinophils and are essential for the growth and differentiation of eosinophils [29].

As mast cells and eosinophils are the main cells observed in the conjunctival allergic response, the role of IL-4 in the allergic response is very important. It is involved in the switching of B cells from IgM to IgE, T cell growth and Th2 differentiation. The IL-4 gene cluster is on chromosome 5 which includes IL-3, IL-4, IL-5 and IL-13 [32].

The medical treatment of SAC and PAC includes topical vasoconstrictors and the H_1 receptor blocker, olopatadine. The combined treatment with both of these agents provides greater relief. The mast cell stabilizer sodium cromoglycate is used for prevention rather than treatment, inhibiting the initial release of inflammatory mediators. The use of steroids remains limited to serious symptoms and its long-term use could result in cataract and glaucoma.

Vernal and Atopic Keratoconjunctivitis

VKC and AKC are the most severe atopic disorders because of their chronicity and their potential to involve the cornea and subsequently impair vision. The role of genetic and environmental factors remains unclear. Vernal disease is commonly seen in pediatric patients and it is characterized by intense pruritus and copious mucus secretion, giant papillae in the upper tarsus and the presence of gelatinous nodules around the limbus, with or without Trantas dots [1].

Although the pathogenesis of this disorder remains unknown, there is a contribution of both type I and type IV hypersensitivity reactions [33]. There is a genetic predisposition to this disease leading to an imbalance between Th2 and Th1 cells, which favors IgE synthesis [34].

AKC is found in atopic dermatitis patients and is the most severe of the allergic conjunctival diseases [34, 35]. Occasionally, these patients may have episcleritis, scleritis and even uveitis – whether these disorders are related to atopy or are just chance associations remains unknown. Individuals suffering from generalized allergic disorders are at a greater risk of contact lens-induced allergy.

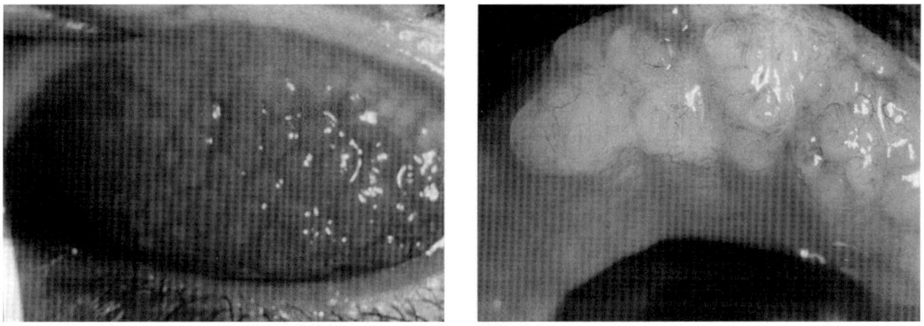
a b

Fig. 1. ***a*** Upper tarsal conjunctiva in a contact lens-wearing patient showing giant papillary reaction. ***b*** Upper fornix (double eversion of upper lid) showing giant papillary conjunctival reaction.

Local Contact Lens-Induced Allergic Conjunctivitis

Contact lens-induced papillary conjunctivitis (GPC) appears to be an allergic response to the contact lens, to the preservatives in the contact lens solution or to deposits on the contact lens [36].

Giant Papillary Conjunctivitis

GPC is a chronic inflammatory process leading to the production of giant papillae (>0.3 mm) on the tarsal conjunctiva lining the upper eye lids (fig. 1). The condition occurs in patients who wear soft contact lenses, an ocular prosthesis or have unburied sutures after surgery [37]. The etiology is uncertain and probably multifactorial, but the clinical picture resembles that of VKC [38]. It seems to be a delayed-type hypersensitivity reaction. The symptoms are pseudoptosis, redness, irritation, mucoid discharge, blurring of vision, tearing and photophobia. The eye is dry and the upper eye lid will show the characteristic giant papillae on the tarsal, and sometimes in the forniceal, conjunctiva (fig. 1). Mucous, cell debris and microorganisms are frequently found on the lenses and play a pathogenic role in GPC [39]. The immune privilege of the eye may reduce the incidence of intraocular inflammation. However, the lens produces a continuous antigenic stimulus evoking a localized allergic reaction in the upper tarsal conjunctiva [40]. Hard contact lenses wearers are rarely affected and GPC appears to occur after longer periods, up to 8 years [38]. Allergic and dry eye symptoms improve by switching to a disposable form of soft contact lenses [41]. The condition is more common in patients with a history of asthma, rhinitis or hay fever-type allergic reaction (SAC).

Pathogenesis of Giant Papillary Conjunctivitis

GPC is due to a combination of mechanical irritation and hypersensitivity [42]. A history of generalized allergy and/or allergy to disinfectant solutions is relatively frequent [43]. The allergy correlates with high levels of IgE and IgG in tears, IgM deposits on lenses and conjunctival infiltration by eosinophils. An increase in eotaxin levels in tears also correlates with GPC [44]. A high level of mucosal mast cells and a significant increase in tear concentrations of leukotriene C_4 levels have been found in patients with contact lens-associated GPC [45]. Thus, leukotriene-inhibitory therapy may be beneficial to patients. The presence of neutrophil chemotactic factors in the tears of patients with GPC is also important, as the release of these factors from the injured conjunctiva may play an important role [46]. The reduction in lactoferrin levels in tears would favor microbial deposition on the contact lens [47].

The lens coatings from GPC patients induced a tear IgE response and cellular infiltration at the epithelial-stromal junction in tarsal conjunctival biopsy specimens [48]. Such allergic responses in the eye are late phase reactions, and increased levels of IL-1 have been found [49]. Contact lens wear can cause a change in corneal physiology which can lead to epithelial, stromal and endothelial compromise [50].

The inflammatory response in allergic disease is caused by the recruitment of leukocytes by chemokines and the upregulation of adhesion factors. IL-1 increases chemokine production, adhesion factors, macrophage infiltration and activity, and lymphocyte proliferation [50]. The presence of eosinophils at the site of allergic reactions is due to increased levels of RANTES, eotaxin and macrophage inflammatory protein-1α. These chemokines are also chemotactic for activated T cells, eosinophils, basophils and monocytes/macrophages [51, 52]. Eotaxin has a potent and selective chemotactic effect for eosinophils. All of these soluble factors are known to interact through a CC chemokine receptor (CCR3), which is mainly expressed on eosinophils, basophils and Th2 cells [53].

Other Forms of Contact Lens-Related Allergy

Contact lens-related allergic conjunctivitis can also occur from preservatives in the lens care solutions or eye drops. This allergic reaction is secondary to the antigen deposit on the surface of the contact lens [54, 55]. Rarely, subepithelial, nummular peripheral opacities may be seen in allergic conjunctivitis [49]. The signs and symptoms are the same as in other forms of allergic conjunctivitis.

Contact lens preservative solutions such as chlorhexidine, thimerosal, benzalkonium chloride and ethylenediamine tetraacetate can bind on the plastic material of the soft contact lens causing delayed-type hypersensitivity reactions

[56–58]. Preservative deposits build up on the lens surface with time and contain minerals, organic material, e.g. mucin, lipid and protein, and microorganisms. These deposits also become barriers to the permeation of oxygen and carbon dioxide [59].

In the case of contact lens wear, the immune privilege of the eye may be compromised as a result of changes in the conjunctiva and cornea. Minimization of the risk of corneal infection and a hypersensitivity reaction can be achieved by the safe use of contact lenses and related products. As the use of contact lenses for refractive, cosmetic and therapeutic purposes is increasing, the prevalence of these allergic disorders of the conjunctiva should be found to increase.

References

1 Ono SJ: Vernal keratoconjunctivitis: evidence in immunoglobulin E-dependent and immunoglobulin E-independent eosinophilia. Clin Exp Allergy 2003;33:279–281.

2 Stahl JL, Barney NP: Ocular allergic disease. Curr Opin Allergy Clin Immunol 2004;4:455–459.

3 Bonini S, Bonini S: Pathogenesis of allergic conjunctivitis; in Denburg JA (ed): Allergy and Allergic Diseases: The New Mechanism and Therapeutics. Totowa, Humana Press, 1998.

4 Bisgaard H, Ford-Hutchison AW, Charleson S, Taudorf E: Production of leukotrienes in human skin and conjunctiva after specific allergen challenge. Allergy 1985;40:417–423.

5 Metcalfe DD, Baram D, Mekori YA: Mast cells. Physiol Rev 1997;77:1033–1079.

6 Leu G, Keane-Myers A, Miyazaki D, Tai A, Ono SJ: Molecular and Cellular Aspects of Allergic Conjunctivits; in Streilein JW (ed): Immune Response and the Eye. Chem Immunol. Basel, Karger, 1999, vol 73, pp 39–58.

7 Ono SJ, Abelson MB: Allergic conjunctivitis: update on pathophysiology and prospects for future treatment. J Allergy Clin Immunol 2005;115:118–122.

8 Irani AMA, Butrus SI, Tabbara KF, Schwartz LB: Human conjunctival mast cell distribution of MCT and MCTC in vernal conjunctivitis and giant papillary conjunctivitis. J Allergy Clin Immunol 1990;86:34–40.

9 Collum LMT, Kilmartin DJ: Acute allergic conjunctivitis; in Abelson MB (ed): Allergic Diseases of the Eye. Philadelphia, Saunders, 2000, pp 108–132.

10 Proud D, Sweet J, Stein P, Settipane RA, Kagey-Sobotka A, Friedland MH, Lichtenstein LM: Inflammatory mediator release on conjunctival provocation of allergic subjects with allergen. J Allergy Clin Immunol 1990;85:896–905.

11 Bielory L, Ghafoor S: Histamine receptors and the conjunctiva. Curr Opin Allergy Clin Immunol 2005;5:437–440.

12 Anderson DF, Zhang S, Bradding P, McGill JI, Holgate ST, Roche WR: The relative contribution of mast cell subsets to conjunctival TH2-like cytokines. Invest Ophthalmol Vis Sci 2001;42:995–1001.

13 Leonardi A, Borghesan F, Faggian D, Depaoli M, Secchi AG, Plebani M: Tear and serum soluble leukocyte activation markers in conjunctival allergic diseases. Am J Ophthalmol 2000;129:151–158.

14 Fahy GT, Easty DL, Collum LMT, et al: Double masked trial of lodoxamide and sodium cromoglycate in allergic eye disease. A multicentered study. Eur J Ophthamol 1992;2:144–149.

15 Leino M, Ennevaara K, Latvala AL, Nordgren P, Posti AM, Suves R, Takalo E: Double-blind group comparative study of 2% nedocromil sodium eye drops with 2% sodium cromoglycate and placebo eye drops in the treatment of seasonal allergic conjunctivitis. Clin Exp Allergy 1992;22:929–932.

16 Abelson MB, Smith LM: Levocabastine. Evaluation in the histamine and compound 48/80 models of ocular allergy in humans. Ophthalmology 1988;95:1494–1497.

17 McGill JI, Holgate ST, Church MK, Anderson DF, Bacon A: Allergic eye disease mechanisms. Br J Ophthalmol 1998;82:1203–1214.
18 Ono SJ, Nakamura T, Miyazaki D, Ohbayashi M, Dawson M, Toda M: Chemokines: role in leukocyte development, trafficking and effector function. J Allergy Clin Immunol 2003;111:1185–1199.
19 Abelson MB, Madiwale N, Weston JH: Conjunctival eosinophils in allergic ocular disease. Arch Ophthalmol 1983;101:555–556.
20 Trocme SD, Kephart G, Bourne WM, Buckley RJ, Gleich GJ: Eosinophil major basic protein deposition in human corneal shield ulcers. Invest Ophthalmol Vis Sci 1992;33(suppl):984.
21 Foster CS, Calonge MD: Atopic keratoconjunctivitis. Ophthalmology 1990;97:992–1000.
22 Anderson DF, Zhang S, MacLeod JDA, McGill JI, Roche WR, Holgate ST: Conjunctival mast cells are heterogenous with respect to cytokine storage. Invest Ophthalmol Vis Sci 1997;36:57–62.
23 Bacon AS, McGill JI, Anderson DF, Baddeley S, Lightman SL, Holgate ST: Adhesion molecules and relationship to leukocyte levels in allergic eye disease. Invest Ophthalmol Vis Sci 1998;39: 322–330.
24 Yanni JM, Weimer LK, Sharif NA, Xu SX, Gamache DA, Spellman JM: Inhibition of histamine-induced human conjunctival epithelial cell responses by ocular allergy drugs. Ann Allergy Asthma Immunol 1997;79:541–545.
25 Bacon AS, Tuft SJ, Metz DP, McGill JI, Buckley RJ, Baddeley S, Lightman SL: The origin of keratopathy in chronic allergic eye disease: a histopathological study. Eye 1993;7(suppl):21–25.
26 Morgan SJ, Williams JH, Walls AF, Church MK, Holgate ST, McGill JI: Mast cell numbers and staining characteristics in the normal and allergic human conjunctiva. J Allergy Clin Immunol 1991;87:111–116.
27 Uchio E, Ono S, Ikezawa Z, Ohno S: Serum levels of soluble intercellular adhesion molecules-1, vascular cell adhesion molecule-1, and interleukin-2 receptor in patients with vernal keratoconjunctivitis and allergic conjunctivitis. Allergy 1999;54:135–141.
28 Zhang S, Anderson DF, McGill JI, Holgate ST, Roche WR: Human mast cells express stem cell factor. J Pathol 1998;186:59–66.
29 Cook EB: Tear cytokines in acute and chronic ocular allergic inflammation. Curr Opin Allergy Clin Immunol 2004;4:441–445.
30 Graziano FM: Conjunctival mast cells in ocular allergic disease. Allergy Asthma Proc 2001;22: 121–126.
31 Allansmith MR, O'Connor GR: Immunoglobulin: structure, function and relation to the eye. Surv Ophthalmol 1970;14:367–402.
32 Ryan JJ: Interleukin-4 and its receptor: essential mediator of the allergic response. J Allergy Clin Immunol 1997;99:1–5.
33 Horan RF, Schneider LC, Sheffer AL: Allergic skin disorders and mastocytosis. JAMA 1992;268: 2858–2868.
34 Beltrani VS: The clinical spectrum of atopic dermatitis. J Allergy Clin Immunol 1999;104: S87–S98.
35 Tuft SJ, Kemeny DM, Dart JKG, Buckley RJ: Clinical features of atopic keratoconjunctivitis. Ophthalmology 1991;98:150–158.
36 Lemp MA: Contact lenses and associated anterior segment disorders: dry eye, blepharitis, and allergy. Ophthalmol Clin North Am 2003;16:463–469.
37 Robin JB, Regis-Pacheco LF, May WN, Schanzlin DJ, Smith RE: Giant papillary conjunctivitis associated with an extruded buckle. Arch Ophthalmol 1987;105:619–624.
38 Allansmith MR, Korb DR, Grenier JV, Henriquez AS, Simon MA, Finnemore VM: Giant papillary conjunctivitis in contact lens wearers. Am J Ophthalmol 1977;83:697–708.
39 Fowler SA, Korb DR, Finnemore VM, Allansmith MR: Surface deposits on worn hard contact lenses. Arch Ophthalmol 1984;112:757–759.
40 Hart DE: Contact lens/tear film interactions: deposits and coatings; in Dabezies OH (ed): Contact Lenses: The CLAO Guide to Basic Science and Clinical Practice, update 7. Boston, Little Brown, 1990, vol 45, pp A-1–A-127.
41 Boswall GJ, Ehlers WH, Liustro A, Worall M, Donshik PC: A comparison of conventional and disposable extended wear contact lenses. CLAO J 1993;19:158–165.

42 Heidemann DG, Dunn SP, Siegal MJ: Unusual causes of giant papillary conjunctivitis. Cornea 1993;12:78–80.
43 Begley CG, Riggle A, Tuel JA: Association of giant papillary conjunctivitis with seasonal allergies. Optom Vis Sci 1990;67:192–195.
44 Moschos MM, Eperon S, Guex-Crosier Y: Increased eotaxin in tears of patients wearing contact lenses. Cornea 2004;23:771–775.
45 Irkec MT, Orhan M, Erdener U: Role of tear inflammatory mediators in contact lens-associated giant papillary conjunctivitis in soft contact lens wearer. Ocul Immunol Inflamm 1999;7:35–38.
46 Elgebaly SA, Donshik PC, Rahhal F, Williams W: Neutrophil chemotactic factors in the tears of giant papillary conjunctivitis patients. Invest Ophthalmol Vis Sci 1991;32:208–213.
47 Sac RA, Jones B, Antignani A, Libow R, Harvey H: Specificity and biological activity of the protein deposits on the hydrogel surface: relationship of polymer structure to biofilm formation. Invest Ophthalmol Vis Sci 1987;28:842–849.
48 Ballow M, Donshik PC, Rapacz P, Maenza R, Yamase H, Muncy L: Immune responses in monkeys to lenses from patients with contact lens induced giant papillary conjunctivitis. CLAO J 1989;15: 64–70.
49 Dinarello C: Biologic basis for inteleukin-1 in disease. Blood 1996;87:2095–2147.
50 Robboy MW, Comstock TL, Kalsow CM: Contact lens-associated corneal infiltrates. Eye Contact Lens 2003;29:146–154.
51 Baggiolini M, Dewald B, Moser B: Human chemokines: an update. Annu Rev Immunol 1997;15: 675–705.
52 Moschos MM, Eperon S, Guex-Crosier Y: Increased eotaxin in tears of patients wearing contact lenses. Cornea 2004;23:771–775.
53 Ono SJ, Nakamura T, Miyazaki D, Ohbayashi M, Dawson M, Toda M: Chemokines: role in leukocyte development, trafficking and effector function. J Allergy Clin Immunol 2003;111:1185–1199.
54 Refojo MF, Holly FJ: Tear protein absorption on hydrogels: a possible cause of contact lens allergy. Contact Intraoc Lens Med J 1977;23:3–11.
55 Nancy A, McNamara. Innate defense of the ocular surface. Eye Contact Lens 2003;29:S10–S13.
56 Holden BA, Markides AJ: On the desirability and efficiency of chemical sterilization of hydrophilic lenses. Aust J Optom 1971;54:325–336.
57 Baudouin C: Allergic reaction to topical eye drops. Curr Opin Allergy Clin Immunol 2005;5:459–463.
58 Tripathi RC, Tripathi BJ, Ruben M: The pathology of soft contact lens spoilage. Ophthalmology 1980;87:369–378.
59 Rubin M, Khoo CY: Contact Lenses, medical aspects. Pittsburgh, PG Publishing, 1989, pp 15–18.

Dr. Mohammad Siddique
Department of Ocular Immunology
Institute of Ophthalmology and Moorfields Eye Hospital
University College London, Bath Street
London EC1V 9EL (UK)
Tel. +44 20 7608 6882, Fax +44 20 7608 4044, E-Mail drmsiddique@hotmail.com

Niederkorn JY, Kaplan HJ (eds): Immune Response and the Eye.
Chem Immunol Allergy. Basel, Karger, 2007, vol 92, pp 176–184

Dry Eye Syndromes

Stefano Barabino[a,b], *M. Reza Dana*[a]

[a]Laboratory of Immunology, Schepens Eye Research Institute, and Cornea Service, Massachusetts Eye and Ear Infirmary, Department of Ophthalmology, Harvard Medical School, Boston, Mass., USA; [b]Department of Neurosciences, Ophthalmology, and Genetics, University of Genoa, Genoa, Italy

Abstract

Over the past 20 years it has become clear that dry eye syndrome (DES) or keratoconjunctivitis sicca (KCS) is a complex multifactorial disease characterized by an immune and inflammatory process that affects the lacrimal glands and ocular surface. In this paradigm, inflammation is seen as both the cause and consequence of conjunctival and corneal cell damage. In this chapter, we identify the unique characteristics of the lacrimal gland, the role of epithelial cells, regulatory T cells, and cytokines in maintaining ocular surface homeostasis and tear secretion function. We analyze the factors inducing loss of the lacrimal gland homeostasis and its consequences, and in so doing hope to provide a picture of the role of the immune system in the pathophysiology of KCS and useful information to help understand the complexity of DES.

Dry eye syndrome (DES), or keratoconjunctivitis sicca (KCS), affects tens of millions of people worldwide, including the US, representing one of the most common ocular pathologies [1]. The term 'dry eye syndrome' includes different forms of dry eye. The National Eye Institute/Industry Workshop on Clinical Trials in Dry Eyes produced a classification which essentially separates DES into two major types: (a) *tear-deficient* (including Sjögren's syndrome and non-Sjögren's tear-deficient) and (b) *evaporative forms* [2].

Even while it is not presently known what triggers the pathogenic mechanisms that lead to dry eye, a growing body of evidence suggests that chronic KCS is characterized by an inflammatory process affecting the functional unit of the lacrimal gland-ocular surface [3]. Sjögren's syndrome, representing the classic form of exocrine (lacrimal) deficiency associated with KCS, is characterized by a chronic inflammatory infiltration of the lacrimal and salivary glands. All the forms of dry eye are characterized by variable degrees of ocular surface inflammation [4]. In fact, inflammation is the key mechanism of corneal and conjunctival cell damage, which is responsible for many of the symptoms reported by patients and for the signs of ocular surface pathology.

Here we review the immunological aspects of the lacrimal gland and the ocular surface, and how the loss of local immunohomeostasis can lead to KCS.

Lacrimal Gland Inflammation

The lacrimal and salivary glands of many patients with primary or secondary (e.g. to rheumatoid arthritis) Sjögren's syndrome, and similarly graft-versus-host disease, have signs of autoimmune disease evidenced by focal periductal and perivascular lymphocytic infiltrates, which consist primarily of CD4+ T cells and B cells. The infiltrates usually begin around a high endothelial venule, a vascular structure expressing adhesive molecules that facilitate homing of lymphocytes. Lacrimal gland biopsies from Sjögren's syndrome patients show a marked expression of intercellular adhesion molecule-1 (ICAM-1), which interacts with its receptor lymphocyte function-associated antigen (LFA-1), and plays an important role in lymphocyte transmigration into inflammatory sites [5]. The activated immune cells in the inflammatory infiltrate release pro-inflammatory cytokines, such as interleukins IL-1β and IL-2, interferon-γ and tumor necrosis factor-α, which lead to the destruction of the secretory architecture of the glands and dysfunction of the surviving tissue, thereby contributing to a significant decrease in fluid production, and induce the symptoms and signs of KCS. Another sign of autoimmune disease is the presence of antibodies to a number of different autoantigens in the sera of Sjögren syndrome patients, including Ro/SSA, La/SSB, 120-kDa α-fodrin, and the M_3 muscarinic acetylcholine receptor (M_3AchR) [6]. Autoantibodies are also present in the serum of the nonobese diabetic and MRL/lpr mouse models of Sjögren's syndrome, even though the pattern of expression may be different compared to that observed in man [7]. The presence of secretory and intracellular proteins in the sera leads to the question of how they get exposed to the immune system in order to initiate and maintain an autoimmune response which generates lacrimal gland infiltrates.

Recently, Zhu et al. [8] induced an autoimmune disease in rabbits resembling Sjögren's syndrome by injecting into the lacrimal gland autologous peripheral blood lymphocytes stimulated in culture with epithelial cells obtained from the contralateral excised gland. Interestingly, the histopathological picture of the lacrimal glands so treated was similar to the findings in Sjögren patients, showing predominantly CD4+ T cells infiltrates. A continuous decrease in tear production and stability and an increase in rose Bengal staining of the ocular surface were recorded in eyes injected with activated lymphocytes, and in the contralateral lacrimal gland-excised eyes by 2 weeks, indicating a generalized autoimmune phenomenon. Even if an important remaining point to verify in this model is whether the acinar cell preparation [the putative antigen-presenting cells (APCs) of this model] is completely devoid of any professional bone marrow-derived APCs, which can stimulate the T cells, the epithelial cells seem to have an important role in the immunohomeostasis of the lacrimal gland.

In non-Sjögren's dry eye, the lacrimal gland dysfunction is attributed to senile atrophy with lobular and periductal fibrosis, resulting in part from loss of hormonal support, in particular to low levels of androgens. However, in a study of lacrimal glands obtained at autopsy, lymphocytic infiltration was observed to increase with age and to be accompanied by fibrosis and acinar atrophy [9]. Such finding suggest that the tear volume and protein content changes observed with aging are not due only to senescent atrophy but also to immune dysfunction of the lacrimal gland.

Understanding the mechanisms of the homeostasis of the lacrimal gland and its failure will provide a rationale approach to pathophysiological and therapeutic studies of the different forms of DES.

Immunohomeostasis of the Lacrimal Gland

The lacrimal gland normally contains small populations of plasma cells, T lymphocytes (with a ratio of 2:1 of CD8+/CD4+ cells), and a limited array of dendritic cells, macrophages, and B cells. The normal population of T lymphocytes includes regulatory cells of CD8+ and CD4+, which play a critical role in maintaining the local immunohomeostasis. In fact, it has been demonstrated that lacrimal gland epithelial cells from healthy rabbits can be induced to begin expressing major histocompatibility complex (MHC) class II molecules when they are isolated and placed in primary culture, and lacrimal glands from human cadaver frequently contain large numbers of MHC class I-expressing acinar cells [10]. Class II molecules traffic through a system of endomembrane compartments that contain autoantigens, i.e. La/SSB, and enzymes capable of proteolytically processing autoantigen, i.e. cathepsins B and D [11]. All of these observations together with the fact that epithelial cells come in contact with lymphocytes, suggest that epithelial cells constitutively process and expose potentially pathogenic autoantigens in the same way that professional APCs process and present antigens. This confirmation comes from the work of Zhu et al. [8] who have shown that lacrimal gland acinar cells can stimulate lymphocyte proliferation when cocultured with peripheral blood lymphocytes from the same rabbit [12].

The fact that lacrimal glands are primed for an autoimmune response that normally does not occur is due to regulatory processes including regulatory lymphocytes and immunomodulatory factors such as TGF-β.

The Role of Regulatory T Cells

'Suppressor' or regulatory T cells (T_{reg}) are potent immunoregulatory cells that suppress T cell receptor-induced proliferation of CD4+ and CD8+ T cells in vitro by a cell contact-dependent mechanism. The modern era of regulatory T cells began with the observation by Asano et al. [13] that the adoptive transfer of CD4+ CD25+-depleted T cells induced several organ-specific autoimmune diseases in recipient immunodeficient animals. CD4+ CD25+ T cells also prevented the development of organ-specific autoimmunity observed when certain strains of mice were thymectomized on day 3 of life. Taken together, these studies demonstrate that CD4+ CD25+ T_{reg} cells play an important role in the generation and maintenance of peripheral self-tolerance. Piccirillo and Shevach [14] proposed two general categories of CD4+ CD25+ T_{reg} cells which differ in their origin, antigen specificity and effector mechanism. One T_{reg} subset develops during the normal process of T cell maturation in the thymus, resulting in the generation of a naturally occurring population of CD4+ CD25+ T_{reg} (nT_{reg}) cells that survive in the periphery poised to prevent potential autoimmune responses. The second subset of induced CD4+ CD25+ T_{reg} (iT_{reg}) cells, whose precursor is also thymically derived, develops as a consequence of ex vivo peripheral activation of classical naive CD4+ CD25+ T cell populations under different stimulatory conditions including antigen in the presence of immunosuppressive cytokines, such as IL-10 and TGF-β_1, vitamin D_3 and dexamethasone, CD40-CD40L blockade or immature dendritic cell populations [14]. Currently, it is not clear whether nT_{reg} and iT_{reg} cells preferentially function alone or in synchrony in the autoimmune lacrimal gland and ocular surface disease. Additionally, it is important to emphasize that other cell subsets (e.g. CD8+ or γδ T cells) may also function as regulatory cells. However, further studies are necessary to clarify their role in Sjögren's syndrome.

The Role of TGF-β

TGF-β seems to play a crucial role in maintaining local immunohomeostasis in the lacrimal gland. Mice homozygous for a nonfunctional TGF-β_1 gene develop inflammatory lesions, predominantly lymphocytic, in the lacrimal glands between the ages of 2 and 4 weeks, disrupting their structure and function and severely limiting their ability to generate tears [15]. In anterior chamber-associated immune deviation, CD4+ T_{reg} cells, termed Th3, are a possible source of TGF-β in the lacrimal gland, which could induce APCs to become TGF-β-secreting cells that prevent lymphocytes from differentiating into effector cells, and may direct them to differentiate into regulatory cells, as hypothesized by Mircheff [16]. Sex hormones can significantly influence TGF-β production. In a mouse model of Sjögren's syndrome, the MRL/lpr, Rocha et al. [17] demonstrated that subcutaneous administration of dihydrotestosterone increased TGF-β expression by lacrimal epithelial cells in the lacrimal gland, elicited a dramatic suppression of the inflammation, and increased the functional activity of the lacrimal gland.

Loss of Immunohomeostasis of the Lacrimal Gland

According to Mircheff [16], the loss of immunohomeostasis in the lacrimal gland could be caused by environmental or physiological perturbations, which lead epithelial cells to begin exposing or presenting epitopes that formerly were cryptic, or to a decrease in regulatory cell numbers. The potential exposure of cryptic antigens by epithelial cells has been shown by studies reporting that the autoantigens Ro/SSA and La/SSB can be expressed on the surface membrane after viral infection, cytokine stimulation, or oxidative stress [18]. Overcoming the relative crypticity has not been elucidated so far – this may be due to increased rates of apoptosis, alterations in basal-lateral endomembrane traffic, or by MHC class II direct presentation of autoantigen epitopes to CD4+ T cells [17].

Apoptosis is a rare physiological process in the normal lacrimal gland. Apoptotic bodies containing Ro/SSA, La/SSB, M_3aChR and fodrin are processed by macrophages and dendritic cells and presented to CD4+ T cells. This process is controlled by androgens and estrogens, which maintain low levels of apoptosis. In animal models, the decrease in sex hormones induced by ovariectomy can trigger lacrimal gland apoptosis as well as lymphocytic infiltration, while treatment with androgen and estrogen seems to play a role to maintain lacrimal gland structure and function.

Lacrimal gland epithelial cells secrete IgA_2 and a number of tear proteins which are subject to a complex basal-lateral membrane/endomembrane traffic. The secretory process can be influenced by various physiological and environmental factors. Chronic muscarinic receptor stimulation with carbachol, for example, causes secretory products to reflux in endosomes and could be a source of secretion of autoantigens to the interstitial space. Decreases in neural stimulation and viral infection with Epstein-Barr virus, hepatitis C, or human T cell leukemia virus type 1, have been hypothesized to have a similar effect on lacrimal gland epithelial secretion.

Further studies are necessary to clarify the mechanisms of the loss of immunohomeostasis in the lacrimal gland, but the use of T_{reg} cells and the modulation of TGF-β may have important effects on the treatment of Sjögren's syndrome.

Ocular Surface Inflammation

The ocular surface acts as an anatomical and functional unit able to keep an immunosilent environment in continuously challenging environmental conditions. Even after stimulation with pathogens, the intracellular expression of Toll-like receptors (TLR-2 and -4) by corneal epithelial cells has not been demonstrated [19].

Recently, a growing body of evidence has suggested that DES is associated with variable degree of ocular surface inflammation, and immunomodulatory drugs such as cyclosporine and steroids have been found to reduce markers of inflammation, and to improve symptoms and signs of KCS. The exact pathogenesis of inflammation has not been firmly established. The first step in the generation of inflammation is an inciting stimulus which can alter ocular surface homeostasis. A desiccating environmental stress, alterations in the tear film compositions secondary to lacrimal gland inflammation, interruption of neuronal stimulation for tear secretion, hyperosmolarity, and microtrauma from eyelids during blinking are some of the factors which could play a role in inducing loss of ocular surface immunohomeostasis and triggering DES.

Loss of Immunohomeostasis of the Ocular Surface

In DES, ocular surface inflammation at the tissue level is characterized by vascular engorgement and variable degrees of matrix edema, accompanied by extravasation of protein and fluid from leaky vessels, and loss of epithelial barrier function. At the molecular level, ample data demonstrate enhanced expression of pro-inflammatory cytokine (e.g. IL-1, IL-6, IL-8, and TNF-α) and chemokine (e.g. IL-8) mRNA and protein by the ocular surface epithelium and tear film [20]. Epithelial cell proliferation, impaired epithelial surface production of mature protective surface molecules, including the membrane-spanning mucin, MUC-1, keratinization, and angiogenesis can result from an increased concentration of these proinflammatory cytokines. Furthermore, in an experimental dry eye model, increased expression of matrix metalloproteinase-9 in tear fluid and corneal and conjunctival epithelia has been reported [21]. This enzyme could break tight junction proteins, and therefore the corneal epithelial barrier responsible for fluorescein staining of the cornea, a diagnostic sign of DES.

Another set of molecules recently implicated in the ocular surface disease of patients with dry eye are chemokines. Chemokines are proteins of low molecular weight that play a crucial role in leukocyte activation and recruitment, and as such play a critical role in homeostatic mechanisms as well as regulation of inflammatory responses. In vitro studies have shown that stimulation of human conjunctival epithelial cells with TNF-α, IL-1β and IFN-γ induces the release of RANTES and IL-8, chemokine ligands that are critical for the recruitment of T cells and neutrophils, respectively. Interestingly, recent data from our laboratory have shown that conjunctival epithelial cells of patients with various forms of dry eye uniformly overexpress a CC chemokine receptor (CCR5), implicating epithelial cells in the regulation of bone marrow-derived cell recruitment in dry eyes [22].

KCS has also been associated with a significantly increased level of HLA-DR and ICAM1 expression by conjunctival epithelial cells, as demonstrated by histological and flow-cytometric analysis [23]. Recently, Gao et al. [24] demonstrated that conjunctival epithelial cells not only express ICAM-1, but they are capable of synthesizing ICAM-1 mRNA and protein, thereby emphasizing their active role in DES inflammation. These epithelial cells may acquire antigen-presenting capability, and the immunologically activated epithelial cells may be the target of lymphocytes or they may participate directly in the recruitment of inflammatory cells, thus perpetuating inflammation and immune responsiveness. However, to date, there is no conclusive proof in the literature of a possible role of ocular surface epithelial cells serving as 'non-professional' APCs and priming CD4+ T cells, as has been shown for lacrimal gland epithelia. Although the inflammatory features of DES are similar to other ocular surface diseases, such as atopic diseases or cicatrizing conjunctivitis, a causal role for inflammation in DES has still to be elucidated.

T-lymphocytic infiltration has been observed in conjunctival biopsy specimens of patients with moderate-to-severe Sjögren's syndrome [25], and DES has been related to a delayed-type hypersensitivity reaction (type IV hypersensitivity). This is supported by the observation that T cells are predominantly CD4+ with increased expression of CD11a+ and CD23+, indicating an activated phenotype. CD4+ T_H1 cells recognize antigenic peptides in association with MHC class II molecules on the surface of APCs, and release pro-inflammatory cytokines that increase vascular permeability and recruit other inflammatory cells to the site of injury. One critical area for further studies in DES is to determine the role of professional (bone marrow-derived) APCs of the ocular surface in activating T cells. As demonstrated by Hamrah et al. [26], the cornea is endowed with several resident distinct subpopulations of (mostly monocytic CD11b+) CD45+ bone marrow-derived cells whose numbers increase during ocular surface inflammation and who acquire an activated phenotype (high MHC class II antigen expression). Preliminary data from our laboratory [27] have shown that in an experimental model of dry eye the cornea demonstrates a significant increase in the number of activated CD45+ CD11b+ monocytes, suggesting that not only the conjunctiva but also the cornea plays a pivotal role in the immunopathogenesis of KCS.

Conclusion

Lacrimal gland and ocular surface inflammation are certainly important factors in DES pathophysiology. Considerable work remains to be done to elucidate the interface between immunity and ocular surface in DES. Further studies in human and animal models of DES incorporating both intrinsic (immune, endocrine, and neuronal) and extrinsic (environmental) factors will offer important advances in the field.

References

1 Schaumberg DA, Sullivan DA, Buring JA, Dana MR: Prevalence of dry eye syndrome among US women. Am J Ophthalmol 2003;136:318–326.
2 Lemp MA: Report of the National Eye Institute/Industry workshop on clinical trials in dry eyes. CLAO J 1995;21:221–232.
3 Stern ME, Beuerman RW, Fox RI, Gao J, Mircheff AK, Pflugfelder SC: The pathology of dry eye: the interaction between ocular surface and lacrimal glands. Cornea 1998;17:584–589.
4 Dana MR, Hamrah P: Role of immunity and inflammation in corneal and ocular surface disease associated with dry eye. Adv Exp Med Biol 2002;506:729–738.
5 Saito I, Terauchi K, Shimuta M, Nishiimura S, Yoshino K, Takeuchi T, Tsubota K, Miyasaka N: Expression of cell adhesion molecules in the salivary and lacrimal glands of Sjögren's syndrome. J Clin Lab Anal 1993;7:180–187.
6 Gordon TP, Bolstad AI, Rischmueller M, Jonsson R, Waterman SA: Autoantibodies in primary Sjögren's syndrome: new insights into mechanisms of autoantibody diversification and disease pathogenesis. Autoimmunity 2001;34:123–132.
7 Barabino S, Shen L, Chen L, Rashid S, Rolando M, Dana MR: The controlled environment chamber: a new mouse model for dry eyes. Invest Ophthalmol Vis Sci 2005;46:2766–2771.
8 Zhu Z, Stevenson D, Schechter JE, Mircheff AK, Atkinson R, Trousdale MD: Lacrimal histopathology and ocular surface disease in a rabbit model of dacryoadenitis. Cornea 2003;22:25–32.
9 Damato BE, Allan D, Murray SB, Lee WR: Senile atrophy of the human lacrimal gland: the contribution of chronic inflammatory disease. Br J Ophthalmol 1984;68:674–680.
10 Mircheff AK, Gierow JP, Lee LM, Lambert RW, Akashi RH, Hofman FM: Class II antigen expression by lacrimal epithelial cells. An updated working hypothesis for antigen presentation by epithelial cells. Invest Ophthalmol Vis Sci 1991;32:2302–2310.
11 Yang T, Zeng H, Zhang J, Okamoto CT, Warren DW, Wood RL, Bachmann M, Mircheff AK: MHC class II molecules, cathepsins, and La/SSB proteins in lacrimal acinar cell endomembranes. Am J Physiol 1999;277:C994–C1007.
12 Guo Z, Azzarolo AM, Schechter JE, Warren DW, Wood RL, Mircheff AK, Kaslow HR: Lacrimal gland epithelial cells stimulate proliferation in autologous lymphocyte preparations. Exp Eye Res 2000;71:11–22.
13 Asano M, Toda M, Sakaguchi N, Sakaguchi S: Autoimmune disease as a consequence of developmental abnormality of a T cell subpopulation. J Exp Med 1996;184:387–396.
14 Piccirillo CA, Shevach EM: Naturally-occurring CD4+ CD25+ immunoregulatory T cells: central players in the arena of peripheral tolerance. Semin Immunol 2004;16:81–88.
15 McCartney-Francis NL, Mizel DE, Frazier-Jessen M, Kulkarni AB, McCarthy JB, Wahl SM: Lacrimal gland inflammation is responsible for ocular pathology in TGF-beta 1 null mice. Am J Pathol 1997;151:1281–1288.
16 Mircheff AK: Sjögren's syndrome as failed local immunohomeostasis: prospects for cell-based therapy. Ocul Surf 2003;1:160–179.

17 Rocha EM, Wickham LA, Huang Z, Toda I, Gao J, da Silveira LA, Sullivan DA: Presence and testosterone influence on the levels of anti- and pro-inflammatory cytokines in lacrimal tissues of a mouse model of Sjögren's syndrome. Adv Exp Med Biol 1998;438:485–491.
18 Clark DA, Lamey PJ, Jarrett RF, Onions DE: A model to study viral and cytokine involvement in Sjögren's syndrome. Autoimmunity 1994;18:7–14.
19 Ueta M, Nochi T, Jang MH, Park EJ, Igarashi O, Hino A, Kawasaki S, Shikina T, Hiroi T, Kinoshita S, Kiyono H: Intracellularly expressed TLR2s and TLR4s contribution to an immunosilent environment at the ocular mucosal epithelium. J Immunol 2004;173:3337–3347.
20 Pflugfelder SC, Jones D, Ji Z, Afonso A, Monroy D: Altered cytokine balance in the tear fluid and conjunctiva of patients with Sjögren's syndrome keratoconjunctivitis sicca. Curr Eye Res 1999;19:201–211.
21 Luo L, Li DQ, Doshi A, Farley W, Corrales RM, Pflugfelder SC: Experimental dry eye stimulates production of inflammatory cytokines and MMP-9 and activates MAPK signaling pathways on the ocular surface. Invest Ophthalmol Vis Sci 2004;45:4293–4301.
22 Gulati A, Sacchetti M, Bonini S, Dana MR: Chemokine receptor CCR5 expression in conjunctival epithelium of patients with dry eye syndrome. Arch Ophthalmol 2006;124:710–716.
23 Brignole F, Pisella PJ, Goldschild M, De Saint Jean M, Goguel A, Baudouin C: Flow cytometric analysis of inflammatory markers in conjunctival epithelial cells of patients with dry eyes. Invest Ophthalmol Vis Sci 2000;41:1356–1363.
24 Gao J, Morgan G, Tieu D, Schwalb TA, Luo JY, Wheeler LA, Stern ME: ICAM-1 expression predisposes ocular tissues to immune-based inflammation in dry eye patients and Sjögrens syndrome-like MRL/lpr mice. Exp Eye Res 2004;78:823–835.
25 Stern ME, Gao J, Schwalb TA, Ngo M, Tieu DD, Chan C, Reis BL, Whitcup SM, Thompson D, Smith JA: Conjunctival T-cell subpopulations in Sjögren's and non-Sjögren's patients with dry eye. Invest Ophthalmol Vis Sci 2002;43:2609–2614.
26 Hamrah P, Huq SO, Liu Y, Zhang Q, Dana MR: Corneal immunity is mediated by heterogeneous population of antigen-presenting cells. J Leukoc Biol 2003;74:172–178.
27 Rashid S, Barabino S, Dana R: Changes in corneal endowment of immune cells in novel dry eye model. Invest Ophthalmol Vis Sci 2005;46:E-3585.

Dr. M. Reza Dana
Schepens Eye Research Institute, Department of Ophthalmology
Harvard Medical School, 20 Staniford Street
Boston, MA 02114 (USA)
Tel. +1 617 912 7404, Fax +1 617 912 0117, E-Mail dana@vision.eri.harvard.edu

Niederkorn JY, Kaplan HJ (eds): Immune Response and the Eye.
Chem Immunol Allergy. Basel, Karger, 2007, vol 92, pp 185–194

Bacterial Infections of the Cornea (*Pseudomonas aeruginosa*)

Linda D. Hazlett

Department of Anatomy and Cell Biology, Wayne State University School of Medicine, Detroit, Mich., USA

Abstract

Pseudomonas aeruginosa is a common organism associated with bacterial keratitis, especially in extended wear contact lens users. Recent advances in the field have been made using animal models, including inbred murine models that are classed as resistant (cornea heals) versus susceptible (cornea perforates). Overall, studies with these inbred mice provide a better understanding of the mechanisms of innate immune responsiveness and abrogation of immune privilege operative after *P. aeruginosa* corneal infection.

Microbial keratitis, which has been associated with complications due to extended wear contact lens usage, has an incidence of 25,000–30,000 cases annually. Treatment cost is approximately USD 15–30 million, a considerable economic and medical impact [1]. *Pseudomonas aeruginosa* is a Gram-negative pathogen that induces keratitis and typically requires corneal injury for invasion [2]. Animal models are produced by topical application of bacteria after epithelial abrasion, intrastromal inoculation, or placement of a contaminated suture or contact lens on the cornea [3–6]. These approaches have increased understanding of innate immune mechanisms and alterations in immune privilege in the bacterially infected cornea.

Microbial Keratitis

MIP-2, IL-1, and PMN

The innate immune response often includes local polymorphonuclear neutrophil (PMN) recruitment, essential to control bacterial replication and host survival, but PMN persistence is also associated with pathology, and, in the cornea, includes stromal scarring and perforation [7–9]. PMN infiltration into inflamed tissue is controlled largely by local production of inflammatory mediators. In the mouse, two members of the CXC family of chemokines – macrophage inflammatory protein-2 (MIP-2), a functional homologue of human interleukin (IL)-8, and KC, the murine homologue of GROα – are potent chemoattractants and activators of PMNs. In corneal infections, MIP-2 is the major chemokine that attracts PMNs into the *P. aeruginosa*-infected cornea, and persistence of PMNs in the susceptible (cornea perforates) C57BL/6 (B6) mouse cornea correlates with higher chemokine levels (mRNA and protein) [10].

IL-1, which is produced by macrophages, monocytes and resident corneal cells [11, 12], also influences PMN influx into tissues [13, 14]. When tested, IL-1α and -1β (mRNA and protein) were elevated in B6 (susceptible) and BALB/c (resistant) mice, and levels peaked 1 day after infection. Significantly greater amounts of IL-1 protein were detected in B6 versus BALB/c mice 1 and 3 days after infection, and 5 days after infection, IL-1α and -1β (mRNA and protein) levels remained elevated in B6 but began declining in BALB/c mice. Neutralization of IL-1β in infected B6 mice [15] reduced disease severity, evidenced by a reduction in PMNs in the cornea (MPO assay), bacterial load, MIP-2 mRNA and protein. The data confirmed IL-1 as important in *P. aeruginosa* keratitis [15].

CD4+ T Cells and Genetic Susceptibility to P. aeruginosa

The role of T cells in *P. aeruginosa* corneal infection was first studied in inbred B6 wild-type and β_2-microglobulin knockout mice (B6 background, knockout of CD8+ T cells) [16]. Corneas of both groups perforated by 7 days after infection, and histopathology was similar with infiltration of PMNs within 24 h after infection. After infection, CD4+ and CD8+ T cells were present in the cornea of wild-type mice by 3 days; by 5 days, activated (IL-2R and CD25+) cells were positively immunostained. Corneas of wild-type mice depleted of CD4+ T cells and infected with *P. aeruginosa* did not perforate 7 days after infection in contrast to mice depleted of CD8+ T cells (i.e. the β_2-microglobulin knockout mice) or treated with an irrelevant antibody. Antibody neutralization of interferon (IFN)-γ before infecting B6 mice also prevented perforation and was associated with a lower delayed-type hypersensitivity response over B6 mice similarly treated with an irrelevant antibody. These data support the notion that a CD4+ T cell (Th1)-dominant response following *P. aeruginosa* infection is associated with genetic susceptibility and corneal perforation in B6 mice [16] and provided initial evidence that CD4+ T cells are important in keratitis.

Mice favoring a Th1 (B6, C57BL/10, and B10.D2/nSn) versus Th2 (BALB/c, BALB/cBy, BALB.B, and BALB.K) response [17] were also evaluated after *P. aeruginosa* infection [18]. Mice favoring a Th1 T cell immune response exhibited a similar course of disease, and the infected eyes of all mice perforated in the week following infection. In contrast, mice favoring a Th2 T immune response exhibited a milder disease course and no corneal perforation. These in vivo studies corroborated that mice favoring Th1-type responses are susceptible (cornea perforates) while mice favoring Th2 responses are resistant (no corneal perforation). Gene array studies confirmed the Th1 versus Th2 bias of B6 versus BALB/c mice [19], but whether T cells similarly contribute to the pathogenesis in human disease remains unknown.

MIP-1α Regulates CD4+ T Cell Chemotaxis

MIP-1α (CC chemokine) is produced by activated T cells, macrophages, Langerhans cells (LCs), PMNs, and B cells [20]. In vitro chemotaxis and MIP-1α receptor studies suggest that the chemokine attracts T and B cells, macrophages [21, 22], and PMNs [23, 24] to inflammatory sites. Ribonuclease protection assay data suggested that mRNA expression levels for MIP-1α were significantly upregulated after *P. aeruginosa* infection in outbred mice [25]. In susceptible (B6) over resistant (BALB/c) mice, greater amounts of MIP-1α (mRNA and protein) were also detected in the infected cornea 1–5 days after infection. BALB/c mice treated with recombinant MIP-1α protein (injected subconjunctivally or systemically) had exacerbated disease associated with a significant increase in PMNs in the cornea. This treatment also induced recruitment of activated (CD25+) CD4+ T lymphocytes into the cornea, converting the resistant to a susceptible (cornea perforates) phenotype [26]. In recombinant MIP-1α-treated BALB/c mice, depletion of CD4+ T cells versus sham depletion significantly decreased PMNs in the infected cornea suggesting that T cells regulate PMN persistence. In complementary studies, B6 mice given a MIP-1α neutralizing antibody showed reduced corneal PMNs and less pathology. Corneal mRNA levels for MIP-2 and IL-1β were also reduced 5 days after infection (1.7- and 2-fold), collectively providing evidence that MIP-1α directly contributed to CD4+ T cell chemotaxis into the infected cornea and that it also indirectly participated in PMN persistence through regulation of IL-1 [15] and MIP-2 [10].

IL-12 and IFN-γ in C57BL/6 Mice

Th1 response development depends upon IL-12 and the ability of T cells to respond [27, 28]. IL-12 may modulate the progress of an infection including production of other immunoregulatory cytokines such as IFN-γ [29, 30]. Therefore, studies investigated whether IL-12 is associated with IFN-γ production and the susceptibility response of B6 mice after *P. aeruginosa* challenge. IL-12 knockout mice (B6 background) were also tested to examine disease progression in the absence of endogenous cytokine. When tested, both groups of mice were susceptible to corneal challenge with *P. aeruginosa*, and corneal perforation was observed 5–7 days after infection. Semiquantitative RT-PCR and ELISA analyses confirmed that IL-12 message and protein levels were elevated after infection in the wild-type cornea compared to knockout mouse cornea [31]. Immunostaining for IL-12 p40 in wild-type B6 mice revealed that stromal PMNs were the cytokine source [31]. Knockout mice showed a significant decrease in corneal IFN-γ (and tumor necrosis factor-α) mRNA and had a significant increase in bacterial load 5 days after infection over wild-type mice, suggesting that with or without IL-12, B6 mice remain susceptible. Data suggest that in the presence of IL-12, its own augmentation and upregulation of IFN-γ production contributes to disease pathogenesis; without IL-12, insufficient amounts of IFN-γ allow unchecked bacterial growth in the cornea and corneal perforation.

IL-18, IFN-γ and NK Cells in BALB/c Mice

IL-18, which is produced by macrophages and dendritic cells, is released as an inactive precursor, requiring cleavage by IL-1β-converting enzyme for maturation [32, 33]. IL-18 provides costimulation, with IL-12, for IFN-γ production and may act synergistically to drive Th1 T cell development [34, 35]. The role of IL-18 and IFN-γ in the resistance response of BALB/c mice was tested. Semiquantitative RT-PCR detected IFN-γ expression levels in the cornea of infected mice 1–7 days after infection. Cytokine levels were significantly upregulated compared with control uninfected normal corneas [36]. Constitutive IL-18 mRNA was detected similarly in the normal, uninfected cornea, and levels were significantly elevated 1–7 days after infection. To test whether IL-18 regulated IFN-γ production, mice were injected with an anti-IL-18 monoclonal antibody. Treatment decreased corneal IFN-γ mRNA [36] levels, and both bacterial load and disease severity increased when compared to IgG-injected mice. These data provide evidence that IL-18 is critical to the resistance response of BALB/c mice by induction of IFN-γ and that IFN-γ is required for bacterial killing/stasis in the cornea [4, 37]. Its killing effect was found to be indirect through regulation of nitric oxide levels [38].

Further study of the resistance response in BALB/c mice examined the role of the neuropeptide, substance P in IFN-γ production. Natural killer cells were required to produce IFN-γ; the cells expressed the neurokinin-1 receptor (the major substance P receptor); they directly regulated IFN-γ through this receptor [39] suggesting a unique link between the nervous system and development of innate immunity in the cornea (fig. 1).

Antigen Presentation: Langerhans Cells and Costimulation

LCs are antigen-presenting cells that constitutively express major histocompatibility class II antigen. Numerous stimuli, including infectious [40, 41],

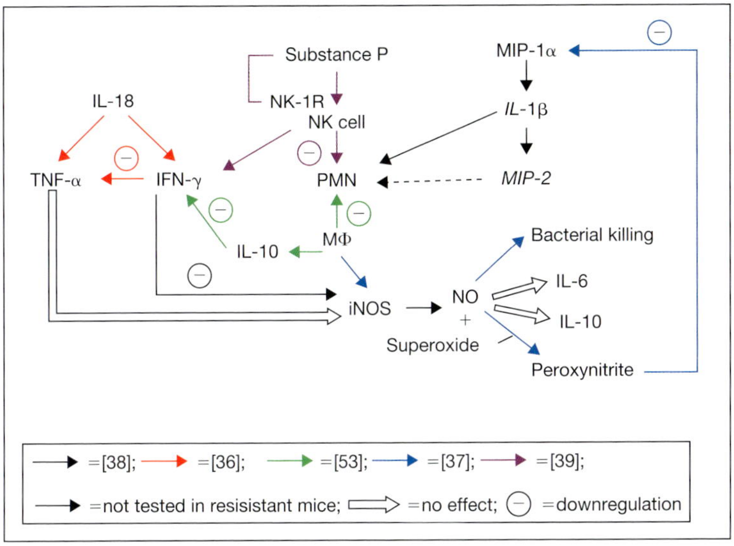

Fig. 1. A working diagram of cell, cytokine and neuropeptide interactions in the infected cornea resulting in resistance (corneal healing). iNOS = Inducible nitric oxide synthase; MΦ = macrophages; NK-1R = neurokinin-1 receptor.

noninfectious [42], and experimental extended wear contact lens usage [43] initiate their centripetal migration from the conjunctiva into the cornea. To test the consequences of LCs in the cornea before infection with *P. aeruginosa*, LCs were induced centripetally by sterile bead application onto the wounded cornea [44] of susceptible B6 and resistant BALB/c mice [45]. We detected no difference in disease response in bead- versus sham-treated B6 mice after infection. However, significant differences leading to corneal perforation were observed in infected, bead-treated BALB/c mice and included an increased number of ADPase-stained [46] LC in the central cornea and enhanced B7-1 co-stimulatory molecule expression. Remarkably, the presence of LCs in the BALB/c cornea before infection was also associated with the presence of activated CD4+ T cells. The cell infiltrate in the stroma of bead- versus sham-treated corneas also differed and was characterized by macrophages [45]. Further study examined the role of LCs and signaling through the B7/CD28 co-stimulatory pathway in the *P. aeruginosa*-infected cornea [47]. Mature, B7 positive-stained LCs in the cornea and *Pseudomonas* antigen-associated cells in draining cervical lymph nodes increased after infection in susceptible versus resistant mice. When B6 mice were treated (subconjunctivally and systemically) with neutralizing B7 (B7-1/B7-2) antibodies, disease severity was reduced, and the number of B7-positive cells, as well as the recruitment and activation of CD4+ T cells in the cornea, were significantly decreased. B6 mice endogenously lacking CD28 also exhibited a less severe disease response (no perforation) when compared with wild-type mice, supporting a critical role for B7/CD28 costimulation in the susceptibility to *P. aeruginosa* ocular infection. To test whether lymph nodes (cervical) were required as the site of antigen presentation by LCs to naïve T cells and whether the subsequent T cell response in the cornea was antigen specific, draining cervical lymph nodes [48] were removed in B6 mice followed by challenge with *P. aeruginosa* and subsequent immunostaining for CD4+ T cells in cornea. Whether or not lymph nodes were present (sham surgery) or surgically removed, CD4+ T cells that were activated (CD25+) remained detectable in the cornea suggesting that T cells in the conjunctiva migrate into the cornea where they are activated locally and at least, in part, nonspecifically.

Macrophages in Innate Response to P. aeruginosa *Ocular Infection*

Macrophages are essential for host defense [49, 50], participating in innate and acquired immunity. Macrophages from Th1 (e.g. B6) T cell responder mice appear more easily activated than those from Th2 (e.g. BALB/c) strains [51, 52], and the cells express distinct metabolic programs [49]. The role of the macrophage in the host response to *P. aeruginosa* ocular challenge was tested in B6-susceptible (cornea perforates) and -resistant (cornea heals) BALB/c mice by cell depletion before infection using subconjunctival injections of clodronate liposomes [53]. This increased the onset and/or severity of disease in both mouse strains. B6 corneas perforated earlier, and eye shrinkage in the macrophage-depleted group was exacerbated. In BALB/c mice, the corneas of macrophage-depleted mice perforated within 7 days after infection, changing their response to susceptibility.

We tested whether depletion of macrophages affected other inflammatory cell populations, such as the PMNs. PMNs were quantitated by the myeloperoxidase (MPO) assay in the cornea of both mouse strains after injection of clodronate liposomes or PBS liposomes. In B6 mice, no difference in PMN number was observed 1 day after infection, but by 3 days after infection, the cornea of clodronate liposome-injected mice had significantly elevated MPO levels. In BALB/c mice, MPO assays showed that after macrophage depletion, PMN number was significantly elevated 1 and 3 days after infection, suggesting that macrophages participate in regulating the number of PMNs in the cornea in both mouse groups but that regulation is reduced/delayed in B6 mice. Depletion of macrophages also resulted in dysregulation of cytokines that attract PMNs into the cornea in both mouse groups, confirming that cytokine production is at least one mechanism by which the macrophage regulates PMN influx into the bacterially infected cornea.

Increased expression levels for IFN-γ were detected in the cornea of BALB/c mice injected with clodronate liposomes 3 and 5 days after infection. However, no difference was seen in mRNA expression levels for TNF-α or IL-4 in the macrophage-depleted versus PBS liposome-injected group. In contrast, mRNA expression levels of IL-10 were significantly lower in the cornea of BALB/c mice treated with clodronate liposomes 1–5 days after infection. IL-10 protein levels paralleled the molecular data, were significant 5 days after infection, and supported a biologically functional role for IL-10 in balancing corneal pro-inflammatory cytokine levels.

Toll-Like Receptors in Bacterial Keratitis

The Toll family of receptors (TLR), conserved throughout evolution from flies to humans, is central in initiating innate immune responses. This family of receptors, composed of transmembrane molecules, links the extracellular compartment where contact and recognition of microbial pathogens occurs and the intracellular compartment, where signaling cascades leading to cellular responses are initiated. Gene array data showed that the expression of TLRs and related molecules – including CD14, soluble IL-1 receptor antagonist, TLR-6, and IL-18 receptor accessory protein – were significantly elevated in susceptible versus resistant mice [19]. In a sterile keratitis model [1], when C3H/HeJ (TLR-4 point mutation) versus control mice were treated with lipopolysaccharide from *P. aeruginosa*, a significant increase in stromal thickness and haze was seen in the cornea of control mice but not in TLR-4 mutant mice; the severity of disease coincided with PMN stromal infiltration. Another study showed that the corneal epithelium has functional TLR-2 and -9 and that TLR-2, -4 and -9 signal through myeloid differentiation factor 88 [54]. In human corneal epithelial cells, TLR-5, that recognizes bacterial flagellin, was detected at the corneal cell surface of deeper but not superficial epithelial cells [55]. TLR-5 signaling elicits an epithelial response by activating NF-κB signaling, producing pro-inflammatory cytokines such as IL-6 and IL-8.

Overall, these and other animal studies have provided provocative clues as to the mechanisms operative in the abrogation of immune privilege by a bacterial pathogen such as *P. aeruginosa*. The significance of these data, particularly their correlation with human disease, awaits resolution.

Acknowledgment

The study was supported by NIH grants R01EY02986, R01EY16058 and P30EY04068.

References

1 Khatri S, Lass JH, Heinzel FP, et al: Regulation of endotoxin-induced keratitis by PECAM-1, MIP-2, and toll-like receptor 4. Invest Ophthalmol Vis Sci 2002;43:2278–2284.
2 Hazlett LD, Rosen DD, Berk RS: Age-related susceptibility to *Pseudomonas aeruginosa* ocular infection in mice. Infect Immun 1978;20:25–29.
3 Kernacki KA, Hobden JA, Hazlett LD: Murine model of bacterial keratitis; in Zak O, Sande M (eds): Handbook of Animal Models of Infection. London, Academic Press, 1999, pp 361–366.
4 Hazlett LD: Pathogenic mechanisms of *P. aeruginosa* keratitis: a review of the role of T cells, Langerhans cells, PMN, and cytokines. DNA Cell Biol 2002;21:383–390.
5 Szliter EA, Morris CA, Carney F, et al: Development of a new extended-wear contact lens model in the rat. CLAOJ 2002;28:119–123.
6 Szliter E, Barrett R, Gabriel M, et al: *Pseudomonas aeruginosa*-induced inflammation in the rat extended wear contact lens model. Eye Contact Lens 2006;32:12–18.
7 Steuhl KP, Doring G, Henni A, et al: Relevance of host-derived and bacterial factors in *Pseudomonas aeruginosa* corneal infection. Invest Ophthalmol Vis Sci 1987;28:1559–1568.
8 Hazlett LD, Rosen D, Berk RS: Experimental *Pseudomonas* eye infection in cyclophosphamide-treated mice. Invest Ophthalmol Vis Sci 1977;16:649–652.
9 Hazlett LD: Corneal response to *Pseudomonas aeruginosa* infection. Progr Retin Eye Res 2004;23:1–30.
10 Kernacki KA, Barrett RP, Hobden JA, et al: Macrophage inflammatory protein-2 is a mediator of polymorphonuclear neutrophil influx in ocular bacterial infection. J Immunol 2000;164:1037–1045.
11 Niederkorn JY, Peeler JS, Mellon J: Phagocytosis of particulate antigens by corneal epithelial cells stimulates interleukin-1 secretion and migration of Langerhans cells into the central cornea. Reg Immunol 1989;2:83–90.
12 Dinarello CA: Biological basis for interleukin-1 in disease. Blood 1996;87:2095–2147.
13 Dinarello CA, Wolff SM: The role of interleukin-1 in disease. N Engl J Med 1993;328:106–113.
14 Arend WP, Malyak M, Guthridge CJ, et al: Interleukin-1 receptor antagonist: role in biology. Annu Rev Immunol 1998;16:27–32.
15 Rudner XL, Kernacki KA, Barrett RP, et al: Prolonged elevation of IL-1 in *Pseudomonas aeruginosa* ocular infection regulates macrophage-inflammatory protein-2 production, polymorphonuclear neutrophil persistence, and corneal perforation. J Immunol 2000;164:6576–6582.
16 Kwon B, Hazlett LD: Association of CD4+ T cell-dependent keratitis with genetic susceptibility to *Pseudomonas aeruginosa* ocular infection. J Immunol 1997;159:6283–6290.
17 Gorham JD, Güler ML, Steen RG, et al: Genetic mapping of a murine locus controlling development of T helper 1/T helper 2 type responses. Proc Natl Acad Sci 1996;93:12467–12472.
18 Hazlett LD, McClellan S, Kwon B, et al: Increased severity of *Pseudomonas aeruginosa* corneal infection in strains of mice designated as Th1 versus Th2 responsive. Invest Ophthalmol Vis Sci 2000;41:805–810.
19 Huang X, Hazlett LD: Analysis of *Pseudomonas aeruginosa* corneal infection using oligonucleotide microarray. Invest Ophthalmol Vis Sci 2003;44:3409–3416.
20 Haelens A, Wuyts A, Proost P, et al: Leukocyte migration and activation by murine chemokines. Immunobiology 1996;195:499–521.
21 Baggiolini M, Dewald B, Moser B: Interleukin-8 and related chemotactic chemokines – CXC and CC chemokines. Adv Immunol 1994;55:97–179.
22 DiPietro A, Burdick M, Low AE, et al: MIP-1α as a critical macrophage chemoattractant in murine wound repair. J Clin Invest 1998;101:1693–1698.
23 Shanley TP, Schmal H, Friedl HP, et al: Role of macrophage inflammatory protein-1α (MIP-1α) in acute lung injury in rats. J Immunol 1995;154:4793–4802.
24 Bonecchi R, Polentarutti N, Luini W, et al: Up-regulation of CCR1 and CCR3 and induction of chemotaxis to CC chemokines by IFN-gamma in human neutrophils. J Immunol 1999;162:474–479.
25 Kernacki KA, Goebel DJ, Poosch M, et al: Early cytokine and chemokine gene expression during *Pseudomonas aeruginosa* corneal infection in mice. Infect Immun 1998;66:376–379.

26 Kernacki KA, Barrett RP, McClellan S, et al: MIP-1α regulates CD4+ T cell chemotaxis and indirectly enhances PMN persistence in *Pseudomonas aeruginosa* corneal infection. J Leukoc Biol 2001;70:911–919.
27 O'Garra A: Cytokines induce the development of functionally heterogenous T helper cell subsets. Immunity 1998;8:275–283.
28 Abbas AK, Murphy KM, Sher A: Functional diversity of helper T lymphocytes. Nature 1996;383:787–793.
29 Locksley RM: Interleukin 12 in host defense against microbial pathogens. Proc Natl Acad Sci 1993;90:5879–5880.
30 Bohn E, Autenrieth IB: IL-12 is essential for resistance against *Yersinia enterocolitica* by triggering IFN-gamma production in NK cells and $CD4^+$ T cells. J Immunol 1996;156:1458–1468.
31 Hazlett LD, Rudner XL, McClellan SA, et al: Role of IL-12 and IFN-γ in *Pseudomonas aeruginosa* corneal infection. Invest Ophthalmol Vis Sci 2002;43:419–424.
32 Ghayur T, Banerjee S, Hugunin M, et al: Caspase-1 processes IFN-γ-inducing factor and regulates LPS-induced IFN-γ production. Nature 1997;386:619–623.
33 Lu H, Shen C, Brunham RC: *Chlamydia trachomatis* infection of epithelial cells induces the activation of caspase-1 and release of mature IL-18. J Immunol 2000;165:1463–1469.
34 Shibuya K, Robinson D, Zonin F, et al: IL-1α and TNF-α are required for IL-12-induced development of Th1 cells producing high levels of IFN-γ in BALB/c but not C57BL/6 mice. J Immunol 1998;160:1708–1716.
35 Netea MG, Fantuzzi G, Kullberg BJ, et al: Neutralization of IL-18 reduces neutrophil tissue accumulation and protects mice against lethal *Escherichia coli* and *Salmonella typhimurium* endotoxemia. J Immunol 2000;164:2644–2649.
36 Huang X, McClellan SA, Barrett RP, et al: IL-18 contributes to host resistance against infection with *Pseudomonas aeruginosa* through induction of IFN-gamma production. J Immunol 2002;68: 5756–5763.
37 Hazlett LD, McClellan S, Goshgarian C: The role of nitric oxide in resistance to *P. aeruginosa* ocular infection. Ocul Immunol Inflamm 2005;13:279–288.
38 McClellan SA, Lighvani S, Hazlett LD: IFN-gamma: regulation of nitric oxide in the *P. aeruginosa*-infected cornea. Ocul Immunol Inflamm 2006;14:21–28.
39 Lighvani S, Huang X, Trivedi PP, et al: Substance P regulates NK cell IFN-γ production and resistance to *Pseudomonas aeruginosa* infection. Eur J Immunol 2005;35:1567–1575.
40 Hendricks RL, Janowicz M, Tumpey TM: Critical role of corneal Langerhans cells in the CD4- but not CD8-mediated immunopathology in herpes virus-1-infected mouse cornea. J Immunol 1992;148:2522–2529.
41 Hazlett LD, Moon M, Dawisha S, et al: Age alters Langerhans cell response to *P. aeruginosa* ocular challenge. Curr Eye Res 1986;5:343–355.
42 Williamson JSP, Dimarco S, Streilein JW: Immunobiology of Langerhans cells on the ocular surface. I. Langerhans cells within the central cornea interfere with induction of anterior chamber associated immune deviation. Invest Ophthalmol Vis Sci 1987;28:1527–1532.
43 Hazlett LD, McClellan SM, Hume EBH, et al: Extended wear contact lens usage induces Langerhans cell migration into cornea. Exp Eye Res 1999;69:575–577.
44 Peeler JS, Niederkorn JY: Antigen presentation by Langerhans cells in vivo: donor derived Ia^+ Langerhans cells are required for induction of delayed-type hypersensitivity but not for cytotoxic T lymphocyte responses to alloantigens. J Immunol 1986;136:4362–4371.
45 Hazlett LD, McClellan SA, Rudner XL, et al: The role of Langerhans cells in *P. aeruginosa* infection. Invest Ophthalmol Vis Sci 2002;43:189–197.
46 Chaker MB, Tharp MD, Bergestresser PR: Rodent epidermal Langerhans cells demonstrate greater histochemical specificity for ADP than for ATP and AMP. J Invest Dermatol 1984;82:496–500.
47 Hazlett LD, McClellan S, Barrett R, et al: B7/CD28 costimulation is critical in susceptibility to *Pseudomonas aeruginosa* corneal infection: a comparative study using monoclonal antibody blockade and CD28-deficient mice. J Immunol 2001;166:1292–1299.
48 Barrett R, McClellan S, Huang X, et al: Cervical lymph nodes are not required for T cell trafficking to the cornea after Pseudomonas aeruginosa eye infection. Invest Ophthalmol Vis Sci 2003;43: ARVO E-Abstract 716.

49 Mills CD, Kinkaid K, Alt JM, et al: M-1/M2 macrophages and Th1/Th2 paradigm. J Immunol 2000;164:6166–6173.
50 Nathan CF: Secretory products of macrophages. J Clin Invest 1987;79:319–326.
51 Liew FY, Li Y, Moss D, et al: Resistance to *Leishmania major* infection correlates with the induction of nitric oxide synthase in murine macrophages. Eur J Immunol 1991;21:3009–3014.
52 Oswald IP, Afroun S, Bray D, et al: Low response of BALB/c macrophages to priming and activating signals. J Leukoc Biol 1992;52:315–322.
53 McClellan SA, Huang X, Barrett RP, et al: Macrophages restrict *Pseudomonas aeruginosa* growth, regulate polymorphonuclear neutrophil influx and balance pro- and anti-inflammatory cytokines in BALB/c mice. J Immunol 2003;170:5219–5227.
54 Johnson AC, Heinzel FP, Diaconu E, et al: Activation of Toll-like receptor (TLR)2, TLR4, and TLR9 in the mammalian cornea induces MyD88-dependent corneal inflammation. Invest Ophthalmol Vis Sci 2005;46:589–595.
55 Zhang J, Xu K, Ambati B, et al: Toll-like receptor 5-mediated corneal epithelial inflammatory responses to *Pseudomonas aeruginosa* flagellin. Invest Ophthalmol Vis Sci 2003;44:4247–4254.

Dr. Linda D. Hazlett
Department of Anatomy and Cell Biology
Wayne State University School of Medicine
540 East Canfield Avenue
Detroit, MI 48201 (USA)
Tel. +1 313 577 1079, Fax +1 313 577 3125, E-Mail lhazlett@med.wayne.edu

Niederkorn JY, Kaplan HJ (eds): Immune Response and the Eye.
Chem Immunol Allergy. Basel, Karger, 2007, vol 92, pp 195–202

Cicatrizing and Autoimmune Diseases

Saadia Rashid[a,b], *M. Reza Dana*[a–c]

[a]Schepens Eye Research Institute, [b]Harvard Medical School, and [c]Department of Ophthalmology, Massachusetts Eye and Ear Infirmary, Boston, Mass., USA

Abstract

Autoimmune disorders of the ocular surface represent a clinically heterogeneous group of conditions where acute and chronic autoreactive mechanisms can cause significant damage to the eye. When severe and affecting the epithelium and substantia propria of the conjunctiva, cicatrization can ensue, leading to significant mechanical alterations as a result of the fibrosis. These conditions, though generally infrequent, can be the cause of profound pathology and visual disability, and often need systemic immune modulation for therapy.

The ocular surface faces the unique and perpetual challenge of defending the eye against invasion of exogenous substances on one hand, and quenching vigorous vision-threatening inflammatory responses on the other. The balance is maintained by the presence of two immunologically diverse tissues located side by side: the immunologically active conjunctiva with an extensive presence of blood vessels, lymphatics and immune cells (including T cells) located adjacent to the immune-privileged cornea. However, the proximity of the peripheral cornea to the conjunctiva comes with a price: blood vessels derived from the anterior conjunctival and deep episcleral arteries extend 0.5 mm into the clear cornea [1]. These vessels, along with the adjacent subconjunctival lymphatics that drain into the regional lymph nodes, provide a route for the afferent arc of corneal immune reactions. The vasculature also allows for diffusion of immunoglobulins and complement components into the cornea. By virtue of higher molecular weight, IgM and C1 are present in higher concentrations in the corneal periphery [1]. Furthermore, the antigen-presenting cells (APCs), namely corneal epithelial Langerhans cells and stromal macrophages and dendritic cells, are present in higher numbers in the periphery compared to the central cornea, with a majority expressing an activated phenotype in the periphery [2]. These factors make the peripheral cornea more susceptible to breakdown of immune privilege leading to a variety of autoimmune disorders such as Mooren's ulcer and the collagen vascular diseases discussed below. Furthermore, the cornea as a whole can get secondarily affected by cicatrizing diseases of the conjunctiva, due to their anatomical proximity. This chapter discusses the immunopathogenesis of Mooren's ulcer and peripheral ulcerative keratitis (PUK) as illustrative examples of the two most common autoimmune diseases of the peripheral cornea, and ocular cicatricial pemphigoid (OCP), the prototype cicatrizing disorder of the conjunctiva.

Mooren's Ulcer

Mooren's ulcer is a chronic, progressive, painful, idiopathic ulceration of the peripheral corneal stroma and epithelium that can lead to extensive corneal vascularization and fibrosis. The ulcer starts in the periphery of the cornea and spreads both centripetally and towards the sclera. Evidence suggests that it is an autoimmune disease although the exact mechanism is unknown. The possible autoimmune mechanisms involved in the pathogenesis of Mooren's ulcer are discussed below.

The process may be initiated by alterations in corneal antigens by a systemic disease, infection or trauma stimulating both humoral and cellular responses [3]. A cornea-associated autoantigen, identical in sequence to human neutrophil calgranulin [4], has been detected in the corneal stroma [5], and autoantibodies to this autoantigen have been found in the sera of the affected patients [4]. Furthermore, it has been shown that pro-inflammatory cytokines IL-1 and TNF-α, that are produced in response to trauma or inflammation, can upregulate calgranulin gene expression by corneal stromal keratocytes [5]. Hence environmental insults may lead to the expression of autoantigens in the cornea as an early step in the breakdown of corneal immune privilege in genetically susceptible individuals. HLA-DR17 (3) and/or DQ2 may increase genetic susceptibility to Mooren's ulcer [6].

A large number of infiltrating macrophages and CD4+ T lymphocytes are reported in the affected cornea and adjacent conjunctiva [7]. Recently, bone marrow-derived multipotential progenitor cells have been reported in the cornea, especially in the superficial stroma [8]. Strong expression of CD34 (marker of hematopoietic progenitor cells and endothelium), c-kit (marker of hematopoietic and stromal progenitor cells) and STRO-1 (a differentiation antigen present on bone marrow fibroblast cells) has been reported in the effected corneas and may be involved in the disease pathogenesis by synergizing with other factors to amplify autoimmune destructive reactions and contributing to the regenerative process [8]. There is also an aberrant expression of major histocompatibility complex (MHC) class II (HLA-DR antigen) by a large number of keratoconjunctival epithelial cells and corneal stromal keratocytes [9]. Both macrophages and corneal keratocytes can act as APCs, and the upregulation of MHC class II molecules on their surface suggests an activated phenotype for antigen presentation (presumably the autoantigen described above) to the CD4+ T helper cells and subsequent T cell priming and proliferation. Cell-mediated immunity against the corneal antigens has been demonstrated by cytokine production (macrophage migration inhibition factor) in response to corneal antigens presented to lymphocytes from Mooren's ulcer patients [3]. Foster [3] has also demonstrated blastogenic transformation and lymphocytic proliferation in response to normal corneal stroma in a patient with the disease.

Humoral immunity has also been implicated. Patients with the disease have been reported to have circulating IgG antibodies to human corneal and conjunctival epithelium, elevated serum IgA levels, circulating immune complexes, and antibodies and complement bound to conjunctival epithelium [3]. It is postulated that unregulated T helper cell response (as manifest by systemic decrease in the number of suppressor T cells relative to the number of T helper cells in Mooren's ulcer patients) leads to T helper cell-mediated activation and proliferation of B cells, antibody overproduction, and subsequent immune complex deposition and complement activation [10]. The perpetuation of the ulcerative process may occur when complement activation leads to neutrophil chemotaxis and degranulation, release of collagen and proteoglycan-degrading matrix metalloproteinases (MMPs), further altering and exposing corneal antigens, leading to a vicious cycle of antigen recognition, presentation and destruction until the target autoantigen is nearly consumed [11]. Indeed, activated degranulating neutrophils and high levels of collagenases are reported in the ulcerating cornea suggesting that neutrophils are the source of proteases and collagenases [3].

The immune privilege of the cornea is dependent upon several factors such as avascularity of the normal cornea, reduced expression of MHC class II antigens by resident corneal APCs [2], and expression of apoptosis-inducing Fas ligand on corneal epithelium and endothelium [12]. The extensive vascularization and upregulation of MHC class II by APCs seen in corneal ulcers are examples of loss of immune privilege. Furthermore, inflammatory cells such as neutrophils and activated T cells are especially vulnerable to apoptosis induced by Fas ligand [12]. The inflammatory damage done by the activated T cells and neutrophils present in corneal lesions is another instance of breakdown of immune privilege.

Peripheral Ulcerative Keratitis Associated with Systemic Immune-Mediated Diseases

PUK refers to a crescent-shaped destructive inflammation of the juxtalimbal corneal stroma associated with an epithelial defect, stromal degradation and inflammatory cell infiltration often with concomitant conjunctival, scleral and episcleral inflammation. Autoimmune PUK is seen in patients with collagen vascular diseases/vasculitides, and often occurs in association with rheumatoid arthritis (RA) but may also be seen in Wegener's granulomatosis, systemic lupus erythematosus, polyarteritis nodosa, and other inflammatory diseases. Although the exact pathogenesis of corneal ulceration in PUK is unknown, the possible mechanisms involved are discussed below in the context of RA-associated PUK.

RA is characterized by the formation of IgM antibodies against IgG (rheumatoid factor). These rheumatoid factors lead to immune complex formation and deposition in the joints and vessels (a type III hypersensitivity reaction), with complement/macrophage activation and the resultant secretion of pro-inflammatory cytokines, particularly IL-1 and TNF-α [13]. Convincing experimental evidence of one single joint-specific endogenous antigen in the synovial lesions is still lacking, and the finding of disease predisposition in HLA-DR4+ individuals lends support to the notion that RA is caused by recognition of self-antigen [14].

The pathogenesis of scleral and corneal inflammation may be the same as that for the joint disease [15]. IgG antibody may be produced in response to an unknown antigenic stimulus by the cells associated with synovial tissue (and by analogy scleral or corneal collagen). The IgG antibody may be altered, leading to the development of autoantibodies and immune complexes with the abnormal IgG, and the subsequent deposition of immune complexes in the synovium (or sclera and limbus) [15]. These complexes activate the complement cascade that attracts neutrophils and macrophages. The corneal ulcers in patients with RA-associated PUK have been shown to have infiltrating APCs, mainly macrophages, with an activated phenotype (HLA-DR+) [16]. Upregulation of gene expression of pro-inflammatory cytokines TNF-α and IL-6 have also been reported in corneal keratocytes surrounding the ulcer [17], suggesting that corneal keratocytes, which may potentially serve as nonprofessional APCs, are also activated in this condition. These cytokines can cause MMP production causing collagenolytic corneal damage. Activated MMP-1 (the enzyme that hydrolyzes fibrillar type 1 collagen, the major component of corneal stroma) has been found in ulcerating corneas, presumably produced either by infiltrating macrophages or activated corneal keratocytes, along with reduced or absent tissue inhibitor of metalloproteinases [16]. Furthermore, accumulation of

MMP-9 in tears (produced by infiltrating granulocytes), and MMP-2 overexpression by cultured keratocytes from perforated corneas have been reported [18]. Activated MMP-2 and MMP-9 target type IV basement membrane collagen and may initiate perforation by breaching the corneal basement membranes (epithelial cell and Descemet's) [19]. Apparently O^- and NO^- may be generated by activated macrophages and neutrophils, as a result of immunological responses to pro-inflammatory cytokines, and these free radicals may activate MMPs, inactivate tissue inhibitors of metalloproteinases, and breach epithelial cell barriers if these cells were already the target of an inflammatory cell attack in systemic disease [18]. Given the evidence that corneal epithelial cell surface proteins may be targeted by circulating antibodies in RA patients [20], the authors suggest that once the corneal basement membranes have been disrupted by activated MMP-9/MMP-2, the corneal stroma may be freely invaded by macrophages which freely liberate matrix-degrading MMP-1 that causes PUK progression [18].

The presence of activated APCs, MMPs and pro-inflammatory cytokines in the cornea with PUK is an example where autoimmunity may cause breakdown of immune privilege in the cornea causing extensive corneal meltdown.

Cicatrizing Conjunctivitis

Having discussed the two common autoimmune diseases of the cornea, we now turn our attention to a spectrum of clinical disorders that causes conjunctival fibrosis and scar formation, collectively called chronic cicatrizing conjunctivitis (CCC). The list of autoimmune causes of CCC is exhaustive and include, among others, OCP, linear IgA disease, Stevens-Johnson syndrome and graft-versus-host disease. Although the conjunctiva is not an immune-privileged site per se, in many cases the end stage of CCC causes corneal scarring and hence may lead to blindness. We therefore discuss the immunopathogenesis of OCP below as a prototype CCC and the sequence of immune events ultimately affecting the immune-privileged cornea.

Ocular Cicatricial Pemphigoid

OCP is a chronic progressive inflammatory disease that causes bilateral progressive subconjunctival fibrosis eventuating in a blind scarred eye in untreated cases. It is characterized by autoantibodies, most commonly IgG, that bind to corneal epithelial basement membrane zone (BMZ) autoantigens, namely β4 protein of the α6β4 integrin [21] and epiligrin [22]. The autoantibody formation may be triggered in genetically predisposed individuals by environmental triggers such as ocular exposure to epinephrine, idoxuridine, and phospholine iodide [23]. The HLA-DQB1*0301 gene (DQw7) confers an increased genetic predisposition to OCP possibly by having a role in T cell recognition of basement membrane antigens, resulting in anti-BMZ autoantibody production [23]. Binding of autoantibody to the target autoantigen at the epithelial BMZ leads to the development of a type II hypersensitivity reaction involving complement activation, deposition and inflammatory cell infiltration [23]. The conjunctiva of OCP patients has been shown to be infiltrated with predominantly T cells (activated phenotype; surface IL-2 expression), with a 3-fold increase in the epithelium and a 20-fold increase within the substantia propria [24], along with an increased number of macrophages, dendritic cells and neutrophils [24].

The infiltrating macrophages and conjunctival fibroblasts have been implicated in subepithelial fibrosis, which is a key event in the extensive conjunctival cicatrization seen in this disease. Fibrogenic and angiogenic cytokines, such as TGF-β, platelet-derived growth factor, and basic fibroblast growth factor are produced by the conjunctival macrophages which leads to fibroblast migration and proliferation, as evident by the abnormally hyperproliferative conjunctival fibroblasts of patients with OCP [25]. These activated fibroblasts produce an abnormal new extracellular matrix and collagen, thus causing the subepithelial fibrosis that characterizes OCP [23].

Progression of subepithelial conjunctival fibrosis in OCP leads to the formation of symblepharon (fibrotic bands between palpebral and bulbar conjunctiva) and ankyloblepharon (fusion of the lower eyelid to the bulbar conjunctiva) resulting in restriction of ocular mobility. Scarring also causes trichiasis and distichiasis due to alterations in eyelash follicle orientation, and this together with severe dry eye due to scar-induced blockage of tear gland openings causes damage to the corneal epithelium. Advanced OCP is hence accompanied by blinding keratopathy, corneal neovascularization, pseudopterygium formation, and progressive thinning and perforation. Bacterial superinfection follows due to several factors including use of topical steroids, bandage contact lenses, chronic irritation due to trichiasis, meibomitis and lagophthalmos. OCP is an example of an immune-mediated disorder with the primary pathology in the conjunctiva with collateral damage to the neighboring cornea and adnexa as extensive cicatrization spills over into the neighboring structures.

Conclusion

Maintenance of ocular surface homeostasis is essential for corneal clarity and normal vision. Immune-mediated ocular surface disorders constitute a challenging and heterogeneous group of disorders, with a common end-stage denominator: loss of corneal transparency clinically, and loss of corneal immune privilege at the cellular and molecular levels. Whatever the inciting stimulus might be, once the immune system is challenged to mount an inflammatory attack against its own tissue, a vicious cycle ensues, ultimately resulting in compromise of the ocular surface integrity. Much needs to be explored regarding the exact immunopathogenesis of various ocular surface autoimmune diseases, which is fundamental to preventing blindness in these patients.

References

1 Foster CS, Streilein JW: Basic immunology; in Foster CS, Azar DT, Dohlman CH (eds): The Cornea. Scientific Foundations and Clinical Practice, ed 4. Philadelphia, Lippincott Williams & Wilkins, 2005, pp 59–102.

2 Hamrah P, Huq SO, Liu Y, Zhang Q, Dana MR: Corneal immunity is mediated by heterogeneous population of antigen-presenting cells. J Leukoc Biol 2003;74:172–178.

3 Foster CS: Mooren's ulcer; in Foster CS, Azar DT, Dohlman CH (eds): The Cornea. Scientific Foundations and Clinical Practice, ed 4. Philadelphia, Lippincott Williams & Wilkins, 2005, pp 551–557.

4 Gottsch JD, Liu SH: Cloning and expression of human corneal calgranulin C (CO-Ag). Curr Eye Res 1998;17:870–874.

5 Gottsch JD, Li Q, Ashraf F, O'Brien TP, Stark WJ, Liu SH: Cytokine-induced calgranulin C expression in keratocytes. Clin Immunol 1999;91:34–40.

6 Taylor CJ, Smith SI, Morgan CH, et al: HLA and Mooren's ulceration. Br J Ophthalmol 2000;84:72–75.

7 Xie H, Chen J, Zheng H, Li Y, Liu W: A histochemical and immunohistochemical study of cornea and adjacent bulbar conjunctiva in Mooren's ulcer (in Chinese). Yan Ke Xue Bao 2000;16:139–142.

8 Ye J, Chen J, Kim JC, Yao K: Bone marrow-derived cells are present in Mooren's ulcer. Ophthalmic Res 2004;36:151–155.

9 Wang Z, Chen J, Zheng H: Changes in local immune functions in Mooren's ulcer. Yan Ke Xue Bao 1996;12:33–35.

10 Murray PI, Rahi AH: Pathogenesis of Mooren's ulcer. Br J Ophthalmol 1984;68:182–187.

11 Martin NF, Stark WJ, Maumenee AE: Treatment of Mooren's and Mooren's-like ulcer by lamellar keratectomy: report of six eyes and literature review. Ophthalmic Surg 1987;18:564–569.

12 Griffith TS, Brunner T, Fletcher SM, Green DR, Ferguson TA: Fas ligand-induced apoptosis as a mechanism of immune privilege. Science 1995;270:1189–1192.

13 Weyand CM, Goronzy JJ: The molecular basis of rheumatoid arthritis. J Mol Med 1997;75: 772–785.

14 Stastny P: Association of the B-cell alloantigen DRw4 with rheumatoid arthritis. N Engl J Med 1978;298:869–871.

15 Friedlaender MH: Ocular allergy and immunology. J Allergy Clin Immunol 1979;63:51–60.

16 Riley GP, Harrall RL, Watson PG, Cawston TF, Hazleman BL: Collagenase (MMP-1) and TIMP-1 in destructive corneal disease associated with rheumatoid arthritis. Eye 1995;9:703–718.

17 Prada J, Noelle B, Baatz H, Hartmann C, Pleyer U: Tumor necrosis factor alpha and interleukin 6 gene expression in keratocytes from patients with rheumatoid corneal ulceration. Br J Ophthalmol 2003;87:548–550.

18 Smith VA, Rishmawi H, Hussein H, Easty DL: Tear film MMP accumulation and corneal disease. Br J Ophthalmol 2001;85:147–153.

19 Smith VA, Hoh HB, Easty DL: Role of ocular matrix metalloproteinases in peripheral ulcerative keratitis. Br J Ophthalmol 1999;83:1376–1383.

20 Reynolds I, John SL, Tullo AB, et al: Characterization of two corneal epithelium-derived antigens associated with vasculitis. Invest Ophthalmol Vis Sci 1998;39:2594–2601.
21 Kumari S, Bhol KC, Simmons RK, et al: Identification of ocular cicatricial pemphigoid antibody binding site(s) in human β4 integrin. Invest Ophthalmol Vis Sci 2001;42:379–385.
22 Hsu RC, Lazarova Z, Lee HG, Tung YC, Yu HS: Antiepiligrin cicatricial pemphigoid. J Am Acad Dermatol 2000;42:841–844.
23 Akpek EK, Ilhan-Sarac O: Cicatrizing conjunctivitis; in Foster CS, Azar DT, Dohlman CH (eds): The Cornea. Scientific Foundations and Clinical Practice, ed 4. Philadelphia, Lippincott Williams & Wilkins, 2005, pp 477–502.
24 Sacks EH, Jakobiec FA, Wieczorek R, Donnenfeld E, Perry H, Knowles DM Jr: Immunophenotypic analysis of the inflammatory infiltrate in ocular cicatricial pemphigoid. Further evidence for a T cell-mediated disease. Ophthalmology 1989;96:236–243.
25 Roat MI, Sossi G, Lo CY, Thoft RA: Hyperproliferation of conjunctival fibroblasts from patients with cicatricial pemphigoid. Arch Ophthalmol 1989;107:1064–1067.

Dr. M. Reza Dana
Schepens Eye Research Institute
Harvard Medical School, 20 Staniford Street
Boston, MA 02114 (USA)
Tel. +1 617 912 7404, Fax +1 617 912 0117, E-Mail dana@vision.eri.harvard.edu

Niederkorn JY, Kaplan HJ (eds): Immune Response and the Eye.
Chem Immunol Allergy. Basel, Karger, 2007, vol 92, pp 203–212

How Herpes Simplex Virus Type 1 Rescinds Corneal Privilege

Andrew J. Lepisto[a], *Gregory M. Frank*[b,d], *Robert L. Hendricks*[a–c]

Departments of [a]Immunology, [b]Ophthalmology, and [c]Molecular Genetics and Biochemistry, and [d]Graduate Program in Immunology, School of Medicine, University of Pittsburgh, Pittsburgh, Pa., USA

Abstract

Properties of the cornea such as a lack of blood and lymphatic vessels, a lack of professional antigen-presenting cells, and exposure to immunosuppressive factors in the aqueous humor contribute to a relative state of immune privilege. Ironically, corneal damage and the accompanying visual morbidity following herpes simplex virus type 1 (HSV-1) infection does not results from uncontrolled viral replication, but from an immunoinflammatory process referred to as herpes stromal keratitis (HSK). This review highlights changes in the immune-privileged status of the cornea following HSV-1 infection that contribute to HSK.

Role of T Cells

Good vision is critically dependent on the clarity of the cornea and other tissues that comprise the visual axis. Among the factors that contribute to corneal clarity is an optimal geometric arrangement of collagen fibrils in the corneal stroma, an absence of blood vessels, and a relative lack of hematopoietic cells within the corneal stroma. However, the angiogenesis and edema that typically accompany inflammatory responses can transiently disrupt corneal clarity through neovascularization and disorganization of collagen fibrils. Moreover, inflammatory mediators can effect changes in the keratocytes that produce the extracellular matrix of the corneal stroma, leading to scarring and permanent loss of vision. To avoid these causes of transient or permanent opacity, the cornea has adopted a variety of active and passive mechanisms to inhibit inflammation.

Most of our knowledge on the mechanisms that give rise to corneal immune privilege is derived from studies of corneal transplantation. Indeed, corneal grafts that are placed on an avascular corneal bed enjoy a very high rate of acceptance without the aid of tissue typing and systemic immunosuppression. Although our understanding of these mechanisms remains somewhat rudimentary, it appears that immune responses in the cornea are inhibited by immunosuppressive factors, including transforming growth factor-β (TGF-β), α-melanocyte-stimulating hormone, and Fas ligand (CD95L) expression on corneal cells. Additionally, the lack of blood and lymphatic vessels and antigen-presenting cells (APC) in the normal cornea limits antigen presentation to the immune system. Together, these features of the cornea inhibit immunoinflammatory reactions by limiting the afferent delivery of antigens from the cornea to the lymphoid organs and by neutralizing T cell effector mechanisms within the cornea.

Given the impressive array of anti-inflammatory mechanisms employed by the cornea, and its direct interface with the environment, one might predict that this tissue would frequently fall prey to a variety of environmental pathogens. This is clearly not the case. Moreover, when corneal infections do occur, immunopathology rather than immune deficiency is often the primary cause of the permanent tissue destruction associated with the infection. In this chapter we will discuss one such example involving infection of the cornea with herpes simplex virus type 1 (HSV-1), and the ensuing immunopathologic process that is referred to as herpes stromal keratitis (HSK). We will emphasize how many of the aforementioned aspects of corneal immune privilege are overcome during HSV-1 corneal infections, but will also document distinct differences in the way the immune system handles the virus in the cornea and other tissues.

HSV-1 corneal infection in mice causes a transient epithelial lesion, resulting from HSV-1 replication in and destruction of epithelial cells. These lesions typically heal within 1 week of infection concomitant with elimination of replicating virus from the cornea. The high regenerative capacity of the corneal epithelium permits rapid healing of these lesions with no permanent visual compromise. However, within a week of infection HSK develops in the corneal stroma and is characterized by neovascularization and corneal opacity.

While replicating in the corneal epithelium, HSV-1 gains access to the termini of sensory neurons and is transported by retrograde axonal transport to the neuronal nuclei within the ophthalmic branch of trigeminal ganglia. A brief period of viral replication occurs 2–8 days after corneal infection, followed by establishment of a latent infection. During latency, one or more copies of HSV-1 genome are retained in sensory neurons but no infectious virions are produced. Once latency is established, latent viral genomes are retained within neurons for the life of the individual. However, in some individuals, HSV-1 periodically reactivates from latency in a limited number of infected neurons, and virion components are transported down the nerve axons for assembly and release at the cornea. The recurrent disease experienced by certain individuals results not from re-infection from an external source but rather from reactivation of latent virus in sensory ganglia. Periodic shedding of virus in the cornea can give rise to recurrent bouts of HSK with progressive scarring and visual compromise.

Murine models have provided most of our current understanding of the immunologic involvement in HSK. HSK begins approximately 7 days after HSV-1 infection of mouse corneas, progresses through 21 days after infection, and corneal opacity and neovascularization persists at least through 40 days after infection. Seminal studies by Metcalf et al. [1] established that T cells play a critical role in HSK since T cell-deficient nude mice did not develop disease following corneal infection. Subsequent studies showed that CD4+ T cells orchestrated HSK following corneal infection of BALB/c mice with the RE strain of HSV-1 [2, 3]. Several studies have demonstrated that in HSV-1-infected corneas of BALB/c mice, CD4+ T cells greatly outnumber CD8+ T cells. The reason for the preferential infiltration or retention of CD4+ T cells in the cornea is not clear. Involvement of the corneal microenvironment is suggested by an equivalent infiltration of CD4+ and CD8+ T cells in the infected trigeminal ganglia of mice that exhibit a predominantly CD4+ T cell corneal infiltrate. Thus, even when corneal immune privilege is overcome, marked differences in the composition of the inflammatory infiltrate are observed.

Antigen Presentation

As noted above, corneal immune privilege is thought to derive in part from a lack of professional APCs in the cornea. Although macrophage-like cells have been described in the normal mouse cornea, most lack detectable major histocompatibility complex (MHC) class II and their APC function is questionable and untested [4]. The presence of CD11c-positive dendritic cells (DCs) in the normal cornea is contentious, and even when observed, these cells were found to be abnormal in that they lacked detectable MHC class II [4–6]. Thus, the concept that the normal cornea is devoid of professional APCs remains tenable despite the presence of a network of F4/80-expressing macrophage-like cells. However, the limbal region between the cornea and conjunctiva is heavily populated with Langerhans cells (a type of DC), and these cells have been shown to migrate into the central cornea following a variety of insults including HSV-1 infection [7]. Thus, any potential immune privilege that derives from a lack of corneal APCs is rapidly lost following HSV-1 infection. Studies from several laboratories have established an important role for corneal DCs in HSK. Studies in which Langerhans cells were eliminated from the surface of one eye by exposure to ultraviolet light followed by bilateral corneal infection revealed a role for DCs not only in the inductive phase of the T cell response in lymphoid organs, but also in the effector phase of the response within the infected cornea [7]. The latter conclusion was based on the observation that HSK developed normally in the eye with Langerhans cells, but failed to develop in the Langerhans cell-depleted cornea. Replicating HSV-1 was eliminated normally (by day 5 after infection) from the Langerhans cell-depleted corneas and the corneas appeared normal thereafter. Thus, the capacity of HSV-1 infection to induce DC migration into the cornea can rapidly convert immune privilege to immunopathology.

The possibility that DCs might influence the preferential accumulation of CD4+ over CD8+ T cells arose from studies comparing HSK induction by two different laboratory strains (KOS and RE) of HSV-1 in A/J mouse corneas [3]. HSK resulting from KOS HSV-1 infection had a low incidence (50%), tended to be milder, and was characterized by a predominantly mononuclear infiltrate in which CD8+ T cells outnumbered CD4+ T cells by a 2:1 ratio. In contrast, HSK induced by RE HSV-1 was characterized by a high incidence (80–100%), a predominantly neutrophilic infiltrate, and a preponderance of CD4+ over CD8+ T cells. An important observation in that study was that KOS HSV-1 was a poor inducer of Langerhans cell migration into the cornea. Moreover, when Langerhans cell migration into the cornea was induced prior to infection, KOS HSV-1 induced a high incidence of HSK that was characterized by a predominantly neutrophilic infiltrate in which CD4+ T cells greatly outnumbered CD8+ T cells. Though not conclusive, these findings suggest that the early infiltration of Langerhans cells into the HSV-1-infected cornea favors CD4+ T cell accumulation. The mechanism of this putative preferential attraction of CD4+ T cells by Langerhans cells is not clear but would likely involve a unique set of chemokines and/or homing receptors. These possibilities are currently under investigation.

Cytokines

Following RE HSV-1 corneal infection, CD4+ T cells regulate the migration of neutrophils into the cornea, resulting in damage to the corneal architecture and progressive opacity. Neutrophilic infiltration is regulated in part by the Th1 cytokines interleukin (IL)-2 and interferon (IFN)-γ, which are preferentially produced by CD4+ T cells in the infected cornea [8, 9]. How these cytokines regulate neutrophilic infiltration into the cornea is not entirely clear.

IFN-γ appears to favor neutrophilic extravasation from corneal blood vessels by increasing the expression of platelet endothelial cell adhesion molecule-1 on corneal blood vessels [9]. IL-2 appears to orchestrate neutrophil migration into the central cornea following extravasation into the perivascular space in the peripheral cornea and regulates their survival within the cornea [8].

In contrast to the detrimental role of Th1 cytokines in HSK, there is evidence that Th2 cytokines may play a role in the resolution of disease. For instance, IL-10 and IL-4 appear to be expressed during late stages of HSK concordant with diminishing inflammation [10]. Moreover, IL-10-deficient mice exhibit more severe HSK [11], and HSK is alleviated by topical administration of recombinant IL-10 [11, 12].

Other cytokines with known roles in HSK include tumor necrosis factor (TNF)-α, IL-1, IL-6, IL-12, and IL-17. TNF-α and IL-1 are pluripotent cytokines that influence several aspects of HSK [13], including the infiltration of neutrophils, MHC class II-positive DCs and T cells following HSV-1 infection. Their infiltration is directed by chemokines that are produced in response to IL-1 and TNF-α by both corneal cells (epithelial cells and stromal keratocytes) and by infiltrating bone marrow-derived cells. While these cells appear to be important in the initial elimination of the virus from the infected cornea, they may also create a microenvironment that is conducive to the subsequent development of HSK. Recent studies established that IL-17 is expressed in human corneas with HSK, and that the IL-17 receptor is constitutively expressed by corneal fibroblasts [14]. IL-17, TNF-α, and IFN-γ synergistically induced production of IL-6, the neutrophil-attracting chemokines IL-8 and macrophage inflammatory protein (MIP)-1α, and the DC chemokine MIP-3α by cultured human corneal fibroblasts. IL-17 also synergistically induces the production of the matrix metalloproteinase (MMP)-1 by corneal fibroblasts, which results in the degradation of the collagen matrix of the cornea. Thus, the combined effect of IFN-γ, TNF-α, and IL-17 might produce a microenvironment within the infected cornea that would favor the infiltration of neutrophils and DCs, and damage the corneal stroma architecture leading to opacity and ultimately to scarring during the remodeling process.

Angiogenesis

Among the important elements of corneal immune privilege is the avascular nature of the normal tissue. The lack of blood and lymphatic vessels limits access of the cornea to both the afferent and efferent limbs of the immune response. However, HSK is characterized by a rapid ingrowth of blood vessels into the previously avascular cornea, which appears to be a requisite step in the development of HSK in mice [15]. The proximal mediators of neovascularization in mouse corneas with HSK include vascular endothelial growth factor, angiogenic chemokines, and MMP-9. The production of vascular endothelial growth factor and MMP-9 is regulated by the cytokines IL-1 and IL-6 [16]. Neovascularization is also regulated through a balance of the angiogenic chemokines IL-8 and MIP-2, and angiostatic chemokines such as CXCL10.

Once the cornea is exposed to the efferent arm of the immune system through neovascularization, any immune privilege it previously enjoyed is rapidly lost. Thus, controlling angiogenesis in the cornea might be a useful approach to treating patients with necrotizing HSK. However, the complex interaction of angiogenic and angiostatic factors will render such approaches quite challenging.

Disease Models

At least three hypothetical mechanisms for the involvement of CD4+ T cells in HSK have been advanced and supported by published data. These include: (1) bystander activation of CD4+ T cells by cytokines that are produced in the cornea in response to infection [17–19]; (2) autoimmune reactivity to corneal tissue resulting from molecular mimicry by a viral protein [20–23], and (3) virus-specific activation. Bystander activation of CD4 T cells as a mechanism for HSK development is supported by data obtained from mice expressing a transgenic T cell receptor specific for ovalbumin. Although the CD4+ T cells of these mice were incapable of recognizing viral antigens, the mice developed severe corneal inflammation following HSV-1 infection. CD4 T cells expressing the ovalbumin-specific T cell receptor were recovered from the HSK lesions, and CD4+ T cell depletion abrogated inflammation [24]. These studies provided proof of principle that HSK-like disease can develop in the absence of HSV-1-reactive CD4+ T cells. However, important aspects of the model system employed prevent a direct assessment of the involvement of bystander activation in HSK. For instance, in the absence of an HSV-1-specific adaptive immune response, HSV-1 was never cleared from the corneas, and the mice died at a time when HSK has not fully developed. In fact, when HSV-1 replication was controlled in the corneas of these mice with antiviral drugs, inflammation did not develop [17]. Thus, while bystander activation of CD4+ T cells by cytokines produced in response to uncontrolled virus replication can induce inflammation similar to that seen in HSK, it appears that HSV-1-specific CD4+ T cells are required to trigger the inflammation when virus replication is controlled in corneas of immunologically normal mice. Nonetheless, it remains quite possible that bystander activation of CD4+ T cells contributes to chronic inflammation in HSK.

The potential involvement of an autoaggressive CD4+ T cell attack on corneal tissue during HSK was suggested by studies from the laboratory of Cantor [20–23]. In this model, the HSV-1 UL6 coat protein contains an epitope in common with a normal corneal protein. It is proposed that CD4+ T cells reactive to the UL6 epitope (and cross-reactive to a corneal protein) are generated during infection. These autoreactive CD4+ T cells then infiltrate the infected cornea and mediate tissue destruction. For an as yet unexplained reason, this autoimmune involvement in HSK occurred after corneal infection with the KOS but not the RE strain of HSV-1. Moreover, a study by another group failed to confirm cross-reactivity between the UL6 protein and corneal proteins or the capacity of UL6-specific CD4+ T cells to induce HSK [25]. Additionally, analysis of the specificity of T cell clones isolated from human corneas with HSK has not revealed reactivity to either UL6 or corneal antigens [26]. Thus, the involvement of molecular mimicry-induced autoimmunity in HSK remains contentious.

A view favored by our group and others is that HSV-1-specific CD4+ T cells play a requisite role in the induction and progression of HSK. HSV-1-specific CD4+ T cell clones have been isolated from human [26] and mouse [our unpublished observation] corneas at various stages of HSK. Perhaps the best evidence for an involvement of HSV-1-specific T cells in HSK came from studies in which mice were tolerized to HSV-1 antigens. Injection of HSV-1 into the ocular anterior chamber induces a deviant form of immunity referred to as anterior chamber-associated immune deviation [27]. Preferential inhibition of CD4+ T cell functions, such as delayed-type hypersensitivity and production of Th1 cytokines, characterizes this immune deviation [28]. Induction of cell-mediated immune tolerance of HSV-1 antigens at the time of HSV-1 corneal infection was found to protect the cornea from HSK [29].

Conclusion

It is somewhat ironic that within the immune-privileged cornea, immunopathology is the most devastating manifestation of HSV-1 infection. One might predict that the restrictions placed on the immune system within the cornea would instead result in uncontrolled viral cytopathology. Perhaps because the cornea imposes restrictions on the adaptive immune response, the innate immune system appears to operate effectively to eliminate HSV-1 from the cornea. Unfortunately, some of the key components of corneal immune privilege (e.g. lack of blood vessels and professional APCs) are altered during the course of viral elimination, setting the stage for subsequent immunopathology.

The resulting inflammation is a complex process. What drives the chronic inflammation is not clear. If HSV-1-specific CD4+ T cells drive the inflammation, what is the source of viral antigens? In the mouse model, HSV-1 is eliminated from the cornea by day 7 after infection but inflammation progresses through 21 days after infection and can persist for months. Do APCs that infiltrate the cornea during virus replication maintain antigen presentation for prolonged periods? Are undetectable levels of virus or viral antigens constantly or intermittently shed into the cornea from sensory neurons? Alternatively, does initial virus-specific T cell activation give way to persistent activation by cytokines or autoantigens? Although many such questions await answers, the available evidence suggests that immunology-based therapy is feasible. Despite the complex nature of HSK, it appears that individual modulation of certain components of the immunopathological process can dramatically reduce inflammation in the infected cornea. Neutralizing the Th1 cytokines IL-2 and IFN-γ [8, 9], inhibiting production of the chemokines MIP-1α and MIP-2 [30, 31], and blocking B7 [32] and 4-1BB [33] costimulation can each dramatically reduce inflammation in the infected cornea. Perhaps a combination of these treatments will be effective in reducing inflammation in corneas with HSK, and reestablish the immune-privileged nature of the tissue.

Acknowledgment

This work was supported by grants: RO1 EY010359 (R.L.H.), RO1 EY11850, P30-EY08098 (R.L.H.), and P30-EY02687 from the National Eye Institute, NIH, Bethesda, Md., USA; by an unrestricted research grant (R.L.H) from Research to Prevent Blindness, Inc., New York, N.Y., USA, and by a grant from the Eye and Ear Foundation of Pittsburgh, Pa., USA (R.L.H.).

References

1 Metcalf JF, Hamilton DS, Reichert RW: Herpetic keratitis in athymic (nude) mice. Infect Immun 1979;26:1164–1171.
2 Newell CK, Martin S, Sendele D, Mercadal CM, Rouse BT: Herpes simplex virus-induced stromal keratitis: role of T-lymphocyte subsets in immunopathology. J Virol 1989;63:769–775.
3 Hendricks RL, Tumpey TM: Contribution of virus and immune factors to herpes simplex virus type 1-induced corneal pathology. Invest Ophthalmol Vis Sci 1990;31:1929–1939.
4 Brissette-Storkus CS, Reynolds SA, Lepisto AJ, Hendricks RL: Identification of a novel macrophage population in the normal mouse corneal stroma. Invest Ophthalmol Vis Sci 2002;43:2264–2271.
5 Hamrah P, Liu Y, Zhang Q, Dana MR: The corneal stroma is endowed with a significant number of resident dendritic cells. Invest Ophthalmol Vis Sci 2003;44:581–589.
6 Hamrah P, Zhang Q, Liu Y, Dana MR: Novel characterization of MHC class II-negative population of resident corneal Langerhans cell-type dendritic cells. Invest Ophthalmol Vis Sci 2002;43:639–646.
7 Hendricks RL, Janowicz M, Tumpey TM: Critical role of corneal Langerhans cells in the CD4- but not CD8-mediated immunopathology in herpes simplex virus-1-infected mouse corneas. J Immunol 1992;148:2522–2529.

8 Tang Q, Chen W, Hendricks RL: Proinflammatory functions of IL-2 in herpes simplex virus corneal infection. J Immunol 1997;158:1275–1283.
9 Tang Q, Hendricks RL: Interferon gamma regulates platelet endothelial cell adhesion molecule 1 expression and neutrophil infiltration into herpes simplex virus-infected mouse corneas. J Exp Med 1996;184:1435–1447.
10 Babu JS, Kanangat S, Rouse BT: T cell cytokine mRNA expression during the course of the immunopathologic ocular disease herpetic stromal keratitis. J Immunol 1995;154:4822–4829.
11 Keadle TL, Stuart PM: Interleukin-10 (IL-10) ameliorates corneal disease in a mouse model of recurrent herpetic keratitis. Microb Pathog 2005;38:13–21.
12 Tumpey TM, Elner VM, Chen SH, Oakes JE, Lausch RN: Interleukin-10 treatment can suppress stromal keratitis induced by herpes simplex virus type 1. J Immunol 1994;153:2258–2265.
13 Keadle TL, Usui N, Laycock KA, Miller JK, Pepose JS, Stuart PM: IL-1 and TNF-alpha are important factors in the pathogenesis of murine recurrent herpetic stromal keratitis. Invest Ophthalmol Vis Sci 2000;41:96–102.
14 Maertzdorf J, Osterhaus AD, Verjans GM: IL-17 expression in human herpetic stromal keratitis: modulatory effects on chemokine production by corneal fibroblasts. J Immunol 2002;169: 5897–5903.
15 Zheng M, Deshpande S, Lee S, Ferrara N, Rouse BT: Contribution of vascular endothelial growth factor in the neovascularization process during the pathogenesis of herpetic stromal keratitis. J Virol 2001;75:9828–9835.
16 Biswas PS, Rouse BT: Early events in HSV keratitis – setting the stage for a blinding disease. Microbes Infect 2005;7:799–810.
17 Deshpande S, Zheng M, Lee S, Banerjee K, Gangappa S, Kumaraguru U, Rouse BT: Bystander activation involving T lymphocytes in herpetic stromal keratitis. J Immunol 2001;167:2902–2910.
18 Gangappa S, Deshpande SP, Rouse BT: Bystander activation of CD4+ T cells accounts for herpetic ocular lesions. Invest Ophthalmol Vis Sci 2000;41:453–459.
19 Gangappa S, Deshpande SP, Rouse BT: Bystander activation of CD4+ T cells can represent an exclusive means of immunopathology in a virus infection. Eur J Immunol 1999;29:3674–3682.
20 Panoutsakopoulou V, Sanchirico ME, Huster KM, Jansson M, Granucci F, Shim DJ, Wucherpfennig KW, Cantor H: Analysis of the relationship between viral infection and autoimmune disease. Immunity 2001;15:137–147.
21 Huster KM, Panoutsakopoulou V, Prince K, Sanchirico ME, Cantor H: T cell-dependent and -independent pathways to tissue destruction following herpes simplex virus-1 infection. Eur J Immunol 2002;32:1414–1419.
22 Zhao ZS, Granucci F, Yeh L, Schaffer PA, Cantor H: Molecular mimicry by herpes simplex virus-type 1: autoimmune disease after viral infection. Science 1998;279:1344–1347.
23 Avery AC, Zhao ZS, Rodriguez A, Bikoff EK, Soheilian M, Foster CS, Cantor H: Resistance to herpes stromal keratitis conferred by an IgG2a-derived peptide. Nature 1995;376:431–433.
24 Gangappa S, Babu JS, Thomas J, Daheshia M, Rouse BT: Virus-induced immunoinflammatory lesions in the absence of viral antigen recognition. J Immunol 1998;161:4289–4300.
25 Deshpande SP, Lee S, Zheng M, Song B, Knipe D, Kapp JA, Rouse BT: Herpes simplex virus-induced keratitis: evaluation of the role of molecular mimicry in lesion pathogenesis. J Virol 2001;75:3077–3088.
26 Verjans GM, Remeijer L, Mooy CM, Osterhaus AD: Herpes simplex virus-specific T cells infiltrate the cornea of patients with herpetic stromal keratitis: no evidence for autoreactive T cells. Invest Ophthalmol Vis Sci 2000;41:2607–2612.
27 Whittum JA, Niederkorn JY, McCulley JP, Streilein JW: Intracameral inoculation of herpes simplex virus type I induces anterior chamber associated immune deviation. Curr Eye Res 1983;2:691–697.
28 Streilein JW: Immune regulation and the eye: a dangerous compromise. FASEB J 1987;1:199–208.
29 Ksander BR, Hendricks RL: Cell-mediated immune tolerance to HSV-1 antigens associated with reduced susceptibility to HSV-1 corneal lesions. Invest Ophthalmol Vis Sci 1987;28:1986–1993.
30 Tumpey TM, Fenton R, Molesworth-Kenyon S, Oakes JE, Lausch RN: Role for macrophage inflammatory protein 2 (MIP-2), MIP-1α, and interleukin-1α in the delayed-type hypersensitivity response to viral antigen. J Virol 2002;76:8050–8057.

31 Yan XT, Tumpey TM, Kunkel SL, Oakes JE, Lausch RN: Role of MIP-2 in neutrophil migration and tissue injury in the herpes simplex virus-1-infected cornea. Invest Ophthalmol Vis Sci 1998;39:1854–1862.
32 Chen H, Hendricks RL: B7 costimulatory requirements of T cells at an inflammatory site. J Immunol 1998;160:5045–5052.
33 Seo SK, Park HY, Choi JH, Kim WY, Kim YH, Jung HW, Kwon B, Lee HW, Kwon BS: Blocking 4-1BB/4-1BB ligand interactions prevents herpetic stromal keratitis. J Immunol 2003;171:576–583.

Dr. Robert L. Hendricks
Eye and Ear Institute, University of Pittsburgh
Room 922, 203 Lothrop Street
Pittsburgh, PA 15213 (USA)
Tel. +1 412 647 5754, Fax +1 412 647 5880, E-Mail hendricksrr@msx.upmc.edu

Niederkorn JY, Kaplan HJ (eds): Immune Response and the Eye.
Chem Immunol Allergy. Basel, Karger, 2007, vol 92, pp 213–220

Intraocular Diseases – Anterior Uveitis

Nalini S. Bora[a], *Henry J. Kaplan*[b]

[a]Department of Ophthalmology, Jones Eye Institute, University of Arkansas for Medical Sciences, Little Rock, Ark., [b]Department of Ophthalmology and Visual Science, Kentucky Lions Eye Center, University of Louisville, Louisville, Ky., USA

Abstract

Uveitis is a general term for inflammatory disorders of the uveal tract and encompasses a wide range of underlying etiologies. It may be idiopathic, associated with systemic diseases or result from a variety of infectious agents. Uveitis is responsible for over 2.8% of blindness in the United States. Each year, 17.6% of active uveitis patients experience a transient or permanent loss of vision. Anterior uveitis (AU), which refers to inflammation within the anterior segment of the eye, is the most common form of uveitis. Experimental autoimmune AU (EAAU) is an organ-specific autoimmune disease of the eye, which serves as an animal model of idiopathic human AU. Recently, type I collagen was identified as the target autoantigen in EAAU. Thus, human AU may be an example of autoimmunity to local ocular collagen.

Uveitis

Uveitis is a general term for inflammatory disorders of the uveal tract and encompasses a wide range of underlying etiologies. It may be idiopathic, associated with systemic diseases or result from a variety of infectious agents. Until recently, although uveitis was proposed to be frequently an autoimmune disease, repeated attempts to induce experimental uveitis with uveal antigens met with failure. Additionally, the early work of Wacker et al. [1] and Wacker [2], in which it was demonstrated that retinal antigens were effective immunopathogens, unfortunately focused research on the cause of autoimmune anterior uveitis (AU) to novel retinal antigens instead of iris and ciliary body (CB) antigens. With the discovery of the type I collagen α-2 chain as the target of the immune response in experimental autoimmune AU (EAAU) in rodents [3], the suspicion that acute AU was an autoimmune collagen disease has been confirmed.

Epidemiology and Classification of Uveitis

Uveitis is responsible for over 2.8% of blindness in the United States. Each year, 17.6% of active uveitis patients experience a transient or permanent loss of vision, with 12.5% developing glaucoma [4]. The incidence and prevalence of uveitis has been difficult to determine because the disease is not reportable to the health authorities and is treated in an ambulatory setting. More recently, the epidemiology of the disease in the US has been affected by the aging of the population, racial diversity and an increasing incidence of autoimmune disease. Historically, an incidence rate of 17/100,000 person-years and a prevalence ratio of 204/100,000 over a 10-year period has been reported [5]. However, a recent report from the Northern California Epidemiology of Uveitis Study [6] suggested a higher disease rate for the older population, particularly women, with a higher incidence of chronic disease. Recurrence rates after an initial episode of uveitis in Great Britain showed that 11.3% of patients had at least one recurrence within 5 years, with 2.5% experiencing a second recurrence during this period [7].

In an attempt to more precisely clarify this group of diseases, the International Uveitis Study Group proposed both an anatomic and etiologic classification of uveitis, as well as other descriptive terms of the disease [8]. The location of the primary focus of inflammation, taking into account spillover either to the anterior or posterior segment of the eye, is used to describe the inflammation as anterior (e.g. iritis and iridocyclitis), intermediate (e.g. pars planitis), posterior (e.g. toxoplasmosis) or panuveitis (e.g. diffuse). Other ocular on non-ocular findings do not influence the anatomic classification of uveitis. Important descriptive terms to accurately describe uveitis include the duration of the disease – i.e. acute, <3 months in duration, or chronic, >3 months in duration – and the recurrence of the disease – i.e. with multiple episodes; the term *recurrence* is used to signal the return of intraocular inflammation after a period of quiescence.

Uveitis is etiologically classified as either infectious or non-infectious. The predominant form of the disease is felt to be non-infectious – specifically, autoimmune for AU. HLA-B27-associated acute AU is the most common form of non-infectious uveitis that occurs in genetically predisposed individuals. This allele is frequently associated with acute AU in conjunction with a spondyloarthropathy, such as anklyosing spondylitis. Although the B27 AU is felt to be autoimmune in origin, there is some evidence that a microbial trigger for the disease may exist – specifically, certain species of *Klebsiella*, *Salmonella*, *Shigella*, *Yersinia* and *Chlamydia trachomatis* have been implicated [9]. This has recently focused attention on the role of Toll-like receptors (TLRs) within the eye and the pathogen-associated molecular patterns on these and other microorganisms [10]. For example, the resistance of C3H/HeN mice to endotoxin-induced uveitis (EIU) by lipopolysaccharide (LPS) resides in a point mutation within the coding region of the Tlr4 gene, which results in a functional disruption of Tlr4 signalling [11, 12].

Infectious causes of uveitis include viruses, bacteria, protozoa, parasites and rickettsiae. Typical organisms involve *Toxoplasma gondii*, *Histoplasma capsulatum*, *Toxocara canis*, cytomegalovirus, *Borrelia burgdorferi*, and *Mycobacterium tuberculosis*, for example. Most recently, a presumed viral etiology (i.e. rubella) for a form of AU, namely Fuchs heterochromic cyclitis, has been reported [13]. There is a lingering suspicion that many cases of AU are the result of infection with a pathogen that has not been recognized or is difficult to identify.

Anterior Uveitis

As mentioned, AU is a term which refers to inflammation within the anterior segment of the eye and can be further subdivided anatomically into either iritis and/or iridocyclitis. It is the most common form of uveitis and accounts for approximately 75% of cases. Inflammation occurs in either the iris or the CB, with spillover of vitreous inflammatory cells into the space behind the lens. Retinal involvement is not a component of AU [14, 15]. A single episode of AU does not cause permanent visual loss. It may be uncomfortable for the patient but rarely results in significant visual damage. However, it is the recurrent nature of many of the forms of AU, which ultimately results in the loss of vision secondary to cataract, cystoid macular edema, or glaucoma [14, 15]. The major signs of AU are keratitic precipitates, as well as inflammatory cells and protein flare within the aqueous humor. Most of the disorders associated with AU are not differentiated by the clinical appearance of inflammation within the anterior chamber (AC), but rather by their associated systemic findings – e.g. ankylosing spondylitis, juvenile rheumatoid arthritis, and Kawasaki syndrome. However, the most common form of AU is of unknown (i.e. idiopathic) etiology [6].

Animal Models of Uveitis

Several animal models of uveitis have been reported in the literature [1, 16–38]. The most studied model of intraocular inflammation is experimental autoimmune uveoretinitis (EAU). In EAU, the disease is induced in inbred rodents with various retinal proteins, such as retinal soluble antigen, interphotoreceptor retinoid binding protein, rhodopsin or phosducin [1, 18, 19].

Unfortunately, EAU induced by soluble retinal proteins does not have the clinical characteristics of EAAU. Although the severity of EAU can be altered by the dose of retinal protein used for sensitization, as well as the accompanying adjuvant, the inflammation produced is primarily confined to the posterior segment of the eye [1, 18, 19].

Animal Models of Anterior Uveitis

EIU and EAAU serve as the most frequently studied animal models of AU.

Endotoxin Induced Uveitis

EIU is an animal model of acute AU [22–25]. EIU can be induced in rodents, rabbits and guinea pigs and is characterized by leakage of proteins and infiltration of polymorphonuclear cells into the AC of the eye. The inflammation peaks 24 h after the endotoxin injection and resolves by 48 h [22–25].

EIU can be induced by local or systemic injection of endotoxin. Lipopolysaccharide is a major cell wall component of Gram-negative bacteria and is implicated in their uveitogenicity in EIU. Several factors including E and P selectins have been reported to play an important role in EIU [39]. Tlr4 has been shown to be expressed in the anterior uveal tract and is believed to be responsible for the sensitivity of the iris and CB to bacterial endotoxin, as observed in animal models of EIU [40].

Collagen-Induced Anterior Uveitis – Experimental Autoimmune Anterior Uveitis

EAAU is an organ-specific autoimmune disease of the eye, which serves as an animal model of idiopathic human AAU [3, 28–38]. It was originally described by Broekhuyse et al. [28] in 1991. Bora et al. [33] have extensively characterized this model and have shown that severe inflammation occurs in the anterior segment of the eye of Lewis rats after the foot pad injection of the antigen isolated from bovine iris and CB [3, 33, 34, 36–38]. In EAAU there is no damage to the retina. Thus, EAAU is representative of human AAU in contrast to EAU. EAAU is characterized histologically by lymphocytic infiltration in the iris and CB. Antigen-specific CD4+ T cells can adoptively transfer disease into naïve syngeneic recipients and are the predominant inflammatory cells within the uvea [3, 37]. Study of the cytokine profile of the host during EAAU suggests that the inflammation is mediated by both Th1- and Th2-type CD4+ T cells [38].

Recently, the pathogenic antigen in EAAU has been purified to homogeneity by Bora et al. [3]. The uveitogenic antigen is a 22-kDa fragment of bovine type I collagen α-2 chain and was referred to as CI-α2 (22 kDa) in this report. This antigen was pathogenic only when CI-α2 chain underwent proteolysis and if the bound carbohydrates were intact. Thus, it was suggested that the pathogenic antigen in EAAU is tissue specific because the peptide sequence and/or the posttranslational modification of CI-α2 is novel within the eye. Although human AU has been historically characterized as a collagen disease [41], this was the first time collagen was identified as the target autoantigen in uveitis. It has been suggested that local ocular disease involving collagen may occur without systemic disease – namely, without involvement of systemic collagen [3]. Idiopathic AAU may be an example of autoimmunity to local ocular collagen.

Experimental Melanin Induced Uveitis (EMIU)

Chan et al. [32] and Broekhuyse et al. [35] proposed the term experimental melanin protein-induced uveitis (EMIU) to replace the previous term EAAU for their rodent model of intraocular inflammation. Although this disease, EMIU, is induced by sensitization to a melanin-associated antigen derived from choroid, it is different from EAAU, which is produced by immunization with the melanin-insoluble fraction of the iris/CB. Specifically, EAAU is predominantly AU (i.e. iritis) with mild choroiditis [3, 33, 34, 36–38], whereas EMIU is a panuveitis associated with a severe choroiditis, as well as an iritis [32, 35]. The human disease, AAU, most closely resembles EAAU, while panuveitis is more like EMIU. Further evidence of the difference in both animal disease models is the spontaneous recurrence which is observed in EMIU within 1 week of resolution [32], whereas EAAU is not associated with recurrent disease unless the host is reexposed to the pathogenic antigen [33].

Tolerance Induction for the Treatment of Anterior Uveitis

The AC of the eye is an immune-privileged site [42]. The immune privilege of the AC has been shown to be the result of a number of protective mechanisms including the immunosuppressive properties of ocular cells and immunosuppressive factors in ocular fluid [42]. AC-associated immune deviation [43], initially described by Kaplan and Streilein [44, 45] as F1 lymphocyte immune deviation, refers to the deviant systemic immune response resulting in the generation of antigen-specific suppressor T cells and suppression of delayed-type hypersensitivity after the introduction of antigen into the AC of the eye. The clinical importance of AC-associated immune deviation is unknown; however, animals immunized through the AC with retinal autoantigens (e.g. S-antigen or interphotoreceptor retinoid binding protein) are protected from experimental autoimmune uveitis [46, 47]. Suppression of immunological responsiveness by single or multiple doses of autoantigens via oral, intranasal and intravenous routes has been demonstrated to suppress uveitis in rodent models [48–51].

References

1 Wacker WB, Donoso LA, Kalsow CM, Yankeelov JA Jr, Organisciack DT: Experimental allergic uveitis. Isolation, characterization and localization of a soluble uveitopathogenic antigen from the bovine retina. J Immunol 1977;119:1949–1958.

2 Wacker WB: Experimental allergic uveitis. Investigations of retinal autoimmunity and the immunopathologic responses evoked. Invest Ophthalmol Vis Sci 1991;32:3119–3129.

3 Bora NS, Sohn JH, Kang SG, Cruz JM, Nishihori H, Suk HJ, Wang Y, Kaplan HJ, Bora PS: Type I collagen is the autoantigen in experimental autoimmune anterior uveitis. J Immunol 2004;172: 7086–7094.

4 Nussenblatt RB: The natural history of uveitis. Int Ophthalmol 1990;14:303–308.

5 Darrell RW, Wagener HP, Kurland LT: Epidemiology of uveitis: incidence and prevalence in a small urban community. Arch Ophthalmol 1962;68:502–514.

6 Gritz DC, Wong IG: Incidence and prevalence of uveitis in Northern California: the Northern California Epidemiology of Uveitis Study. Ophthalmology 2004;111:491–500.

7 Knox EG, Mayho A, Cant W, Truelove P: Iridocyclitis: incidence, distribution and health service usage. Community Med 1980;2:97–101.

8 Bloch-Michel E, Nussenblatt RB: International Uveitis Study Group recommendations for the evaluation of intraocular inflammatory disease. Am J Ophthalmol 1987;103:234–235.

9 Chang JH, McCluskey PJ, Wakefield D: Acute anterior uveitis and HLA-B27. Surv Ophthalmol 2005;50:364–388.

10 Takeda K, Akira S: Toll-like receptors in innate immunity. Int Immunol 2005;17:1–14.

11 Poltorak A, He X, Smirnova I, Liu MY, van Huffel C, Du X, Birdwell D, Alejos E, Silva M, Galanos C, Freudenberg M, Ricciardi-Castagnoli P, Layton B, Beutler B: Defective LPS signaling in C3H/HeJ and C57BL/10ScCr mice: mutations in Tlr4 gene. Science 1998;282: 2085–2088.

12 Li Q, Peng B, Whitcup SM, Jang SU, Chan CC: Endotoxin induced uveitis in the mouse: susceptibility and genetic control. Exp Eye Res 1995;61:629–632.

13 de Groot-Mijnes JDF, de Visser L, Rothova A, Schuller M, van Loon AM, Weersink AJL: Rubella virus is associated with Fuchs heterochromic iridocyclitis. Am J Ophthalmol 2006;141:212–214.

14 Nussenblatt RB, Whitcup SM, Palestine AG: Uveitis: Fundamentals and Clinical Practice. St. Louis, Mosby, 1996, p 413.

15 Wakefield D, Dunlop I, McClusky PJ, Penny R: Uveitis: aetiology and disease associations in an Australian population. Aust NZ J Ophthalmol 1986;14:181–187.

16 Caspi RR: Basic mechanisms in immune-mediated uveitic disease; in Lightman SL (ed): Immunology of Eye Disease. Lancaster, Kluwer, 1989, pp 61–86.

17 Caspi RR: Immunogenetic aspects of clinical and experimental uveitis. Reg Immunol 1992;4: 321–330.

18 Gery I, Wiggert B, Redmond RM, Kuwabara T, Crawford MA, Vistica BP, Chader GJ: Uveoretinitis and pinealitis induced by immunization with interphotoreceptor retinoid-binding protein. Invest Ophthalmol Vis Sci 1986;27:1296–1300.

19 Schalken JJ, Winkens HJ, Van Vugt AH, Bovee-Geurts PHM, deGrip WJ, Broekhuyse RM: Rhodopsin-induced experimental autoimmune uveoretinitis: dose-dependent clinicopathological features. Exp Eye Res 1988;47:135–145.
20 Donoso LA, Dua HS, Forrester JV, Lee RH: Immunogenicity of a retinal photoreceptor cell protein, phosducin. Invest Ophthalmol Vis Sci 1993;34:1476.
21 Ichikawa T, Taguchi O, Takahashi T, Ikeda H, Takeuchi M, Tanaka T, Usui M, Nishizuka Y: Spontaneous development of autoimmune uveoretinitis in nude mice following reconstitution with embryonic rat thymus. Clin Exp Immunol 1991;86:112–117.
22 Rosenbaum JT, McDevitt HO, Guss RB, Egbert PR: Endotoxin-induced uveitis in rats as a model for human disease. Nature 1980;286:611–613.
23 Bhattacherjee P, Williams RN, Eakins KE: An evaluation of ocular inflammation following the injection of bacterial endotoxin into the rat foot pad. Invest Ophthalmol Vis Sci 1983;24:196–202.
24 Okumura A, Mochizuki M: Endotoxin-induced uveitis in rats: morphological and biochemical study. Jpn J Ophthalmol 1988;32:457–465.
25 Herbort CP, Chan CC, Nussenblatt RB: Endotoxin-induced uveitis in the rat: a hypothesis for preferential involvement of the anterior uvea. Curr Eye Res 1990;9:119–124.
26 Fujino Y, Hum QL, Hikita N, Nussenblatt RB, Gery I, Chan CC: Immunopathology of experimental autoimmune uveoretinitis in primates. Autoimmunity 1992;13:303–309.
27 Rao NA, Wacker WB, Marak GE Jr: Experimental allergic uveitis: clinicopathologic features associated with varying doses of S antigen. Arch Ophthalmol 1979;97:1954–1958.
28 Broekhuyse RM, Kuhlmann ED, Winkens HJ, Van Vugt AH: Experimental autoimmune anterior uveitis (EAAU), a new form of experimental uveitis. I. Induction by a detergent-insoluble, intrinsic protein fraction of the retina pigment epithelium. Exp Eye Res 1991;52:465–474.
29 Broekhuyse RM, Kuhlmann ED, Winkens HJ: Experimental autoimmune anterior uveitis (EAAU). II. Dose-dependent induction and adoptive transfer using a melanin-bound antigen of the retina pigment epithelium. Exp Eye Res 1992;55:401–411.
30 Broekhuyse RM, Kuhlmann ED, Winkens HJ: Experimental autoimmune anterior uveitis (EAAU). III. Induction by immunization with purified uveal and skin melanins. Exp Eye Res 1993;56:575–583.
31 Broekhuyse RM, Kuhlmann ED: Experimental autoimmune anterior uveitis. The preparation of uveitogenic ocular melanin. Invest Ophthalmol Vis Sci 1993;34:698–700.
32 Chan CC, Hikita N, Dastgheib K, Whitcup SM, Gery I, Nussenblatt RB: Experimental melanin-protein-induced uveitis in the Lewis rat: immunopathologic processes. Ophthalmology 1994;101: 1275–1280.
33 Bora NS, Kim MC, Kabeer NH, Simpson SC, Tandhasetti MT, Cirrito TP, Kaplan AD, Kaplan HJ: Experimental autoimmune anterior uveitis: induction with melanin-associated antigen from the iris and ciliary body. Invest Ophthalmol Vis Sci 1995;36:1056–1066.
34 Kim MC, Kabeer NH, Tandhasetti MT, Kaplan HJ, Bora NS: Immunohistochemical studies on melanin associated antigen (MAA) induced experimental autoimmune anterior uveitis (EAAU). Curr Eye Res 1995;14:703–710.
35 Broekhuyse RM, Winkens HJ, Kuhlmann ED: Intraperitoneally injected melanin is highly uveitogenic. Exp Eye Res 1996;62:199–200.
36 Simpson SC, Kaplan HJ, Bora NS: Uveitogenic proteins isolated from bovine iris and ciliary body. Eye 1997;11:206–208.
37 Bora NS, Woon MD, Tandhasetti MT, Cirrito TP, Kaplan HJ: Induction of experimental autoimmune anterior uveitis (EAAU) by a self-antigen: melanin complex without adjuvant. Invest Ophthalmol Vis Sci 1997;38:2171–2175.
38 Woon MD, Kaplan HJ, Bora NS: Kinetics of cytokine production in experimental autoimmune anterior uveitis (EAAU). Curr Eye Res 1998;17:955–961.
39 Whitcup SM, Kozhich AT, Lobanoff M, Wolitzky BM, Chan CC: Blocking both E-selectin and P-selectin inhibits endotoxin-induced leukocyte infiltration into the eye. Clin Immunol Immunopathol 1997;83:45–52.
40 Brito BE, Zamora DO, Bonnah RA, Pan Y, Planck SR, Rosenbaum JT: Toll-like receptor 4 and CD14 expression in human ciliary body and TLR-4 in human iris endothelial cells. Exp Eye Res 2004;79:203–208.

41 Woods AC: Uveitis associated with collagen disease; in Endogenous Inflammation of the Uveal Tract. Baltimore, Williams & Wilkins, 1992, p 275.
42 Streilein JW: Immunologic privilege of the eye. Springer Semin Immunopathol 1999;21:95–111.
43 Streilein JW, Niederkorn JY: Induction of anterior chamber-associated immune deviation requires an intact, functional spleen. J Exp Med 1981;153:1058–1067.
44 Kaplan HJ, Streilein JW: Immune response to immunization via the anterior chamber of the eye. I. F1-lymphocyte-induced immune deviation. J Immunol 1977;118:809–814.
45 Kaplan HJ, Streilein JW: Immune response to immunization via the anterior chamber of the eye. II. An analysis of F1 lymphocyte-induced immune deviation. J Immunol 1978;120:689–693.
46 Roberge FG, De Kozak Y, Utsumi T, Faure JP, Nussenblatt RB: Immune response to intraocular injection of retinal S-antigen in adjuvant. Graefes Arch Clin Exp Ophthalmol 1989;227:67–71.
47 Hara Y, Capsi RR, Wiggert B, Chan CC, Streilein JW: Use of ACAID to suppress interphotoreceptor retinoid binding protein-induced experimental autoimmune uveitis. Curr Eye Res 1992; 11(suppl):97–100.
48 Thurau SR, Chan CC, Suh E, Nussenblatt RB: Induction of oral tolerance to S-antigen induced experimental autoimmune uveitis by a uveitogenic 20mer peptide. J Autoimmun 1991;4:507–516.
49 Nussenblatt RB, Caspi RR, Mahdi R, Chan CC, Roberge F, Lider O, Weiner HL: Inhibition of S-antigen induced experimental autoimmune uveoretinitis by oral induction of tolerance with S-antigen. J Immunol 1990;144:1689–1695.
50 Sasamoto Y, Kawano YI, Bouligny R, Wiggert B, Chader GJ, Gery I: Immunomodulation of experimental autoimmune uveoretinitis by intravenous injection of uveitogenic peptides. Invest Ophthalmol Vis Sci 1992;33:2641–2649.
51 Dua HS, Abrams MS, Barrett JA, Donoso LA: The effect of retinal autoantigens and their peptides on the inhibition of experimental autoimmune uveitis. Eye 1992;6:447–452.

Dr. Nalini S. Bora
Department of Ophthalmology, Pat and Willard Walker Eye Research Center
Jones Eye Institute, University of Arkansas for Medical Sciences
4301 West Markham, 523
Little Rock, AR 72205–7199 (USA)
Tel. +1 501 686 8293, Fax +1 501 686 8316, E-Mail NBora@UAMS.edu

Niederkorn JY, Kaplan HJ (eds): Immune Response and the Eye.
Chem Immunol Allergy. Basel, Karger, 2007, vol 92, pp 221–227

Glaucoma

Gülgün Tezel[a], *Martin B. Wax*[b]

[a]Kentucky Lions Eye Center, University of Louisville School of Medicine, Louisville, Ky., [b]Alcon Research Ltd., Fort Worth, Tex. and University of Texas, Southwestern Medical Center, Dallas, Tex., USA

Abstract

Glaucoma is a chronic neurodegenerative disease of the optic nerve, in which apoptosis of retinal ganglion cells (RGCs) and progressive loss of optic nerve axons result in structural and functional deficits in glaucoma patients. This neurodegenerative disease is indeed a leading cause of blindness in the world. The glaucomatous neurodegenerative environment has been associated with the activation of multiple pathogenic mechanisms for RGC death and axon degeneration. Growing evidence obtained from clinical and experimental studies over the last decade also strongly suggests the involvement of the immune system in this neurodegenerative process. Paradoxically, the roles of the immune system in glaucoma have been described as either neuroprotective or neurodestructive. A balance between beneficial immunity and harmful autoimmune neurodegeneration may ultimately determine the fate of RGCs in response to various stressors in glaucomatous eyes. Based on clinical data in humans, it has been proposed that one form of glaucoma may be an autoimmune neuropathy, in which an individual's immune response facilitates a somatic and/or axonal degeneration of RGCs by the very system which normally serves to protect it against tissue stress.

Aberrant T Cell Immunity

Growing evidence supports an aberrant activity of the immune system in glaucoma patients [1–3]. In fact, glaucomatous injury sites, namely the retina and the optic nerve, are 'immune privileged' as are other tissues in the central nervous system (CNS). This requires the deletion and active regulation of immune responses for the control of potentially damaging and sight-threatening autoimmune diseases [4, 5]. Similar to the anterior segment of the eye [6], apoptotic elimination of T cells is likely an essential protective mechanism to prevent inflammation and antigen encounter in the retina and optic nerve.

Despite immune privilege, however, autoreactive T cells are able to enter normal, uninjured brain with an intact blood-brain barrier [7] as part of the constitutive immune surveillance [8]. Although there is no evidence of T cell accumulation in the retina or optic nerve head tissues of glaucomatous eyes, which may be due to the transitory nature of sentinel T cells, episodic disruptions of the blood-eye barrier may facilitate their access into these tissues. The site-specific stromal recruitment of T cells may initially play an important role as a protective mechanism, since it allows early contact of the immune system with cellular debris, destruction of damaged cells, and the removal of pathogenic agents from the CNS. This elicits what has been called 'protective immunity', in which the recruited T cells mediate the protection of neurons from degenerative conditions by providing a source of cytokines, including IFN-γ and possibly neurotrophins [9–11]. Protective immunity has been suggested to occur as a homeostatic response to injury to reduce the secondary degeneration of retinal ganglion cells (RGCs). This has been induced experimentally in rodents by active or passive immunization with self-antigens [12, 13].

While T cell-mediated immune responses may initially be beneficial and even necessary to optimally limit neurodegeneration as evidenced in rodents, compelling evidence in humans obtained during the past decade suggests the conversion of protective immunity or self-limited inflammatory responses into the chronic autoimmune neurodegeneration seen in glaucoma. Despite the neuroprotective features of the immune system, an autoimmune component, resulting from a failure to properly control an aberrant, stress-induced immune response, likely accompanies the progression of neurodegeneration in a cohort of glaucoma patients. This occurs primarily in glaucoma patients in whom the intraocular pressure is in the 'normal' range (i.e. so-called 'normal pressure' or 'low tension' glaucoma). The presentation of neuronal antigens to the immune system may initiate further immune responses followed by the expansion and secondary recruitment of circulating, pathogenic T cells that may lead to antigen-mediated neurotoxicity through an 'autoimmune neurodegenerative disease'.

Support for such a T cell-mediated component of the neurodegenerative immune response in glaucoma is evidenced by abnormal T cell subsets in many glaucoma patients [14]. Recent experimental studies have also provided evidence that antigen-stimulated T cells may directly be cytotoxic to RGCs, mostly through the Fas/Fas ligand-dependent pathway. Although retinal microglia are involved in the apoptotic elimination of T cells from the retina and optic nerve head, similarly via Fas/Fas ligand interactions, RGCs progressively undergo apoptosis in antigen-immunized animals, which results in a pattern of neuronal damage similar to human glaucoma [Tezel and Wax, unpublished data]. These data suggest that T cell-mediated neurodegeneration not only depends on aberrant activation of autoreactive T cells but may also reflect a dysfunction in the apoptotic termination of the T cell response in the retina and a loss of immune privilege in this site.

Humoral Immune Response

The evidence that the humoral immune response also favors the onset and/or progression of neurodegeneration in some glaucoma patients is found in studies of autoantibodies in glaucoma patient sera or tissues and studies of autoantibody-mediated toxicity to RGCs in experimental models. For example, there is an increased prevalence of monoclonal gammopathy [15] and elevated serum titers of autoantibodies to many optic nerve [16] and retinal antigens [17–20] in patients with glaucoma. There is also evidence of immune globulin deposition in the glaucomatous retina [21]. It has been proposed that peripapillary chorioretinal atrophy, commonly present in glaucomatous eyes [22], may be the site for a facilitated access of serum antibodies to the retina [21], since the blood-retina barrier is disrupted in these areas. Increased autoantibodies in the serum of glaucoma patients include those to heat shock proteins, e.g. hsp60, hsp27, and α-crystallins [18, 19]. The increased titers of serum autoantibodies may reflect a response to tissue stress and/or injury in glaucomatous eyes. However, direct application of antibodies against small heat shock proteins to retinal neurons, at similar concentrations to that found in the serum of many glaucoma patients, has resulted in the apoptotic death of these neurons, in vitro and ex vivo [19, 23, 24]. This apoptotic effect has been found to be associated with the diminished protective abilities of native heat shock proteins, including the attenuation of the ability of native hsp27 to stabilize retinal actin cytoskeleton [24]. These findings suggest that heat shock protein autoantibodies have direct pathogenic potential to facilitate RGC death in glaucoma and that their presence is not just an epiphenomenon. This is further supported by a clinical study in which serum titers of autoantibodies to heat shock proteins did not differ depending on the degree of glaucomatous damage in either American or Japanese patients [25]. On the other hand, antibody-mediated neuronal damage in glaucoma may also occur indirectly by way of a 'mimicked' autoimmune response to a sensitizing antigen [17, 18, 26]. Molecular mimicry as a potential causal mechanism of glaucomatous neurodegeneration is supported by findings of elevated autoantibodies to bacterial heat shock proteins, including hsp60 [18], as well as the increased expression of HLA-DR/CD8 on circulating T cells of normal pressure glaucoma patients [14]. In addition, epitope mapping revealed that the immunogenicity of rhodopsin antibodies in these patients is shared by epitopes of proteins found in common bacterial and viral pathogens [26].

Additional recent reports from several laboratories of elevated serum antibodies against neuron-specific enolase [27] or phosphatidylserine [28], and complex patterns of serum antibodies against retina and optic nerve antigens [29] in glaucoma patients also support the association of serum autoantibodies with glaucomatous neurodegeneration.

Tissue Stress in Glaucoma

What seems to be the most important parameter for the modulation of the immune system in glaucoma is that the retina and optic nerve head are under widespread and long-term tissue stress in glaucomatous eyes. In addition to the clinical evidence of elevated intraocular pressure in glaucoma patients, there is also evidence of hypoxic [30] and oxidative tissue stress [31] in glaucomatous eyes. The tissue stress in glaucoma is best represented by increased expression of stress proteins, including heat shock proteins, in the retina and optic nerve head [32]. While heat shock proteins function as endogenous protectants of retinal neurons in response to a variety of stressors, including those associated with glaucoma [24, 33], they also have the ability to elicit an activated immune response. For example, heat shock proteins are known to be highly antigenic, and immune responses to heat shock proteins are implicated in the development of a number of human autoimmune diseases as a consequence of molecular mimicry [34, 35].

Tissue stress is probably a major force that drives a resting immune system over the threshold of antigen-specific activation, since several stress-associated costimulatory factors are required for the activation of resting antigen-presenting cells, including glial cells [35–37]. Glial major histocompatibility complex class II expression is indeed induced under stress conditions [38, 39]. Similarly, optic nerve head and retinal glia, including both macroglia and microglia, prominently respond to glaucomatous tissue stress by exhibiting an activated phenotype [40], which includes the activation of their antigen-presenting ability. Major histocompatibility complex class II molecules on glial cells are upregulated in glaucomatous eyes [41]. Microglial cells [42], and also glial fibrillary acidic protein-positive astrocytes, exhibit HLA-DR immunolabeling in glaucomatous human donor eyes [41]. Thus, glial cells not only function in the innate immune response (by clearing the debris and the deleterious breakdown products from degenerating RGCs and their axons), but are also involved in adaptive immunity through antigen presentation. In addition, despite their many neuroprotective functions, glial cells may also be directly cytotoxic to RGCs through the increased production of neurotoxic cytokines [43]. Due to their diverse functions, glial cells have been implicated in traumatic injuries and chronic neurodegenerative diseases of the CNS [44–47]. The prominent and persistent activation of glial cells in glaucomatous eyes, including the activation of their antigen-presenting ability, point out a similar role of these cells in the activation of an autoimmune neurodegenerative process in glaucoma.

Conclusion

The onset, progression, and termination of tissue-specific immune responses are largely determined by the interactions between the tissue-infiltrating T cells, stromal cells of the CNS (in the case of glaucoma, RGCs, astrocytes, and Müller cells), and tissue macrophages (microglia). Whether the outcome of immune system activity is deleterious or beneficial for tissue integrity and function depends on complex interactions between these cells [48]. Although protective autoimmunity may govern the retina and optic nerve environment under homeostatic conditions, it is proposed that an adverse neurodegenerative component resulting from a failure to properly rectify the initial injury-induced immune response, accompanies neurodegeneration in some glaucoma patients. Tissue stress present in glaucomatous eyes seems to be decisive for the balance between protective immunity and the progression of neurodegeneration by autoimmunity. Alterations in neuron-glia-T cell interactions under glaucomatous stress conditions, along with the increased antigenicity in the damaged tissue and the increased antigen-presenting ability of resident glial cells, appear to be important factors determining the role of the immune system in glaucoma. Continued efforts to better understand the role of the immune system in glaucoma should allow for both the identification of biomarkers that may signal the most advantageous time to intervene in order to minimize disease progression, as well as the development of immunomodulatory strategies that could be utilized for such therapeutic gain.

References

1 Wax MB, Tezel G: Neurobiology of glaucomatous optic neuropathy: diverse cellular events in neurodegeneration and neuroprotection. Mol Neurobiol 2002;26:45–55.
2 Tezel G, Wax MB: The immune system and glaucoma. Curr Opin Ophthalmol 2004;15:80–84.
3 Tezel G, Wax MB: Glial modulation of retinal ganglion cell death in glaucoma. J Glaucoma 2003;12:63–68.
4 Gregerson DS: Immune privilege in the retina. Ocul Immunol Inflamm 1998;6:257–267.
5 Streilein JW, Okamoto S, Sano Y, Taylor AW: Neural control of ocular immune privilege. Ann NY Acad Sci 2000;917:297–306.
6 Griffith TS, Brunner T, Fletcher SM, Green DR, Ferguson TA: Fas ligand-induced apoptosis as a mechanism of immune privilege. Science 1995;270:1189–1192.

7 Raivich G, Jones LL, Kloss CU, Werner A, Neumann H, Kreutzberg GW: Immune surveillance in the injured nervous system: T-lymphocytes invade the axotomized mouse facial motor nucleus and aggregate around sites of neuronal degeneration. J Neurosci 1998;18:5804–5816.
8 Hickey WF, Hsu BL, Kimura H: T-lymphocyte entry into the central nervous system. J Neurosci Res 1991;28:254–260.
9 Schwartz M, Kipnis J: Protective autoimmunity: regulation and prospects for vaccination after brain and spinal cord injuries. Trends Mol Med 2001;7:252–258.
10 Kipnis J, Mizrahi T, Hauben E, Shaked I, Shevach E, Schwartz M: Neuroprotective autoimmunity: naturally occurring CD4+CD25+ regulatory T cells suppress the ability to withstand injury to the central nervous system. Proc Natl Acad Sci USA 2002;99:15620–15625.
11 Schwartz M, Kipnis J: Autoimmunity on alert: naturally occurring regulatory $CD4^+CD25^+$T cells as part of the evolutionary compromise between a 'need' and a 'risk'. Trends Immunol 2002;23: 530–534.
12 Schwartz M: Neuroprotection as a treatment for glaucoma: pharmacological and immunological approaches. Eur J Ophthalmol 2003;13(suppl 3):S27–S31.
13 Schwartz M: Neurodegeneration and neuroprotection in glaucoma: development of a therapeutic neuroprotective vaccine: the Friedenwald lecture. Invest Ophthalmol Vis Sci 2003;44:1407–1411.
14 Yang J, Patil RV, Yu H, Gordon M, Wax MB: T cell subsets and sIL-2R/IL-2 levels in patients with glaucoma. Am J Ophthalmol 2001;131:421–426.
15 Wax MB, Barrett DA, Pestronk A: Increased incidence of paraproteinemia and autoantibodies in patients with normal-pressure glaucoma. Am J Ophthalmol 1994;117:561–568.
16 Tezel G, Edward DP, Wax MB: Serum autoantibodies to optic nerve head glycosaminoglycans in patients with glaucoma. Arch Ophthalmol 1999;117:917–924.
17 Romano C, Barrett DA, Li Z, Pestronk A, Wax MB: Anti-rhodopsin antibodies in sera from patients with normal-pressure glaucoma. Invest Ophthalmol Vis Sci 1995;36:1968–1975.
18 Wax MB, Tezel G, Saito I, Gupta RS, Harley JB, Li Z, Romano C: Anti-Ro/SS-A positivity and heat shock protein antibodies in patients with normal-pressure glaucoma (see comments). Am J Ophthalmol 1998;125:145–157.
19 Tezel G, Seigel GM, Wax MB: Autoantibodies to small heat shock proteins in glaucoma. Invest Ophthalmol Vis Sci 1998;39:2277–2287.
20 Yang J, Tezel G, Patil RV, Romano C, Wax MB: Serum autoantibody against glutathione S-transferase in patients with glaucoma. Invest Ophthalmol Vis Sci 2001;42:1273–1276.
21 Wax MB, Tezel G, Edward PD: Clinical and ocular histopathological findings in a patient with normal-pressure glaucoma (see comments). Arch Ophthalmol 1998;116:993–1001.
22 Tezel G, Kass MA, Kolker AE, Wax MB: Comparative optic disc analysis in normal pressure glaucoma, primary open-angle glaucoma, and ocular hypertension. Ophthalmology 1996;103: 2105–2113.
23 Tezel G, Wax MB: Inhibition of caspase activity in retinal cell apoptosis induced by various stimuli in vitro. Invest Ophthalmol Vis Sci 1999;40:2660–2667.
24 Tezel G, Wax MB: The mechanisms of hsp27 antibody-mediated apoptosis in retinal neuronal cells. J Neurosci 2000;20:3552–3562.
25 Wax MB, Tezel G, Kawase K, Kitazawa Y: Serum autoantibodies to heat shock proteins in glaucoma patients from Japan and the United States. Ophthalmology 2001;108:296–302.
26 Romano C, Li Z, Arendt A, Hargrave PA, Wax MB: Epitope mapping of anti-rhodopsin antibodies from patients with normal pressure glaucoma. Invest Ophthalmol Vis Sci 1999;40:1275–1280.
27 Maruyama I, Ohguro H, Ikeda Y: Retinal ganglion cells recognized by serum autoantibody against gamma-enolase found in glaucoma patients. Invest Ophthalmol Vis Sci 2000;41:1657–1665.
28 Kremmer S, Kreuzfelder E, Klein R, Bontke N, Henneberg-Quester KB, Steuhl KP, Grosse-Wilde H: Antiphosphatidylserine antibodies are elevated in normal tension glaucoma. Clin Exp Immunol 2001;125:211–215.
29 Joachim SC, Pfeiffer N, Grus FH: Autoantibodies in patients with glaucoma: a comparison of IgG serum antibodies against retinal, optic nerve, and optic nerve head antigens. Graefes Arch Clin Exp Ophthalmol 2005;243:817–823.
30 Tezel G, Wax MB: Hypoxia-inducible factor 1α in the glaucomatous retina and optic nerve head. Arch Ophthalmol 2004;122:1348–1356.

31 Tezel G, Yang X, Cai J: Proteomic identification of oxidatively modified retinal proteins in a chronic pressure-induced rat model of glaucoma. Invest Ophthalmol Vis Sci 2005;46:3177–3187.
32 Tezel G, Hernandez MR, Wax MB: Immunostaining of heat shock proteins in the retina and optic nerve head of normal and glaucomatous eyes. Arch Ophthalmol 2000;118:511–518.
33 Tezel GM, Seigel GM, Wax MB: Density-dependent resistance to apoptosis in retinal cells. Curr Eye Res 1999;19:377–388.
34 Young DB: Heat-shock proteins: immunity and autoimmunity. Curr Opin Immunol 1992;4: 396–400.
35 van Noort JM: Multiple sclerosis: an altered immune response or an altered stress response? J Mol Med 1996;74:285–296.
36 Young RA, Elliott TJ: Stress proteins, infection, and immune surveillance. Cell 1989;59:5–8.
37 van Eden W: Heat-shock proteins as immunogenic bacterial antigens with the potential to induce and regulate autoimmune arthritis. Immunol Rev 1991;121:5–28.
38 Maehlen J, Olsson T, Zachau A, Klareskog L, Kristensson K: Local enhancement of major histocompatibility complex (MHC) class I and II expression and cell infiltration in experimental allergic encephalomyelitis around axotomized motor neurons. J Neuroimmunol 1989;23:125–132.
39 Molleston MC, Thomas ML, Hickey WF: Novel major histocompatibility complex expression by microglia and site-specific experimental allergic encephalomyelitis lesions in the rat central nervous system after optic nerve transection. Adv Neurol 1993;59:337–348.
40 Tezel G, Chauhan BC, LeBlanc RP, Wax MB: Immunohistochemical assessment of the glial mitogen-activated protein kinase activation in glaucoma. Invest Ophthalmol Vis Sci 2003;44: 3025–3033.
41 Yang J, Yang P, Tezel G, Patil RV, Hernandez MR, Wax MB: Induction of HLA-DR expression in human lamina cribrosa astrocytes by cytokines and simulated ischemia. Invest Ophthalmol Vis Sci 2001;42:365–371.
42 Neufeld AH: Microglia in the optic nerve head and the region of parapapillary chorioretinal atrophy in glaucoma. Arch Ophthalmol 1999;117:1050–1056.
43 Tezel G, Wax MB: Increased production of tumor necrosis factor-alpha by glial cells exposed to simulated ischemia or elevated hydrostatic pressure induces apoptosis in cocultured retinal ganglion cells. J Neurosci 2000;20:8693–8700.
44 Mitrovic B, Martin FC, Charles AC, Ignarro LJ, Anton PA, Shanahan F, Merrill JE: Neurotransmitters and cytokines in CNS pathology. Prog Brain Res 1994;103:319–330.
45 Streit WJ: The role of microglia in brain injury. Neurotoxicology 1996;17:671–678.
46 Stoll G, Jander S: The role of microglia and macrophages in the pathophysiology of the CNS. Prog Neurobiol 1999;58:233–247.
47 Aloisi F: The role of microglia and astrocytes in CNS immune surveillance and immunopathology. Adv Exp Med Biol 1999;468:123–133.
48 Carson MJ: Microglia as liaisons between the immune and central nervous systems: functional implications for multiple sclerosis. Glia 2002;40:218–231.

Dr. Gülgün Tezel
Kentucky Lions Eye Center, University of Louisville School of Medicine
301 East Muhammad Ali Boulevard
Louisville, KY 40202 (USA)
Tel. +1 502 852 7395, Fax +1 502 852 3811, E-Mail gulgun.tezel@louisville.edu

Niederkorn JY, Kaplan HJ (eds): Immune Response and the Eye.
Chem Immunol Allergy. Basel, Karger, 2007, vol 92, pp 228–243

Intermediate and Posterior Uveitis

John V. Forrester

Department of Ophthalmology, University of Aberdeen Medical School, Aberdeen, UK

Abstract

Sight-threatening intraocular inflammation affecting the posterior segment of the eye may be predominantly located in the peripheral retina and vitreous (intermediate uveitis) or postequatorially where it manifests as inflammation of the retina, retinal vessels and/or optic nerve with cellular infiltration of the choroid and retina and edema particularly at the macula. Involvement of the macula is the main cause for visual loss. Experimental models of posterior uveitis have revealed much concerning the mechanisms of inflammatory cell damage to the retina, implicating CD4 T cells, effector macrophages and pro-inflammatory cytokines. In particular, transgenic and gene deletion models of inflammation have allowed an understanding of how immune privilege in the posterior segment of the eye is disrupted. Importantly, this has led to the development of new treatments with novel immunosuppressants and 'biologics' and the promise of cell-based therapies which may allow customized therapies tailored to the individual's inflammatory profile.

The classification of intraocular inflammatory disease has traditionally presented conceptual difficulties. The uvea (from the Greek *uvea* meaning grape, described as such by early anatomists because of its resemblance to a black grape after dissection of the sclera from the intact globe) is the lymphovascular layer of the eye and becomes engorged after any intraocular inflammatory stimulus. Remarkably, the range of inflammatory processes often respects anatomical boundaries. Thus, anterior inflammation is restricted to the iris and ciliary body (synonyms: anterior uveitis, iridocyclitis, and anterior segment intraocular inflammation) and posterior inflammation is frequently restricted to the choroid (synonyms: choroiditis, chorioretinitis, and posterior segment intraocular inflammation). The difficulty arises when the inflammation crosses boundaries and particularly so when it is restricted to an area of the posterior ciliary body and the anterior or peripheral retina. Clinically, this is recognized by many ophthalmologists by the term intermediate uveitis, and may include a subset of conditions termed specifically pars planitis, since the locus of the disease is predominantly the pars plana ciliaris. In addition, there may be involvement of other ocular sites such as the optic nerve or the sclera and retina in different types of posterior segment intraocular inflammation and to avoid confusion it may be simpler to consider two broad categories of intraocular inflammation: anterior and posterior.

Anterior uveitis is generally considered to present as iridocyclitis (Bora and Kaplan, pp 213–220) while posterior uveitis can be considered to include many different forms of posterior segment intraocular inflammation, of which one subdivision is intermediate uveitis. Related presentations of posterior uveitis include for instance multifocal choroiditis, retinal vasculitis, and vitritis amongst many others (table 1). In addition, central retinal vasculitis and papillitis may be difficult to differentiate from classical optic neuritis due to demyelinating disease, but usually the clinical entities are quite discrete.

Categorization of the many clinical forms of non-infectious posterior segment intraocular inflammation may be based on a relatively simple scientific paradigm, centered on an autoimmune etiology. This notion is drawn from the fact that many of the conditions seen clinically can be reproduced by immunization of a range of animal models with a single autoantigen [1]. Thus different human clinical phenotypes can be mimicked with the same antigen by modifying the conditions such as the animal species and strain, the dose of antigen, the type of adjuvant used and the immune status of the recipient. Clearly not all forms of posterior uveitis can be grouped together in this way, and there are several important specific diseases, e.g. Vogt-Koyanagi-Harada disease (VKH), which have defining features, but as an aid to the management of these diseases this concept is helpful since the protocols for immunosuppression frequently depend on the severity of the disease and the threat to sight rather than the specific diagnosis.

The following sections will demonstrate the scientific underpinning of the clinical approach to diagnosis and management of posterior uveitis.

The Clinical Problem

Infectious versus Non-Infectious Disease

Since many of the posterior uveitic conditions present with a somewhat restricted set of overlapping clinical signs and symptoms, the major clinical dilemma is to decide whether the disease is infectious or non-infectious (table 1). This has important therapeutic implications since many infectious diseases can be worsened by inappropriate use of immunosuppressants, while on the other

Table 1. Classification of posterior segment intraocular inflammation

Infectious
Endophthalmitis
Bacterial infections
Tuberculosis, leprosy, Lyme disease, syphilis, and opportunistic infections (e.g. *Pneumocystis carinii*)
Parasitic infections
Toxoplasmosis, toxocariasis, cysticercosis, diffuse unilateral subacute neuroretinitis
Viral infections
Acute retinal necrosis (herpes simplex), herpes zoster (peripheral outer retinal necrosis), cytomegalovirus, HTLV-1, others
Fungal (Candida, Aspergillus, others)
Non-infectious
Involving eye alone
Pars planitis
Idiopathic vitritis
Idiopathic retinal vasculitis
Idiopathic multifocal retinochoroiditis
Sympathetic ophthalmia
White dot syndromes
Histoplasmosis-like disease
Associated with systemic disease
Behçet's disease
Sarcoidosis
Vogt-Koyanagi-Harada disease
Connective tissue diseases

hand early control of non-infectious, immune-based uveitic disease can preserve vision. Examples of the former conditions include herpes simplex retinitis or cytomegalovirus retinitis, in which the use of immunosuppressants may sharply exacerbate the disease. In contrast, some infectious diseases may induce ocular tissue damage due to the associated immunological reaction and thus the correct treatment would be the combined use of antibiotics and immunosuppressants. Examples of this form of uveitic disease would be miliary tuberculosis and ocular toxoplasmosis.

Once the condition has been confirmed to be non-infectious, and is presumptively autoimmune or at least immune mediated, two major questions present themselves: what is the specific diagnosis and is there a significant threat to vision? In some cases these two questions are linked since the pattern of disease frequently will predict its course. For instance, some diseases such as birdshot retinochoroidopathy (one of the white dot syndromes) carry a poor prognosis despite both the insidious nature of the disease and attempts to intervene with systemic immune suppression. Other disorders such as low-grade pars planitis have a good prognosis and merely require careful clinical observation provided there is no maculopathy. In other cases, the specific diagnosis may be difficult to identify and a careful assessment of the threat to vision is essential. This requires targeted investigation including fundus imaging, electrophysiology and other ocular function tests as well as systemic evaluation of general health to determine the risk of side effects from therapy should immunosuppression be required. These general principles are described in detail in recent monographs and guidelines [2, 3].

Non-Infectious Uveitis: Is Posterior Uveitis One or Several Diseases?

A question testing many ophthalmologists is whether the various clinical forms of non-infectious posterior uveitis represent discrete clinical entities or whether the condition is a single disease entity of varying severity reflecting the initial insult or inciting factors and the immune status of the patient at the time of disease onset. Most ophthalmologists adhere to the former view and recognize many disease entities, each with a site of origin in a specific ocular tissue component with a clear disease pattern and prognostic outcome. For example, pars planitis originates in the pars plana ciliaris and its hallmark is 'snow banking' in the retinal periphery. Snow banking is a clinical term for a dense amorphous exudate incorporating the vitreous base, retina and choroid and is composed of inflammatory cells, degenerating tissue debris and hyaline material [for review see ref. 4]. Sympathetic ophthalmia is a well-recognized condition of autoimmune inflammatory disease in which the second eye develops uveitis following penetrating injury to the first eye. It is characterized by granulomatous inflammation at the level of the outer retina (Dalen-Fuch's nodules) but is considered to spare the choriocapillaris layer [for review see ref. 4]. Serpiginous choroiditis is a spreading inflammation at the level of the retinal pigment epithelium which occurs in the apparent absence of significant inflammatory cell involvement in the vitreous. Recent indocyanine green studies of choroidal inflammatory diseases have allowed a new classification of ocular inflammatory disease, but lack definitive clinicopathological correlative evidence to support each disease entity [5].

In contrast, an alternative view has been proposed that the posterior segment of the eye has a limited set of responses to inflammatory insult, namely: [a] inflammatory cell infiltration of the vitreous (vitreous haze); [b] chorioretinal infiltration (granulomatous deposits, subretinal infiltrates of cells and/or neovascular membranes); [c] inflammation of the retinal vessels (retinal vasculitis); and [d] edema, which is frequently focal and centered on the macula (macular edema) but may be extensive as in the localized detachments of VKH or predominantly involve the optic nerve (optic nerve swelling) [1, 6, 7]. As indicated above, this view is based on data from experimental models using defined retinal autoantigens.

Experimental Models

Historical Overview

Uveitis has long been considered to have an autoimmune basis [8]. Because of the marked involvement of uveal tissue it was assumed that the autoimmune target would reside in the uveal tract. In the first half of the 20th century, experimental models of autoimmune disease were established in many systems using tissue extracts emulsified in various adjuvants, particularly Freund's adjuvant with mycobacterial extract. Janeway [9] has called this the immunologist's 'dirty little secret', since activation of innate immune cell receptors, particularly Toll receptors, was essential to induce a response to inoculated antigen. Models of disease included myelin basic protein-induced experimental autoimmune encephalomyelitis, collagen-induced experimental autoimmune arthritis, and thyroglobulin-induced experimental autoimmune thyroiditis. In all cases, a tissue-specific autoantigen was identified and used to induce the disease [for reviews see ref. 10–12].

Similar studies were performed in uveitis, and initial attempts to extract autoantigen were directed towards uveal tissue. However, inoculation of animals with uveal tissue extracts was not very effective at inducing uveitis. In 1965, Wacker [13] reported that inoculation of guinea pigs with retinal extracts resulted in reproducible uveoretinitis in guinea pigs and this led to the identification of the first retinal autoantigen in 1977 [reviewed in ref. 13]. Since then several other autoantigens have been identified which produce experimental autoimmune uveoretinitis (EAU) in various animal models [for reviews see ref. 14–18] and variations of the basic model (e.g. acute, chronic, and recurrent EAU) system can be used depending on the experimental question under study, similar to the situation in experimental autoimmune encephalomyelitis.

Not all antigens with the ability to induce retinal inflammation are located in the retina. For instance, models of VKH, in which the target cell is thought to be the melanocyte, have shown that the tyrosinase-related protein 1 (Trp 1) can induce a posterior uveitis in rats with similarities to the human disease [19, 20]. In addition, uveal melanin-associated extract contains proteins which can induce experimental models of autoimmune uveitis centered on the anterior segment (experimental autoimmune anterior uveitis, EAAU). Recent studies indicate that the major antigen in this extract is in fact type 1 collagen [21]. In general however, the central theme surrounding autoimmune intraocular inflammation defaults to the notion that eye-restricted autoantigens can lead to variations in the expression of intraocular inflammation which have wide similarity to the range of clinical phenotypes in human disease and importantly that these models are in the main eye specific.

Development of Spontaneous Models of Uveoretinitis

Despite contemporary views that infectious agents may underlie autoimmune disease pathogenesis, a criticism of adjuvant-induced experimental models of disease is that they do not resemble closely enough autoimmune disease in humans in which disease develops in the apparent absence of an inciting stimulus. For trials of disease-modifying agents, spontaneous models of EAU or ocular inflammation would be greatly advantageous. Spontaneous uveitis occurs in veterinary practice particularly in horses, and valuable information has been obtained from immunopathological studies of equine uveitis [22, 23]. However, in practical terms rodent models are necessary to conduct investigative work.

Most models of spontaneously occurring uveoretinitis have been produced in immunologically or genetically modified animals. An early report described the development of spontaneous uveoretinitis in nude (nu/nu) mice reconstituted at 4 weeks of age with rat embryonic thymus [24]. The pathology showed progressive retinal destruction which appeared to be T cell mediated since adoptive transfer of CD4+ T cells from affected mice induced similar disease in syngeneic animals. Interestingly these mice were shown to have antibodies to interphotoreceptor retinoid binding protein but not to retinal S antigen. This has considerable resonance with later findings relating to the now-recognized expression of peripheral antigens in the thymus and their correlation with central tolerance to autoantigens. In a number of studies it has been shown that susceptibility to autoimmune disease correlates inversely with thymic expression of the peripheral tissue antigen, and some elegant quantitative work has revealed this effect in relation to rodent susceptibility to retinal S antigen vs. interphotoreceptor retinoid binding protein [25] and to some extent this has been supported by similar work in humans [26]. These later data would support the view that the spontaneous model of uveoretinitis induced by rat embryonic thymus [24] is interphotoreceptor retinoid binding protein specific.

The role of thymic tolerance in protecting against the development of organ-specific disease and in particular uveoretinitis (EAU) has been further demonstrated in mice in which the autoimmune regulator (AIRE) gene has been deleted [27]. Patients with a rare immunodeficiency disorder, the autoimmune polyendocrinopathy-candidiasis-ectodermal dystrophy syndrome, have defects in the AIRE genes with a tendency to several autoimmune diseases [28]. Mice with the AIRE deletion also have these features, including uveoretinitis. Recent studies have shown that expression of the AIRE gene by thymic medullary epithelial cells is important not only for permitting peripheral antigen expression in the thymus but also for promoting effective antigen presentation by these cells [29].

Szpak et al. [30] earlier developed a spontaneous model of uveoretinopathy in mice in which the susceptibility HLA gene (HLA-A29) was inserted into the mouse genome. Disease developed late usually, after about 12 months, but was present in the majority of A29+ animals (around 80%). The clinical features closely resembled human birdshot retinochoroidopathy. Interestingly, the pathology indicated that there was evidence of retinal vasculitis and inflammatory cells in the inner retina, in addition to the expected granulomatous infiltrate in the choroidal layers. In addition, there were features of retinal pigment epithelial cell migration into the retina with focal areas of serous retinal detachment. These latter findings resemble more closely the severe end-stage phenotype of human birdshot retinochoroidopathy in which subretinal macular edema and exudation can occur [31] and indicate that while the predominant clinical manifestation of the disease can occur at one site, the evolution of the disease can progress to involve most of the intraocular tissues.

Other attempts to develop models of spontaneous uveitis have involved the transgenic expression of foreign antigen in ocular tissues and crossing the single transgenic mice with mice transgenic for the T cell receptor specific for a defined peptide epitope of the foreign antigen [32, 33]. Alternatively, disease was induced by adoptive transfer of antigen-specific T cells similar to T cell transfer models using cell lines to the native antigen (see below).

Examples of this type of model include expression of β-galactosidase in the retina under the rhodopsin, glial fibrillary acidic protein or arrestin promoter to provide varying levels of antigenic expression [34–37]. This has produced evidence to support a role for antigen sequestration in mediating tolerance to retinal antigens [35]. Interestingly, expression of the foreign antigen, hen egg lysozyme, under control of the αA-crystallin promoter has permitted development of a model of spontaneous intraocular inflammation in which there is not only significant damage to lens structure but also a marked retinitis [33]. It has previously been shown that αA-crystallin is present in the retina [38], which may provide an explanation of targeting of this tissue. Crystalllins act as heat shock proteins to control stress responses in non-lens tissues, and the reduction in their content may reflect aging changes in the retina [38].

Spontaneous models of uveoretinitis not only permit investigation of basic immunological mechanisms but also provide good test systems for the evaluation of disease modifiers which can be introduced during active disease without the difficulties of controlling for persisting deposits of autoantigen at sites of antigen inoculation.

Site of Initiation of Disease

An unanswered question in many autoimmune diseases is where and how the disease is initiated. In clinical uveoretinitis, it is assumed that the disease is initiated systemically by some ill-understood mechanism involving molecular mimicry or bystander activation in which autoreactive T cells are activated during invasion of the organism by infectious foreign agents (viruses or bacteria). In some respects this is modelled by specific peptide-adjuvant-induced EAU in which retinal antigen-specific T cells are activated in the secondary lymphoid tissues. The question that follows then is how do these activated T cells find their target antigen. Several studies have addressed this question, mostly using adoptive transfer of in vitro activated antigen-specific T cells rather than active immunization. Initial studies indicated that EAU is CD4+ T cell mediated and requires a certain T cell frequency to mediate inflammation. Prendergast et al. [39] suggest that there is ready access of antigen-specific and non-antigen-specific T cells to the retinal tissues through the retinal vasculature but only antigen-specific T cells are retained, probably due to antigen recognition in situ [40, 41]. In contrast, Xu et al. [40, 41] indicated that T cells, including activated antigen-specific T cells, cannot cross the blood-retinal barrier unless there has been some systemic signal, specific or nonspecific, which renders the retinal endothelial cells susceptible to T cell transmigration. Entry of cells into the retina requires prior upregulation of adhesion molecules on the retinal endothelium and specific interactions between ligand receptor pairs such as intercellular adhesion molecule-1 and lymphocyte function-associated antigen [42]. Furthermore there is preferential recruitment of Th1 T cells in this initial stage of EAU via P-selectin glycoprotein ligand-1 binding [42]. Entry of cells is via the postcapillary venules and is initiated focally in the extreme retinal periphery (pars ciliaris) and around the optic nerve [Xu et al., in preparation]. This has many counterparts in human disease such as the many white dot syndromes which clinically develop lesions around the optic nerve and in the early signs of intermediate uveitis around the retinal periphery.

Mechanism of Tissue Destruction

As the disease progresses, many additional cells are recruited to the retina including nonspecifically activated T cells, granulocytes, macrophages and dendritic cells (DCs) [43]. As indicated above, EAU is CD4+ T cell-mediated but macrophages play a central role in tissue damage. This has been demonstrated in macrophage depletion studies and also in studies in which T cells continue to infiltrate the tissue but the macrophage is disabled and tissue damage is attenuated [for review see ref. 17]. Recent studies have revealed the heterogeneity of macrophage populations, one set of which are pro-inflammatory while another, the alternatively activated macrophage, may have a role in modifying the inflammatory response. Other macrophages, particularly the resident macrophage, may have a scavenging role in clearing dead and dying cells in the absence of a marked inflammatory response [44].

In EAU, infiltrating myeloid cells consist of DCs and activated monocytes many of which express major histocompatibility complex class II antigen. In the later stages of the disease, macrophages lose their major histocompatibility complex class II but express other activation markers such as sialoadhesin [43], Fcγ and CD68. During the peak of EAU, macrophages release large quantities of nitric oxide, one of the mediators inducing tissue damage [45].

The factors regulating macrophage activity are not known. Interferon (IFN)-γ and tumor necrosis factor (TNF)-α, both pro-inflammatory cytokines, are known to be involved in macrophage activation in inflammation generally. However, while transgenic expression of IFN-γ in the rodent eye is associated with increased inflammation [46], IFN-γ-deficient mice also develop EAU through a deviated immune response [47]. Recent studies on accessory molecules involved in antigen presentation, such as CD40 and CD137, indicate a definitive requirement [48, 49], while molecules involved in monocyte adhesion and trafficking, e.g. the chemokine macrophage inflammatory protein-1α, are required at least for T cell entry into the retina [50]. In addition, interleukin (IL)-12 produced by antigen-presenting cells (DCs and macrophages) is central to the development of EAU, although its role as a promoter of inflammation has been undermined by recent data [for review see ref. 15].

Several questions remain, including the nature of the signals which mediate myeloid precursor cells trafficking across the endothelium and the decision to progress towards either a DC or macrophage phenotype; about whether monocytes undergo apoptosis in situ or proliferate, and about programming of macrophages before or after entry into the tissue [45].

Experimental Approaches to Modulating Disease in Experimental Autoimmune Uveoretinitis

EAU is a good model for determining the relationship between the severity of the inflammatory response and its effects, namely the tissue destruction, due to the highly organized structure of the ocular layers in the posterior segment of the eye. Thus, structural damage to the retina and the level of inflammatory cell infiltration can be graded separately. This approach has revealed how treatment of rats with an anti-TNF-α fusion protein can protect the retina from damage despite minimal reduction in the T cell infiltrate. In contrast, this treatment reduced macrophage infiltration [17]. These data suggest that it is possible to disable T cells from performing their usual function of producing macrophage chemoattractant and activation factors without affecting their ability to infiltrate the tissues.

EAU also provides an excellent model for tracking cells in vivo and for evaluating the effects of novel immune modulators. Using the scanning laser ophthalmoscope to track leukocytes in vivo [51], various inhibitors of leukocyte rolling and adhesion have been identified such as antibodies to CD44 (the hyaluronan receptor) and hyaluronan itself [52]. Similarly, inhibitors of chemokines and adhesion molecules have been shown to prevent EAU (see above). Many approaches to immunomodulation have been attempted both at the afferent and efferent limbs of the ocular immune response.

Most of these approaches are directed towards the efferent arm of the immune response in EAU. Attempts to modify the afferent arm, for instance at the level of antigen presentation, have been less frequent. As indicated above, monoclonal antibody therapy against adhesion molecules such as intercellular adhesion molecule-1 or other accessory molecules such as CD40 has been shown to be effective in preventing EAU. A more direct approach is to use DC vaccination therapy. DCs are well known for their antigen presentation capabilities but are now recognized to have a primary function in the unchallenged organism of maintaining tolerance. Such 'tolerogenic' DCs are recognized to be immature in that they fail to express high levels of accessory molecules such as CD40 and CD86, and are more likely to secrete IL-10 than IL-12 [53]. When purified populations of retinal antigen-pulsed immature DCs are inoculated into mice, they inhibit the development of EAU [54]. Similar approaches have been used in other model systems of autoimmune disease and have been attributed to expansion of T regulatory cells, either of the Tr3 variety or the endogenous CD4+ CD25+ T regulatory cells [55–57]. Recent studies in EAU produced similar results, showing that IL-10-producing DCs when administered subcutaneously will induce CD4+ CD25+ T regulatory cells which, when adoptively transferred to syngeneic mice, delay the onset of EAU [Siepman et al., in preparation]. Similar approaches using immune-modified B cells as tolerance-inducing antigen-presenting cells have been successful in modulating EAU [58].

These data open up possibilities for novel approaches to the management of EAU. For instance, it may be possible to customize autologous tolerogenic DCs prepared from the patient's blood for administration to the patient either as a preventive vaccination at the onset of disease or during the course of an attack of uveitis, to downmodulate the inflammation. However, there are several questions to be answered before this can occur: for instance, is specific antigen required to customize DCs and if so which antigens; what degree of immaturity is required for effective tolerance induction; how prolonged is the effect of the treatment, and many other questions?

Translational Studies

Current Therapies

When steroid therapy was introduced in the latter half of the 20th century for various autoimmune conditions, steroids were rapidly applied to sight-threatening uveitis [59, 60], and both topical and systemic preparations are the mainstay of current treatments. However, prolonged use of steroids, particularly systemic steroids, is associated with unacceptable side effects, and many patients return to their pre-treatment vision-losing inflammation as the steroids are tapered. Steroid-sparing agents such as azathioprine and methotrexate are also widely used, but they are less effective and also have side effects.

A major problem in this area of research is the lack of good clinical evidence based on well-controlled randomized clinical trials (RCTs), and this is partly due to difficulties in developing standardized entry and exclusion clinical criteria. In preclinical studies, EAU has provided a benchmark for evaluating the effects of immunosuppressants in autoimmune inflammatory disease and in this respect provides an excellent model for translational research. Early studies in EAU showed the value of this model in developing the use of a wide variety of immunosuppressants for uveitis, including cyclosporine A, FK506, rapamycin, and mycophenolate, all of which are now in clinical use in the treatment of ocular inflammation [61–64]. Direct comparisons of the efficacy of some of these drugs have been reported recently: for instance, FK506 has been shown to be slightly superior to cyclosporine A in the treatment of human uveitis, and to have a better 'quality-of-life' outcome [65].

All of these drugs have major side effects, the most important of which are the life-threatening effects, such as tumor induction, renal toxicity and failure, bone marrow aplasia and hypertension. Accordingly, it is essential in considering the use of these drugs in patients with uveitis to perform a full pretreatment medical assessment including renal, biochemical and hematological function studies. Appropriately trained ophthalmic physicians are necessary to correctly treat these patients.

Newer Approaches to the Management of Sight-Threatening Uveoretinitis

The explosion in the use of 'biologics' in therapy of many human diseases from cancer to aging disorders and autoimmune disease has had significant impact on the treatment of intraocular inflammation/uveitis. Early studies with T cell-depleting drugs, e.g. anti-CD3 and anti-CD52 (Campath 1h), proved to be effective in several conditions, including ocular inflammation [66], but particularly in the latter case, profound effects on marrow function have restricted its use.

Despite the theoretical arguments against the likelihood of a therapy directed against a single cytokine proving effective in inflammatory disorders, the remarkable effectiveness of anti-TNF-α therapy in rheumatoid arthritis generated opportunities for its use in other conditions such as uveitis [67, 68]. Several studies have now reported good therapeutic benefit from anti-TNF-α treatment in uveitis and it has a firm place on the pharmacy shelf despite its high cost. Particular indications include juvenile idiopathic arthritis-associated uveitis with secondary retinal involvement and severe retinal vasculitis with macular disease.

More recently, other biologics have been proposed for use in severe, sight-threatening retinal vasculitis, particularly Behçet's disease. IFN-α therapy was recently reported to have >90% effectiveness in patients with retinal vasculitis who had failed on other therapies, and this has been confirmed in other less extensive studies in both patients with non-Behçet's sight-threatening uveitis [69]. Remarkably, in a bedside-to-bench investigation, patients with uveitis have now been shown to demonstrate a defect in function of circulating plasmacytoid dendritic cells, the constitutive INF-α-producing cells in the body, in which they fail to produce INF-α in response to Toll receptor 9 stimulation [70], perhaps explaining the effectiveness of INF-α treatment in this condition. Problems with IFN-α therapy relate to side effects since many patients feel lassitude and have other side effects such as hair loss, weight loss and depression. In addition, titrating the dose can be difficult since IFN may itself induce a retinopathy which is difficult to differentiate from some of the features of retinal vasculitis. However, in those patients with few or no side effects or who can tolerate the therapy, the effect can transform their lives from the side effects of prolonged use of moderate steroids in combination with one or more immunosuppressants, only just maintaining visual function. In some situations it seems to be more beneficial than anti-TNF-α [71].

The Future: What Is Required for the Development of New and Safer Treatments for Sight-Threatening Posterior and Intermediate Uveitis?

Non-infectious intraocular inflammation (uveitis) and particularly sight-threatening uveoretinitis, is an 'orphan' condition in the sense that it remains ill defined at a clinical level, and as a result presents a problem for regulatory authorities when trying to come to a decision regarding the licensing of new treatment modalities. Disagreement continues to reverberate amongst clinicians concerning whether a general approach to treatment should be developed for intraocular inflammation as a single condition or whether specific therapies should be designed for each clinical entity. As a result, no single therapy or drug has received approval from national or supranational regulatory authorities for use in uveitis, and most drugs are administered 'off label'. In an attempt to develop a minimal set of diagnostic characteristics for uveitis, a consensus paper from a group of experts has been published, setting out a range of clinical symptoms and signs which might form the basis for outcome measures for new drug therapies [72]. In practice, it has been found that direct, robust control of inflammatory sight-threatening disease using an ever increasing range of immunosuppressives, singly or in combination, to minimize side effects has proved highly beneficial in the management of most cases of non-infectious uveitis. There is considerable promise that some of the newer approaches to control of inflammation using 'biologics' will prove valuable. In the meantime, investigation of basic immunological mechanisms both in the experimental models and in patients will shed light on the mechanism of autoimmunity generally and provide insights of value to immunology.

References

1 Forrester JV, Liversidge J, Dua HS, Towler H, McMenamin PG: Comparison of clinical and experimental uveitis. Curr Eye Res 1990;9(suppl):75–84.

2 Forrester JV, Okada A, BenEzra D, Ohno S: Posterior Segment Intraocular Inflammation: Guidelines. The Hague, Kugler, 1998.

3 Whitcup SM, Nussenblatt RB: Uveitis: Fundamentals and Clinical Practice. St. Louis, Mosby, 2005.

4 Boyd SR, Young S, Lightman S: Immunopathology of the noninfectious posterior and intermediate uveitides. Surv Ophthalmol 2001;46:209–233.

5 Bouchenaki N, Cimino L, Auer C, Tao Tran V, Herbort CP: Assessment and classification of choroidal vasculitis in posterior uveitis using indocyanine green angiography. Klin Monatsbl Augenheilkd 2002;219:243–249.

6 Forrester JV: Autoimmunity and autoimmune disease of the eye. Dev Ophthalmol 1999;30:167–186.

7 Forrester JV, McMenamin PG: Immunopathogenic mechanisms in intraocular inflammation; in Streilein JW (ed): Immune Response and the Eye. Chem Immunol. Basel, Karger, 1999, vol 73, pp 159–185.

8 Elschnig A: Studien zur sympathischen Ophhalmis. Die antigene Wirkung des Augenpigmentes. Graefes Arch Ophthalmol 1910;76:509–546.

9 Janeway CA Jr: The immune system evolved to discriminate infectious nonself from noninfectious self. Immunol Today 1992;13:11–16.

10 Stuart JM, Townes AS, Kang AH: Collagen autoimmune arthritis. Annu Rev Immunol 1984;2: 199–218.

11 Wilder RL: Neuroendocrine-immune system interactions and autoimmunity. Annu Rev Immunol 1995;13:307–338.

12 Burkhardt H, Kalden JR: Animal models of autoimmune diseases. Rheumatol Int 1997;17:91–99.

13 Wacker WB: Proctor Lecture. Experimental allergic uveitis. Investigations of retinal autoimmunity and the immunopathologic responses evoked. Invest Ophthalmol Vis Sci 1991;32: 3119–3128.

14 Caspi RR: Immunogenetic aspects of clinical and experimental uveitis. Reg Immunol 1992;4: 321–330.

15 Caspi RR: Th1 and Th2 responses in pathogenesis and regulation of experimental autoimmune uveoretinitis. Int Rev Immunol 2002;21:197–208.

16 Crane IJ, Forrester JV: Th1 and Th2 lymphocytes in autoimmune disease. Crit Rev Immunol 2005;25:75–102.
17 Dick AD, Forrester JV, Liversidge J, Cope AP: The role of tumour necrosis factor (TNF-alpha) in experimental autoimmune uveoretinitis (EAU). Prog Retin Eye Res 2004;23:617–637.
18 Forrester JV, Liversidge J, Dua HS, Dick A, Harper F, McMenamin PG: Experimental autoimmune uveoretinitis: a model system for immunointervention: a review. Curr Eye Res 1992; 11(suppl):33–40.
19 Yamaki K, Takiyama N, Itho N, Mizuki N, Seiya M, Sinsuke W, Hayakawa K, Kotani T: Experimentally induced Vogt-Koyanagi-Harada disease in two Akita dogs. Exp Eye Res 2005;80: 273–280.
20 Yamaki K, Gocho K, Hayakawa K, Kondo I, Sakuragi S: Tyrosinase family proteins are antigens specific to Vogt-Koyanagi-Harada disease. J Immunol 2000;165:7323–7329.
21 Bora NS, Sohn JH, Kang SG, Cruz JM, Nishihori H, Suk HJ, Wang Y, Kaplan HJ, Bora PS: Type I collagen is the autoantigen in experimental autoimmune anterior uveitis. J Immunol 2004;172: 7086–7094.
22 Deeg CA, Thurau SR, Gerhards H, Ehrenhofer M, Wildner G, Kaspers B: Uveitis in horses induced by interphotoreceptor retinoid-binding protein is similar to the spontaneous disease. Eur J Immunol 2002;32:2598–2606.
23 Deeg CA, Ehrenhofer M, Thurau SR, Reese S, Wildner G, Kaspers B: Immunopathology of recurrent uveitis in spontaneously diseased horses. Exp Eye Res 2002;75:127–133.
24 Ichikawa T, Taguchi O, Takahashi T, Ikeda H, Takeuchi M, Tanaka T, Usui M, Nishizuka Y: Spontaneous development of autoimmune uveoretinitis in nude mice following reconstitution with embryonic rat thymus. Clin Exp Immunol 1991;86:112–117.
25 Egwuagu CE, Charukamnoetkanok P, Gery I: Thymic expression of autoantigens correlates with resistance to autoimmune disease. J Immunol 1997;159:3109–3112.
26 Takase H, Yu CR, Mahdi RM, Douek DC, Dirusso GB, Midgley FM, Dogra R, Allende G, Rosenkranz E, Pugliese A, Egwuagu CE, Gery I: Thymic expression of peripheral tissue antigens in humans: a remarkable variability among individuals. Int Immunol 2005;17:1131–1140.
27 Anderson MS, Venanzi ES, Klein L, Chen Z, Berzins SP, Turley SJ, von Boehmer H, Bronson R, Dierich A, Benoist C, Mathis D: Projection of an immunological self shadow within the thymus by the AIRE protein. Science 2002;298:1395–1401.
28 Goldrath AW, Hedrick SM: Central tolerance matters. Immunity 2005;23:113–114.
29 Anderson MS, Venanzi ES, Chen Z, Berzins SP, Benoist C, Mathis D: The cellular mechanism of AIRE control of T cell tolerance. Immunity 2005;23:227–239.
30 Szpak Y, Vieville JC, Tabary T, Naud MC, Chopin M, Edelson C, Cohen JH, Dausset J, de Kozak Y, Pla M: Spontaneous retinopathy in HLA-A29 transgenic mice. Proc Natl Acad Sci USA 2001;98: 2572–2576.
31 Nussenblatt RB, Mittal KK, Ryan S, Green WR, Maumenee AE: Birdshot retinochoroidopathy associated with HLA-A29 antigen and immune responsiveness to retinal S-antigen. Am J Ophthalmol 1982;94:147–158.
32 Ham DI, Kim SJ, Chen J, Vistica BP, Fariss RN, Lee RS, Wawrousek EF, Takase H, Yu CR, Egwuagu CE, Chan CC, Gery I: Central immunotolerance in transgenic mice expressing a foreign antigen under control of the rhodopsin promoter. Invest Ophthalmol Vis Sci 2004;45: 857–862.
33 Zhang M, Vacchio MS, Vistica BP, Lesage S, Egwuagu CE, Yu CR, Gelderman MP, Kennedy MC, Wawrousek EF, Gery I: T cell tolerance to a neo-self antigen expressed by thymic epithelial cells: the soluble form is more effective than the membrane-bound form. J Immunol 2003;170: 3954–3962.
34 Gregerson DS, Dou C: Spontaneous induction of immunoregulation by an endogenous retinal antigen. Invest Ophthalmol Vis Sci 2002;43:2984–2991.
35 Gregerson DS, Xiao JJ: Failure of memory (CD44 high) CD4 T cells to recognize their target antigen in retina. J Neuroimmunol 2001;120:34–41.
36 McPherson SW, Roberts JP, Gregerson DS: Systemic expression of rat soluble retinal antigen induces resistance to experimental autoimmune uveoretinitis. J Immunol 1999;163: 4269–4276.

37 Gregerson DS, Torseth JW, McPherson SW, Roberts JP, Shinohara T, Zack DJ: Retinal expression of a neo-self antigen, beta-galactosidase, is not tolerogenic and creates a target for autoimmune uveoretinitis. J Immunol 1999;163:1073–1080.
38 Kapphahn RJ, Ethen CM, Peters EA, Higgins L, Ferrington DA: Modified alpha A crystallin in the retina: altered expression and truncation with aging. Biochemistry 2003;42:15310–15325.
39 Prendergast RA, Iliff CE, Coskuncan NM, Caspi RR, Sartani G, Tarrant TK, Lutty GA, McLeod DS: T cell traffic and the inflammatory response in experimental autoimmune uveoretinitis. Invest Ophthalmol Vis Sci 1998;39:754–762.
40 Xu H, Forrester JV, Liversidge J, Crane IJ: Leukocyte trafficking in experimental autoimmune uveitis: breakdown of blood-retinal barrier and upregulation of cellular adhesion molecules. Invest Ophthalmol Vis Sci 2003;44:226–234.
41 Xu H, Manivannan A, Liversidge J, Sharp PF, Forrester JV, Crane IJ: Requirements for passage of T lymphocytes across non-inflamed retinal microvessels. J Neuroimmunol 2003;142:47–57.
42 Xu H, Manivannan A, Jiang HR, Liversidge J, Sharp PF, Forrester JV, Crane IJ: Recruitment of IFN-gamma-producing (Th1-like) cells into the inflamed retina in vivo is preferentially regulated by P-selectin glycoprotein ligand 1:P/E-selectin interactions. J Immunol 2004;172:3215–3224.
43 Jiang HR, Lumsden L, Forrester JV: Macrophages and dendritic cells in IRBP-induced experimental autoimmune uveoretinitis in B10RIII mice. Invest Ophthalmol Vis Sci 1999;40: 3177–3185.
44 Taylor PR, Martinez-Pomares L, Stacey M, Lin HH, Brown GD, Gordon S: Macrophage receptors and immune recognition. Annu Rev Immunol 2005;23:901–944.
45 Robertson MJ, Erwig LP, Liversidge J, Forrester JV, Rees AJ, Dick AD: Retinal microenvironment controls resident and infiltrating macrophage function during uveoretinitis. Invest Ophthalmol Vis Sci 2002;43:2250–2257.
46 Zhang M, Fukushima A, Vistica BP, Kim SJ, Hung L, Wawrousek EF, Egwuagu CE, Lee RS, Whitcup SM, Gery I: Skewed abrogation of tolerance to a neo self-antigen in double-transgenic mice coexpressing the antigen with interleukin-1β or interferon-γ. Cell Immunol 2001;207:6–12.
47 Jones LS, Rizzo LV, Agarwal RK, Tarrant TK, Chan CC, Wiggert B, Caspi RR: IFN-gamma-deficient mice develop experimental autoimmune uveitis in the context of a deviant effector response. J Immunol 1997;158:5997–6005.
48 Shao H, Fu Y, Liao T, Peng Y, Chen L, Kaplan HJ, Sun D: Anti-CD137 mAb treatment inhibits experimental autoimmune uveitis by limiting expansion and increasing apoptotic death of uveitogenic T cells. Invest Ophthalmol Vis Sci 2005;46:596–603.
49 Bagenstose LM, Agarwal RK, Silver PB, Harlan DM, Hoffmann SC, Kampen RL, Chan CC, Caspi RR: Disruption of CD40/CD40-ligand interactions in a retinal autoimmunity model results in protection without tolerance. J Immunol 2005;175:124–130.
50 Crane IJ, Xu H, Manivannan A, McKillop-Smith S, Lamont G, Wallace C, Liversidge J, Sharp PF, Forrester JV: Effect of anti-macrophage inflammatory protein-1α on leukocyte trafficking and disease progression in experimental autoimmune uveoretinitis. Eur J Immunol 2003;33:402–410.
51 Xu H, Manivannan A, Goatman KA, Liversidge J, Sharp PF, Forrester JV, Crane IJ: Improved leukocyte tracking in mouse retinal and choroidal circulation. Exp Eye Res 2002;74:403–410.
52 Xu H, Manivannan A, Liversidge J, Sharp PF, Forrester JV, Crane IJ: Involvement of CD44 in leukocyte trafficking at the blood-retinal barrier. J Leukoc Biol 2002;72:1133–1141.
53 Jiang HR, Muckersie E, Robertson M, Xu H, Liversidge J, Forrester JV: Secretion of interleukin-10 or interleukin-12 by LPS-activated dendritic cells is critically dependent on time of stimulus relative to initiation of purified DC culture. J Leukoc Biol 2002;72:978–985.
54 Jiang HR, Muckersie E, Robertson M, Forrester JV: Antigen-specific inhibition of experimental autoimmune uveoretinitis by bone marrow-derived immature dendritic cells. Invest Ophthalmol Vis Sci 2003;44:1598–1607.
55 Gangi E, Vasu C, Cheatem D, Prabhakar BS: IL-10-producing CD4+ CD25+ regulatory T cells play a critical role in granulocyte-macrophage colony-stimulating factor-induced suppression of experimental autoimmune thyroiditis. J Immunol 2005;174:7006–7013.
56 Li Y, Heuser JS, Kosanke SD, Hemric M, Cunningham MW: Protection against experimental autoimmune myocarditis is mediated by interleukin-10-producing T cells that are controlled by dendritic cells. Am J Pathol 2005;167:5–15.

57 Mahnke K, Enk AH: Dendritic cells: key cells for the induction of regulatory T cells? Curr Top Microbiol Immunol 2005;293:133–150.
58 Agarwal RK, Kang Y, Zambidis E, Scott DW, Chan CC, Caspi RR: Retroviral gene therapy with an immunoglobulin-antigen fusion construct protects from experimental autoimmune uveitis. J Clin Invest 2000;106:245–252.
59 Oksala A: The significance of treatment by antibiotics and steroids in acute anterior uveitis. Acta Ophthalmol (Copenh) 1960;38:405–409.
60 Campbell FP: Retina and optic nerve. Arch Ophthalmol 1968;79:789–802.
61 Dick AD, Kreutzer B, Laliotou B, Forrester JV: Phenotypic analysis of retinal leukocyte infiltration during combined cyclosporin A and nasal antigen administration of retinal antigens: delay and inhibition of macrophage and granulocyte infiltration. Ocul Immunol Inflamm 1997;5:129–140.
62 Mochizuki M, Kawashima H: Effects of FK506, 15-deoxyspergualin, and cyclosporine on experimental autoimmune uveoretinitis in the rat. Autoimmunity 1990;8:37–41.
63 Caspi RR, McAllister CG, Gery I, Nussenblatt RB: Differential effects of cyclosporins A and G on functional activation of a T-helper-lymphocyte line mediating experimental autoimmune uveoretinitis. Cell Immunol 1988;113:350–360.
64 Liversidge J, Thomson AW, Sewell HF, Forrester JV: EAU in the guinea pig: inhibition of cell-mediated immunity and Ia antigen expression by cyclosporin A. Clin Exp Immunol 1987;69: 591–600.
65 Murphy CC, Greiner K, Plskova J, Duncan L, Frost NA, Forrester JV, Dick AD: Cyclosporine vs tacrolimus therapy for posterior and intermediate uveitis. Arch Ophthalmol 2005;123:634–641.
66 Dick AD, Meyer P, James T, Forrester JV, Hale G, Waldmann H, Isaacs JD: Campath-1H therapy in refractory ocular inflammatory disease. Br J Ophthalmol 2000;84:107–109.
67 Greiner K, Murphy CC, Willermain F, Duncan L, Plskova J, Hale G, Isaacs JD, Forrester JV, Dick AD: Anti-TNFα therapy modulates the phenotype of peripheral blood CD4+ T cells in patients with posterior segment intraocular inflammation. Invest Ophthalmol Vis Sci 2004;45:170–176.
68 Murphy CC, Greiner K, Plskova J, Duncan L, Frost A, Isaacs JD, Rebello P, Waldmann H, Hale G, Forrester JV, Dick AD: Neutralizing tumor necrosis factor activity leads to remission in patients with refractory noninfectious posterior uveitis. Arch Ophthalmol 2004;122:845–851.
69 Kotter I, Zierhut M, Eckstein AK, Vonthein R, Ness T, Gunaydin I, Grimbacher B, Blaschke S, Meyer-Riemann W, Peter HH, Stubiger N: Human recombinant interferon alfa-2a for the treatment of Behçet's disease with sight threatening posterior or panuveitis. Br J Ophthalmol 2003;87: 423–431.
70 Plskova J, Greiner K, Muckersie E, Duncan L, Forrester JV: Interferon-alpha: a key factor in autoimmune disease? Invest Ophthalmol Vis Sci 2006;47:3946–3950.
71 Kotter I, Deuter C, Stubiger N, Zierhut M: Interferon-α (IFN-α) application versus tumor necrosis factor-α antagonism for ocular Behçet's disease: focusing more on IFN. J Rheumatol 2005;32: 1633–1634.
72 Jabs DA, Nussenblatt RB, Rosenbaum JT: Standardization of uveitis nomenclature for reporting clinical data. Results of the First International Workshop. Am J Ophthalmol 2005;140:509–516.

Dr. John V. Forrester
Department of Ophthalmology, University of Aberdeen
Medical School, Foresterhill
Aberdeen AB25 2ZD (UK)
Tel. +44 1224 681818, Fax +44 1224 685158, E-Mail j.forrester@abdn.ac.uk

Niederkorn JY, Kaplan HJ (eds): Immune Response and the Eye.
Chem Immunol Allergy. Basel, Karger, 2007, vol 92, pp 244–253

Acute Retinal Necrosis

Takeshi Kezuka[a], *Sally S. Atherton*[b]

[a]Department of Ophthalmology, Tokyo Medical University Hospital, Tokyo, Japan;
[b]Department of Cellular Biology and Anatomy, Medical College of Georgia,
Augusta, Ga., USA

Abstract

Acute retinal necrosis (ARN) is a rare disease that is usually caused by one of the three neurotropic human herpesviruses – herpes simplex virus type 1(HSV-1), HSV-2 and varicella-zoster virus (VZV). Although much is known about the clinical course of the disease and its treatment and about the viruses that cause it, comparatively little is known about its pathogenesis. This article will review the history of ARN, the typical clinical findings, and methods of diagnosis. Information from studies of the mouse model of ARN including development of anterior chamber-associated immune deviation (ACAID) and routes of spread will be reconsidered, and the combined information from human and mouse studies will be discussed to suggest mechanisms that contribute to the pathogenesis of ARN in human patients. Finally, puzzles and questions about the disease will be considered.

Acute retinal necrosis (ARN, Kirisawa-Urayama uveitis), a fulminant, viral necrotizing retinitis, was first described in Japan by Urayama et al. [1]. ARN occurs typically in healthy patients but some immunosuppressed patients also develop ARN [2–5]. Although in about two thirds of cases ARN affects only one eye, about one third has bilateral disease. Involvement of the fellow eye may occur coincident with the initial presentation of ARN, or weeks to months or even years later [6–10].

Several members of the human herpesvirus family cause ARN [11]. In 1982, Culbertson et al. [12] observed herpesvirus particles by electron microscopy in the retina of enucleated eyes from patients with ARN. Serum antibodies to herpes simplex virus (HSV), varicella-zoster virus (VZV), cytomegalovirus, and Epstein-Barr virus were demonstrated in these patients. In 1986, they identified VZV in two ARN eyes by immunohistochemistry. They also isolated herpes virus by culture from one of the two eyes [13]. In 2000, Ganatra et al. [11] used PCR and detected VZV and HSV-1 in vitreous specimens of ARN patients older than 25 years, respectively, but found HSV-2 in ARN patients younger than 25 years. In patients with a history of encephalitis, ARN has been associated more often with HSV-1 than HSV-2, whereas HSV-2 ARN is more often observed in patients with a history of meningitis; however, these associations are not absolute [11, 14–17]. Although the neurotropic herpesviruses VZV, HSV-1 and HSV-2 are most frequently associated with ARN, cytomegalovirus has also been identified as a cause of ARN [18, 19].

Patients with ARN usually present with acute loss of vision [1, 20]. As the disease progresses from the acute phase to the chronic phase, patients often have some initial recovery of visual acuity followed by vision loss because of retinal detachment and/or occlusive retinal arteriolitis. Some patients may develop ocular pain due to increased intraocular pressure during the acute phase [21]. Intraocular pressure may be elevated in HSV-associated ARN but may remain normal in VZV-associated ARN. The high intraocular pressure usually returns to normal within 2 months. Three phases of ARN have been described: the acute phase, the chronic phase, and the resolution phase [22]. During the acute phase, patients develop panuveitis and a necrotizing retinitis characterized by white-yellow exudates [21, 23, 24]. In the chronic (retinal detachment) phase, ocular inflammation is reduced, the area of white-yellow retinitis is decreased, and retinal detachment due to vitreous condensation and traction with giant retinal tears are observed [20]. The resolution phase is characterized by lack of inflammation and by stable vitreous condensation. During the resolution phase, macular degeneration, including the presence of preretinal membranes, is observed in more than 70% of the patients with ARN [22].

Clinical Features of Acute Retinal Necrosis

Although numerous clinical findings have been described, none is pathognomonic for ARN. Keratic precipitates that usually appear as white, mutton fat deposits often occur during the onset of HSV or VZV ARN. In the chronic phase, white mutton fat-like precipitates may be replaced by pigmented precipitates (fig. 1). Although anterior granulomatous uveitis is ameliorated within 2 weeks, resolution of the prominent vitritis tends to be delayed compared to the anterior uveitis. The prominent vitreal inflammatory reaction and vitreous opacity usually resolve within 3 weeks, but a vitritis may recur 3–4 weeks later. Fibrotic changes of the vitreous decrease the mobility of vitreous gel, leading to the development of a posterior vitreous detachment which in turn produces vitreous traction on the peripheral retina, resulting in retinal detachment [20].

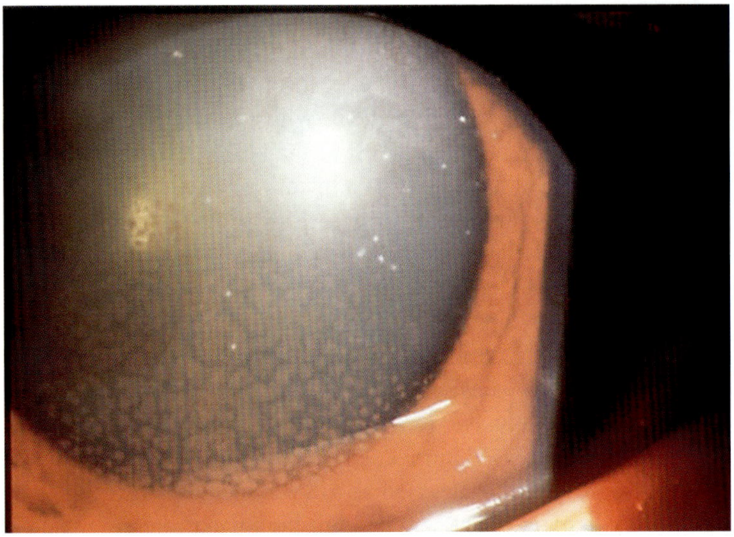

Fig. 1. Pigmented 'mutton fat' keratic precipitates.

During the acute phase of ARN, disk edema is a common finding with occasional disk hemorrhage. Optic neuritis may develop early, and ARN should be suspected if there are optic nerve changes even though typical retinal lesions are not seen. Hemorrhage or distension of the optic nerve may be important signs of viral infiltration via the optic nerve (fig. 2).

White-yellow retinal lesions in the peripheral retina enlarge concentrically in the early phase of ARN. Patchy granular lesions in the retina may fuse to form geographic lesions. In the early phase, the granular lesions in the peripheral retina mimic signs of circulatory blockage (fig. 2). If treated by antiviral therapy, the retinal lesions may become confluent and necrotic due to the immune-mediated attempt to clear the virus. With further progression of the immune reaction, an inflammatory occlusive vasculopathy may develop with arteriolar involvement. The retinal vascular lesion of ARN is an occlusive vasculopathy with arteriolar involvement, and may be divided into an acute phase and a chronic phase. During the acute phase, retinal arteritis and periphlebitis occur with retinal hemorrhage. Fluorescein angiography shows diffuse fluorescein leakage along the retinal artery and areas of early hypofluorescence consistent with ischemic changes. During the chronic phase, venous occlusions develop with severe visual loss. On average, two main arterial occlusions are seen, and ghost vessels occur in severe cases. Visual prognosis is poor when there are two or more ghost vessels.

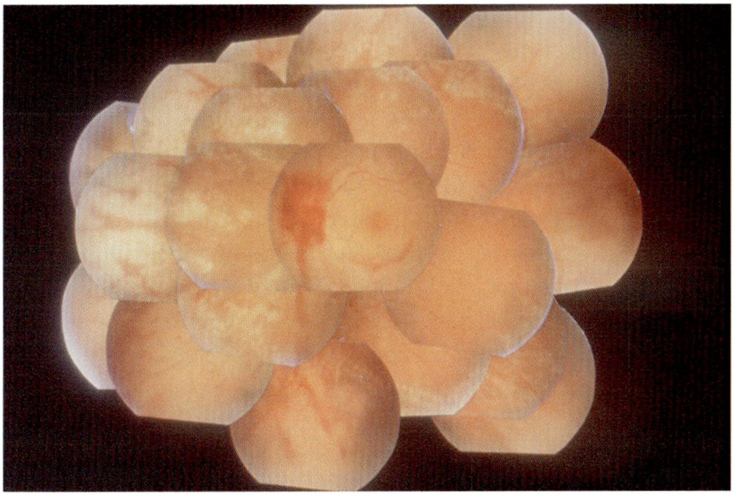

Fig. 2. White-yellow retinal lesions in the peripheral retina and hemorrhage of the optic nerve. Laser surgery was performed posterior to the necrotic peripheral lesions to prevent retinal detachment.

The acute ocular inflammatory changes observed during the acute phase resolve over a period of several months. Vitreal infiltration is composed of fibroblasts and retinal pigment epithelial cells, and these infiltrations form vitreous membranes leading to retinal detachment. In the chronic phase, retinal detachment often occurs because of a giant retinal tear in the area between healthy posterior retina and necrotic peripheral retina. The necrotic retina is very thin, and rhegmatogenous retinal detachments develop because of the strong adhesion between the vitreous and necrotic retina.

Diagnosis and Virus Identification

The initial diagnosis of ARN is usually made on the clinical findings. The Executive Committee of the American Uveitis Society recently published a set of standard diagnostic criteria for the ARN syndrome. The criteria state that the designation of the ARN syndrome should be based on clinical appearance and the course of infection. The mandatory clinical characteristics include the following: (1) one or more foci of retinal necrosis with discrete borders in the peripheral retina; (2) rapid progression of disease if antiviral therapy has not been given; (3) circumferential spread of disease; (4) evidence of occlusive vasculopathy, and (5) a prominent inflammatory reaction in the vitreous and anterior chamber. Optic nerve involvement, scleritis and pain support, but are not required, for the diagnosis of ARN [25].

Even though many cases of ARN can be diagnosed on the basis of the clinical findings, confirmation of the diagnosis and identification of the causative agent are often sought. While viral isolation might intuitively seem like the best approach, recovery of virus is often difficult and time consuming. Herpesvirus particles can be identified by electron microscopy, but this technique cannot differentiate among the herpesvirus types. The most common immunologic approach is to compare the intraocular antibody levels with those in the serum. In normal eyes, a blood-ocular barrier is present in the anterior chamber, and the tight junction between the pigmented and the non-pigmented ciliary epithelium provides an exclusive barrier, preventing passage of interstitial molecules. In ARN patients, the viral antibody titer is higher in intraocular fluids (both aqueous humor and vitreous fluid) than in the serum because of the intraocular production of antibody to the pathogenic virus. Utilizing this understanding, viral antibody titers in intraocular fluid and serum are determined by the fluorescent antibody technique and the antibody quotient equal to (VZV – specific IgG titers in intraocular fluid/total IgG levels in intraocular fluid)/(VZV – IgG titers in sera/total IgG levels in sera) is calculated [26, 27]. A value ≥ 6 is considered diagnostic [27]. Recently, because of increasing availability, PCR of aqueous and/or vitreous fluid is the assay most frequently employed to confirm a diagnosis of ARN and to identify the infectious agent [28–31]. This technique offers many advantages: it is specific (not only for viruses, it can also differentiate between viruses and a large number of other potential intraocular pathogens), it can be done relatively quickly, it is available in most diagnostic laboratories, and it requires only a small amount of sample. Since identification of the causative agent can be done rapidly, the appropriate treatment can be started earlier thereby reducing the potential for vision loss in the infected eye.

Pathogenesis of Acute Retinal Necrosis

Although much is known about the clinical presentation of ARN, about diagnosing ARN, about which among the human herpesviruses cause ARN, and about the biology of those viruses, many of the questions about the pathogenesis of ARN remain to be answered: e.g. by which route(s) does the virus gain access to the retina, how much virus is needed to cause disease, and, since ARN is usually observed in immunocompetent patients, what is the contribution of immune effector cells and/or of immunomodulators to retinal destruction? As with many human diseases, some aspects of the pathogenesis of ARN may be understood by judicious interpretation of results from animal studies. In 1924, von Szily [32] reported that injection of HSV into one eye of a rabbit resulted in retinal destruction in the uninoculated, contralateral eye. Over 50 years later, Whittum et al. [33] described acute retinal necrosis characterized by vasculitis, retinitis and retinal schisis, with loss of the retinal architecture, in the uninoculated eye following injection of HSV-1 into the anterior chamber of one eye of a BALB/c mouse. In addition to the destruction of the retina of the uninoculated eye, mice injected with HSV-1 via the anterior chamber route displayed anterior chamber-associated immune deviation (ACAID) characterized by an impairment in virus-specific delayed hypersensitivity while the humoral immune response to the virus was unaffected. Control mice inoculated with HSV-1 subcutaneously developed vigorous virus-specific delayed hypersensitivity and a high titer of anti-herpesvirus antibody [34].

Some clinical and microscopic features such as vitritis, retinal arteritis, retinal necrosis, and optic neuritis observed in human cases of ARN are replicated in the mouse. Further studies using the mouse model described the route by which injection of virus into one anterior chamber results in virus infection of the retina of the uninoculated eye. From the site of injection in the anterior chamber of one eye, virus spreads via synaptically connected neurons sequentially to the ipsilateral ciliary ganglion, the ipsilateral Edinger-Westphal nucleus, the ipsilateral suprachiasmatic nucleus of the hypothalamus, and finally to the optic nerve and retina of the uninoculated contralateral eye. Although virus infects the contralateral suprachiasmatic nucleus 1–2 days after the ipsilateral suprachiasmatic nucleus, the optic nerve and retina of the injected eye are not infected and the retina of the injected eye is spared [35]. T cells are required for sparing as bilateral retinitis is observed in athymic mice or in mice in which T cells have been depleted [36, 37].

There are several areas where the findings from studies of the mouse model can be extrapolated to understanding the pathogenesis of ARN in patients. Development of ACAID in the mouse suggests that in humans, ARN may be linked to a reduction in delayed hypersensitivity responsiveness. Studies in a small group of ARN patients by Rochet et al. [38] indicated that each patient displayed one or more elements of an abnormal systemic immunologic responsiveness (decreased lymphocyte proliferation, decreased cutaneous reactivity to recall antigens, increased percentage or absolute number of B lymphocytes). Later studies by Kezuka et al. [39] indicated that patients with ARN displayed specific delayed hypersensitivity unresponsiveness to VZV during acute disease and that antigen-specific responsiveness was restored when the patients recovered from ARN. These investigators suggested that patients with ARN develop an ACAID-like response to viral antigens in the intraocular compartment which disappears as the disease is resolved [39, 40]. Although there were differences between the studies by Rochet et al. [38] and Kezuka et al. [39], taken together, the results of these studies support the idea that virus-specific, perhaps systemic, anergy contributes to the pathogenesis of ARN in humans as in the mouse model.

Results of tracing studies using the mouse model show that following anterior chamber inoculation, virus spreads from the site of injection to the retina of the uninjected eye via sequential infection of synaptically connected neurons culminating in infection of the optic nerve and retina of the uninjected eye [35]. Optic neuritis has been reported in some ARN patients, an observation which supports the idea that one route of virus spread to the retina in humans is via the optic nerve [41–44]. Spread via the optic nerve is consistent with the ability of HSV-1, HSV-2 and VZV to spread via neurons. In addition, since ARN has also been described in some patients coincident with or following herpesvirus encephalitis or meningitis, it appears likely that in humans, as has been described in the mouse, one route by which virus enters the eye to infect the retina is by neuronal spread from the central nervous system via the optic nerve.

Although humans with unilateral ARN do not typically have herpetic anterior uveitis in the uninvolved eye, knowledge of the route of spread in the mouse may provide insight into how a virus which is normally found in the trigeminal nerve and trigeminal ganglion could enter pathways synaptically connected to the optic nerve and retina. It is possible that during herpesvirus infection of the cornea and/or anterior segment, virus may not only enter the trigeminal nerves which supply the eye, but also the other nerves which supply the anterior segment of the eye (such as the postganglionic nerves that supply the iris and ciliary body), resulting in latency in non-trigeminal sites. Herpesvirus has been reported in non-trigeminal sites in humans, and results from a recent study suggest that HSV-1 may be latent in the ciliary ganglion [45–48]. Thus, by extrapolating the pathway of virus spread in the mouse to that in humans, HSV-1 (or another neurotropic virus) from an acute or reactivated infection of the ciliary ganglion would have access to neuronal pathways synaptically linked to the optic nerve and retina.

Puzzles and Questions

Although there is a considerable body of knowledge about ARN from studies in human patients and from the mouse model, there remain a number of puzzles and questions about ARN. Since a large percentage of the adult human population is seropositive (and latently infected) with one or more of the neurotropic herpesviruses that cause ARN, it is not known why the incidence of ARN is so low compared with the total number of individuals who are seropositive for these herpesviruses. More information is needed about non-trigeminal sites of herpesvirus latency and also about the role of the immune system in controlling virus replication and spread at synapses, in nerve cell bodies, and in neurons. Such information might be used to design immune-based therapies to limit herpesvirus spread during acute or reactivated infection or to prevent virus reactivation. Since ARN affects only a very small subset of individuals who are acutely or latently infected with herpesvirus and since some or all of the individuals with ARN exhibit impairment in some delayed hypersensitivity responsiveness, understanding how immune suppression is involved in the pathogenesis of ARN may ultimately be employed to predict who among individuals with prior or current herpesvirus infection is at the greatest risk for the development of ARN. In addition, since about one third of ARN patients eventually develops the disease in both eyes, understanding more about the interplay between virus and potential antiviral immune responses in the central nervous system might ultimately be used to predict which ARN patients are at highest risk for involvement of the fellow eye and eliminate the need for long-term prophylactic therapy in patients at low risk for involvement of the fellow eye. In conclusion, continued studies in humans with ARN, combined with judicious interpretation of results of animal models of herpesvirus infection of the eye and brain, will provide additional understanding of the pathogenesis of ARN. Knowledge gained from unraveling the pathogenesis of ARN may ultimately be used to design new pharmacologic or immunologic antiviral therapies to prevent or ameliorate this rare, but potentially, sight-threatening disease.

References

1 Urayama A, Yamada N, Susaki T, Nishiyama Y, Watanabe N, Wakusawa S, Satoh Y: Unilateral acute uveitis with retinal periarteritis and detachment. Jpn J Clin Ophthalmol 1971;25:607–619.
2 Friberg TR, Jost BF: Acute retinal necrosis in an immunosuppressed patient. Am J Ophthalmol 1984;98:515–517.
3 Culbertson WW, Atherton SS: Acute retinal necrosis and similar retinitis syndromes. Int Ophthalmol Clin 1993;33:129–143.
4 Sellitti TP, Huang AJ, Schiffman J, Davis JL: Association of herpes zoster ophthalmicus with acquired immunodeficiency syndrome and acute retinal necrosis. Am J Ophthalmol 1993;116:297–301.
5 Cunningham ET Jr, Short GA, Irvine AR, Duker JS, Margolis TP: Acquired immunodeficiency syndrome-associated herpes simplex virus retinitis. Clinical description and use of a polymerase chain reaction-based assay as a diagnostic tool. Arch Ophthalmol 1996;114:834–840.
6 Price FW, Schlaegel TF: Bilateral acute retinal necrosis. Am J Ophthalmol 1980;89:419–424.
7 Gartry DS, Spalton DJ, Tilzey A, Hykin PG: Acute retinal necrosis syndrome. Br J Ophthalmol 1991;75:292–297.
8 Falcone PM, Brockhurst RJ: Delayed onset of bilateral acute retinal necrosis syndrome: a 34-year interval. Ann Ophthalmol 1993;25:373–374.
9 Ezra E, Pearson RV, Etchells DE, Gregor ZJ: Delayed fellow eye involvement in acute retinal necrosis syndrome. Am J Ophthalmol 1995;120:115–117.

10 Schlingemann RO, Bruinenberg M, Wertheim-van Dillen P, Feron E: Twenty years' delay of fellow eye involvement in herpes simplex virus type 2-associated bilateral acute retinal necrosis syndrome. Am J Ophthalmol 1996;122:891–892.
11 Ganatra JB, Chandler D, Santos C, Kuppermann B, Margolis TP: Viral causes of the acute retinal necrosis syndrome. Am J Ophthalmol 2000;129:166–172.
12 Culbertson WW, Blumenkranz MS, Haines H, Gass DM, Mitchell KB, Norton EW: The acute retinal necrosis syndrome. Part 2: Histopathology and etiology. Ophthalmology 1982;89:1317–1325.
13 Culbertson WW, Blumenkranz MS, Pepose JS, Stewart JA, Curtin VT: Varicella zoster virus is a cause of the acute retinal necrosis syndrome. Ophthalmology 1986;93:559–569.
14 Levinson RD, Reidy R, Chiu MT: Acute retinal necrosis after neonatal herpes encephalitis. Br J Ophthalmol 1999;83:123.
15 Van Gelder RN, Willig JL, Holland GN, Kaplan HJ: Herpes simplex virus type 2 as a cause of acute retinal necrosis syndrome in young patients. Ophthalmology 2001;108:869–876.
16 Tan JCH, Byles D, Stanford MR, Frith PA, Graham EM: Acute retinal necrosis in children caused by herpes simplex virus. Retina 2001;21:344–347.
17 Landry ML, Mullangi P, Nee P, Klein BR: Herpes simplex virus type 2 acute retinal necrosis 9 years after neonatal herpes. J Pediatr 2005;146:836–838.
18 Silverstein BE, Conrad D, Margolis TP, Wong IG: Cytomegalovirus-associated acute retinal necrosis syndrome. Am J Ophthalmol 1997;123:257–258.
19 Tran TH, Rozenberg F, Cassoux N, Rao NA, Lehoang P, Bodaghi B: Polymerase chain reaction analysis of aqueous humour samples in necrotising retinitis. Br J Ophthalmol 2003;87:79–83.
20 Fisher JP, Lewis ML, Blumenkranz MS, Culbertson WW, Flynn HW Jr, Clarkson JG, Gass JD, Norton EW: The acute retinal necrosis syndrome. Part I. Clinical manifestations. Ophthalmology 1982;89:1309–1316.
21 Opremcak EM: Uveitis. A Clinical Manual for Ocular Inflammation, ed 1. New York, Springer, 1995, pp 115–117.
22 Usui N: Acute retinal necrosis. Atarasii Gannka 2003;20:309–320.
23 Culbertson WW, Dix RD: Varicella-zoster virus disease: posterior segment of the eye; in Pepose JS, Holland GN, Wilhelmus KR (eds): Ocular Infection and Immunity. St. Louis, Mosby, 1996, pp 1131–1149.
24 Margolis TP, Atherton SS: Herpes simplex virus diseases: posterior segment of the eye; in Pepose JS, Holland GN, Wilhelmus KR (eds): Ocular Infection and Immunity. St. Louis, Mosby, 1996, pp 1155–1167.
25 Holland GN: Standard diagnostic criteria for the acute retinal necrosis syndrome. Executive Committee of the American Uveitis Society. Am J Ophthalmol 1994;117:663–667.
26 Witmer R: Clinical implications of aqueous humor studies in uveitis. Am J Ophthalmol 1978;86:39–45.
27 Okitsu Y: Diagnostic value of antibody titer and quotient of herpes viruses in intraocular fluids. Jpn J Clin Ophthalmol 1988;42:801–805.
28 Usui M, Usui N, Goto H, Minoda H, Rai T: Polymerase chain reaction for diagnosis of herpetic intraocular inflammation. Ocul Immunol Inflamm 1993;1:105–112.
29 Knox CM, Chandler D, Short GA, Margolis TP: Polymerase chain reaction-based assay of vitreous samples for the diagnosis of viral retinitis. Use in diagnostic dilemmas. Ophthalmology 1998;105:37–44.
30 Asano S, Yoshikawa T, Kimura H, Enomoto Y, Ohashi M, Terasaki H, Nishiyama Y: Monitoring herpesvirus DNA in three cases of acute retinal necrosis by real-time PCR. J Clin Virol 2004;29:206–209.
31 Bonfioli AA, Eller AW: Acute retinal necrosis. Semin Ophthalmol 2005;20:155–160.
32 von Szily A: Experimental endogenous transmission of infection from bulbus to bulbus. Klin Monatsbl Augenheilkd 1924;72:593–602.
33 Whittum JA, McCulley JP, Niederkorn JY, Streilein JW: Ocular disease induced in mice by anterior chamber inoculation of herpes simplex virus. Invest Ophthalmol Vis Sci 1984;25:1065–1073.
34 Whittum JA, Niederkorn JY, McCulley JP, Streilein JW: Intracameral inoculation of herpes simplex virus type 1 induces anterior chamber associated immune deviation. Curr Eye Res 1983;2:691–697.

35 Vann VR, Atherton SS: Neural spread of herpes simplex virus after anterior chamber inoculation. Invest Ophthalmol Vis Sci 1990;32:2462–2472.
36 Azumi A, Atherton SS: Sparing of the ipsilateral retina following anterior chamber inoculation of HSV-1: requirement for either $CD4^+$ or $CD8^+$ T cells. Invest Ophthalmol Vis Sci 1994;34: 3251–3259.
37 Matsubara S, Atherton SS: Spread of HSV-1 to the suprachiasmatic nuclei and retina in T cell depleted BALB/c mice. J Neuroimmunol 1997;80:165–171.
38 Rochat C, Polla BS, Herbort CP: Immunological profiles in patients with acute retinal necrosis. Graefes Arch Clin Exp Ophthalmol 1996;234:547–552.
39 Kezuka T, Sakai J, Usui N, Streilein JW, Usui M: Evidence for antigen-specific immune deviation in patients with acute retinal necrosis. Arch Ophthalmol 2001;119:1044–1049.
40 Kezuka T: Immune deviation and ocular infections with varicella zoster virus. Ocul Immunol Inflamm 2004;12:17–24.
41 Friedlander SM, Rahhal FM, Ericson L, Friedlander SM, Rahhal FM, Ericson L, Arevalo JF, Hughes JD, Levi L, Wiley CA, Graham EM, Freeman WR: Optic neuropathy preceding acute retinal necrosis in acquired immunodeficiency syndrome. Arch Ophthalmol 1996;114:1481–1485.
42 Shayegani A, Odel JG, Kazim M, Hall LS, Bamford N, Schubert H: Varicella-zoster virus retrobulbar optic neuritis in a patient with human immunodeficiency virus. Am J Ophthalmol 1996;122: 586–588.
43 Tornerup NR, Fomagaard A, Nielson NV: HSV-1-induced acute retinal necrosis syndrome presenting with severe inflammatory orbitopathy, proptosis, and optic nerve involvement. Ophthalmology 2000;107:397–401.
44 Maertzdorf J, Van der Lelij A, Baarsma GS, Osterhaus AD, Verjans GM: Herpes simplex virus type 1 (HSV-1)-induced retinitis following herpes simplex encephalitis: indication for brain-to-eye transmission of HSV-1. Ann Neurol 2001;49:104–106.
45 Takasu T, Furuta Y, Sato KC, Fukuda S, Inuyama Y, Nagashima K: Detection of latent herpes simplex virus DNA and RNA in human geniculate ganglia by the polymerase chain reaction. Acta Otolaryngol 1992;112:1004–1011.
46 Mahalingam R, Wellish MC, Dueland AN, Cohrs RJ, Gilden DH: Localization of herpes simplex virus and varicella zoster virus DNA in human ganglia. Ann Neurol 1992;31:444–448.
47 Baringer JR, Pisani P: Herpes simplex virus genome in human nervous system tissue analyzed by polymerase chain reaction. Ann Neurol 1994;36:823–829.
48 Bustos DE, Atherton SS: Detection of herpes simplex virus type 1 in human ciliary ganglia. Invest Ophthalmol Vis Sci 2002;43:2244–2249.

Dr. Sally S. Atherton
Department of Cellular Biology and Anatomy
Medical College of Georgia, R and E Building, CB2915
Augusta, GA 30912 (USA)
Tel. +1 706 721 3731, Fax +1 706 721 6120, E-Mail satherton@mail.mcg.edu

Niederkorn JY, Kaplan HJ (eds): Immune Response and the Eye.
Chem Immunol Allergy. Basel, Karger, 2007, vol 92, pp 254–265

Onchocerca volvulus, Wolbachia and River Blindness

Eric Pearlman, Illona Gillette-Ferguson

Department of Ophthalmology, Case Western Reserve University, Cleveland, Ohio, USA

Abstract

Chronic infection with filarial nematodes results in development of a suppressive response to an immense parasite burden, thereby limiting pathological and clinical manifestations. However, pro-inflammatory responses to dead and degenerating *Onchocerca volvulus* worms and release of endosymbiotic *Wolbachia* bacteria result in corneal opacification, sacrification and visual impairment. This review discusses host and parasite factors implicated in maintaining this balance of pro- an anti-inflammatory responses, and will focus on adaptive and innate immunity to filarial antigens and endosymbiotic *Wolbachia* bacteria.

Over 150 million individuals worldwide are infected with filarial nematodes, which include *Wuchereria bancrofti* and *Brugia malayi* that cause lymphatic filariasis, and *Onchocerca volvulus*, which causes onchocerciasis (river blindness) and infects approximately 17 million individuals. Adult male and female *O. volvulus* worms are present in subcutaneous nodules, and female worms produce millions of first stage larvae (microfilariae) during the 10–14 years that they survive in the human host. Microfilariae migrate through the skin, and the parasite life cycle is continued after ingestion of microfilariae during the blood meal of a *Simulium* blackfly. Microfilariae undergo two molts in the blackfly, migrating through the insect gut, the thorax and into the salivary gland. On a subsequent blood meal, infective third stage larvae are transmitted to the next human host where they undergo a further two molts to become adult males and females.

The host immune response to the immense parasite burden is modulated by suppressive factors produced by the parasites in addition to the host, so that most infected individuals show few signs of clinical disease. Posttreatment studies indicate that clinical responses coincide with parasite death and degeneration, indicating an initial breakdown of the immunosuppressive response to the parasites [1]. These posttreatment observations provide insight into the development of clinical symptoms in chronic infection, where there is continual death and degeneration of parasites. In the skin, clinical responses are manifested as papule formation and severe pruritus, depigmentation and loss of skin elasticity, whereas in the eye, clinical responses include corneal opacification, neovascularization, scarification, resulting in visual impairment and blindness. This review will examine the host and parasite factors that regulate immunosuppression, and which contribute to the pathogenesis of *Onchocerca* keratitis.

Infection and Disease – Host and Parasite Factors Determine the Balance between Pro- and Anti-Inflammatory Responses in Filariasis

Several parasite-derived molecules have been described that have the potential to either block effector responses targeted at the parasites or to modulate the host response. The first group includes antioxidative enzymes and protease inhibitors, whereas the second group includes cytokine homologues and cytokine receptor homologues including migration inhibitory factor, transforming growth factor (TGF)-β, and TGF-β receptor [2], all of which could contribute to suppression of the antiparasite response. Although the cloned proteins have biological activity in vitro, in the absence of a genetic system for these worms, it is difficult to determine their role in the course of infection. Filarial parasites also have glycoproteins that directly suppress or cause deviation of T and B cell responses. For example ES-62, which is secreted by adult parasites, can skew the T cell response to filariae toward a Th2 phenotype by suppressing macrophage interleukin (IL)-12 production [3].

Population-based studies demonstrated an inverse correlation between the number of circulating microfilariae and cell proliferation [4, 5]. Although the underlying mechanisms are not fully understood, IL-10 appears to be involved, as this cytokine is produced by mononuclear cells and T cells of infected individuals [4]. Also, in utero exposure to parasite antigens (comparing infected vs. uninfected mothers) shows elevated levels of IL-10 and TGF-β, and T cells have elevated CTLA4 expression [6]. TGF-β is produced by alternatively activated macrophages and T regulatory cells. Consistent with this notion, T cell clones isolated from peripheral blood of individuals with generalized onchocerciasis have a T regulatory cell phenotype as they selectively produced IL-10 and TGF-β, and not IL-2 [7, 8]. Similarly, T regulatory cells were predominant in experimental models of filarial infection, as CD4+ cells showed elevated CD25, CTLA4 and expression of tumor necrosis factor (TNF) receptor, and reduced cytokine production [9]. Furthermore, in vivo injection of anti-CTLA4 and glucocorticoid-induced TNF receptor restored cytokine production and reduced parasite survival, consistent with a role for these cells in maintaining immunosuppression [9]. Given these findings, it appears that T regulatory cells have a role in regulating the host response to these parasites during chronic infection.

The Pro-Inflammatory Response – Endosymbiotic *Wolbachia* Bacteria

The presence of intracytoplasmic *Rickettsia*-like bacteria in filarial nematodes was first described in 1977 [10], and later identified as *Wolbachia pipientis* [11, 12]. *Wolbachia* infect 25–70% of insect species in addition to crustaceans, and the filarial nematodes are the only group of worms that harbor these bacteria, possibly because they are the only nematode family with an obligate insect host as part of their life cycle. In nematodes, they are present in cells in the hypodermis and uterus, and can be detected in immature microfilariae in the uterus, and in mature microfilariae in the skin [13, 14]. The bacteria are more numerous in the mammalian host than in the insect vector, and appear to have an essential, though poorly understood role in nematode embryogenesis. The symbiotic relationship is revealed by antibiotic treatment of filaria-infected individuals, which effectively sterilizes the adult females, reducing overall microfilaria load and blocking disease transmission [15–17].

The role of *Wolbachia* in the pathogenesis of filarial disease has been implicated from observations made after anti-filarial therapy. Elevated *Wolbachia* DNA and even intact *Wolbachia* are detected in the blood, and are associated with the pro-inflammatory cytokines seen in patients with posttreatment side effects such as fever, edema and headache [18, 19]. Furthermore, *Wolbachia* are required for recruitment of neutrophils to the *Onchocerca* nodules, as the number of neutrophils in nodules from doxycycline-treated individuals is greatly reduced compared with untreated individuals [20].

Production of TNF-α and nitric oxide by mouse macrophages stimulated with filarial extracts is clearly associated with the presence of *Wolbachia* [21], and isolated *Wolbachia* can induce pro-inflammatory cytokine production in infected human and murine cells. The role of *Wolbachia* in a mouse model of ocular onchocerciasis will be discussed below.

Pathogenesis of Ocular Onchocerciasis

Microfilariae invade both the anterior and the posterior eye. In the latter case, they cause uveitis and chorioretinitis, resulting in loss of vision. In the anterior segment, they are present in the anterior chamber and cornea, where they cause sclerosing keratitis.

Eyes from human cases of onchocerciasis are difficult to obtain and show only the late stages of disease; however, in the cornea these manifest as an infiltrate of monocytic and granulocytic cells in the stroma, often surrounding dead and degenerating worms [22]. More revealing are findings from *Onchocerca* dermatitis studies, showing microfilariae surrounded by neutrophils, eosinophils or macrophages [23].

Early experimental models of *O. volvulus* keratitis using guinea pig and murine models demonstrated that prior immunization is essential to develop the corneal opacification and neovascularization characteristic of later stage sclerosing keratitis, which is consistent with responses found in chronically infected individuals [22, 24, 25]. More recent studies from our group and others showed that keratitis is associated with a predominant CD4+, Th2 response both systemically and in the cornea, that IgE and parasite-specific IgG1 were the predominant isotypes produced, and that the predominant cellular infiltrate is neutrophils [26–28]. The use of B cell-deficient μMT mice and FcγR−/− mice revealed that Fc receptors on neutrophils and eosinophils facilitate degranulation of these cells and disruption of corneal clarity [29, 30]. Further studies demonstrated that neutrophil recruitment was mediated by CD31/PECAM-1 and chemokine receptor CXCR2, whereas eosinophil recruitment is dependent on eotaxin, P-selectin and ICAM-1 [27, 31–34].

These findings are consistent with the sequence of events outlined in figure 1: (1) immunization or chronic infection induces a predominant Th2 response, with IL-4 leading to isotype switching to IgE and IgG1, and IL-5 inducing eosinophil differentiation; (2) parasite antigens in the corneal stroma (after microfilaria invasion or injection of parasite antigens) lead to activation of resident cells in the cornea, production of CXC and CC chemokines, elevated expression of adhesion molecules on vascular endothelial cells in the limbus, and infiltration of neutrophils and eosinophils to the corneal stroma, and (3) immune complex-mediated cross linking of Fc receptors on neutrophils and eosinophils results in degranulation and release of cationic proteins and other cytotoxic mediators that disrupt normal corneal clarity. In heavily infected individuals, the response to repeated microfilaria invasion over a number of years results in sclerosis and blindness.

Role of Innate Immunity in O. volvulus *Keratitis*

The role of the innate immune response in *Onchocerca* keratitis has not been investigated in detail for at least two reasons: firstly, as a model for chronically infected individuals who are presumably sensitized prior to ocular involvement, there would be no example of innate immunity in the eye in the

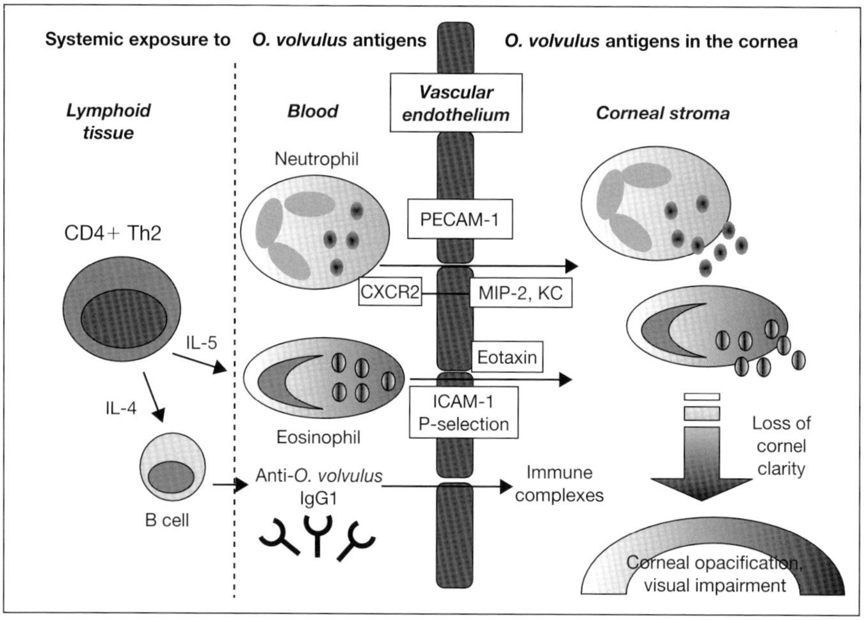

Fig. 1. Proposed sequence of events in adaptive immune response underlying *Onchocerca* keratitis.

absence of an adaptive immune response, and secondly, experimental models showed no detectable corneal opacification or neovascularization unless animals were first immunized [24, 25, 28]. However, in vivo confocal microscopy clearly demonstrated a cellular infiltrate in the corneas of unimmunized mice injected intrastromally with parasite antigens. Further, the cellular infiltrate, which was primarily neutrophils, was associated with an increase in corneal thickness and haze [35]. This approach then allowed examination of innate immunity to *O. volvulus* in the absence of an adaptive immune response.

Using this mouse model of *O. volvulus* keratitis, we demonstrated that endosymbiotic *Wolbachia* bacteria are essential for the pathogenesis of *O. volvulus* keratitis as *O. volvulus* from individuals depleted of *Wolbachia* by antibiotic treatment do not induce corneal inflammation [35]. Furthermore, related filarial species containing *Wolbachia* induce keratitis in contrast to aposymbiotic species lacking *Wolbachia* [35].

To examine the early host responses to *Wolbachia* in the cornea, we injected whole microfilariae into the corneal stroma and followed the fate of *Wolbachia* by immunogold labeling of the major *Wolbachia* surface protein (WSP) [36]. Figure 2 shows the presence of *Wolbachia* in the microfilariae in the cornea, with neutrophils in immediate proximity. Figure 3 shows immunogold labeling in neutrophil vacuoles surrounded by primary granules, supporting the notion that *Wolbachia* are ingested by neutrophils. Furthermore, incubation of neutrophils with *Wolbachia* stimulates release of TNF-α and CXC chemokines KC/CXCL1 and MIP-2/CXCL2 [36].

Wolbachia and Toll-Like Receptors

Toll-like receptors (TLR) are a family of at least twelve pathogen recognition molecules that respond to microbial products such as lipopolysaccharide (LPS; TLR4), bacterial cell wall components (TLR2), DNA-containing unmethylated CG motifs (TLR9) and viral RNA (TLR3, TLR7, and TLR8) [37, 38]. Several reports indicate that *Wolbachia* activate the innate immune responses via TLR-dependent pathways: (1) *Wolbachia* activation of macrophages is decreased in C3H/HeJ mice, which have a point mutation in TLR4 that makes it hyporesponsive to LPS [21]; (2) the severity of *O. volvulus* keratitis was reduced in C3H/HeJ mice [35], and (3) recombinant WSP activates TLR2 and TLR4 [39]. We also show a role for TLR2 in *Wolbachia* and filarial activation [Gillette-Ferguson et al., submitted]. Although initial reports suggested that *Wolbachia* have LPS-like activity, sequencing of the *Wolbachia* revealed no LPS synthase enzymes [40], indicating that TLR2 and TLR4 agonists are more likely to be surface proteins such as WSP and other cell wall components. Our most recent findings show that mice that are deficient in the adaptor molecule myeloid differentiation factor 88 (MyD88), which is common to the signaling pathways of TLR2 and TLR4, do not develop keratitis in response to *O. volvulus* antigens or to isolated *Wolbachia* bacteria [41]. Consistent with this observation, isolated neutrophils from MyD88−/− mice are not activated by *Wolbachia* bacteria or *O. volvulus* antigens, indicating an essential role for this adaptor molecule at two stages of pathogenesis – production of CXC chemokines by resident cells and neutrophil activation [41].

Taken together, findings from our group and others suggest a role for the innate immune response in *Onchocerca* keratitis, as shown in figure 4. As TLR2 and TLR4 are expressed in the cornea [42–44], and activation can induce keratitis, we predict that an inflammatory response to *Wolbachia* is initiated by TLRs on keratocytes, which are likely to be activated after death and degeneration of microfilariae and release of *Wolbachia* into the confined environment of the corneal stroma. Activated keratocytes can mature into stromal fibroblasts, which produce pro-inflammatory cytokines and CXC chemokines [42, 45], and can induce adhesion molecule expression on vascular endothelial cells [32, 33]. Together, these changes mediate neutrophil recruitment from peripheral, limbal vessels into the avascular corneal stroma and migration through the stromal matrix to the site of microfilaria degradation and release of *Wolbachia*. A second

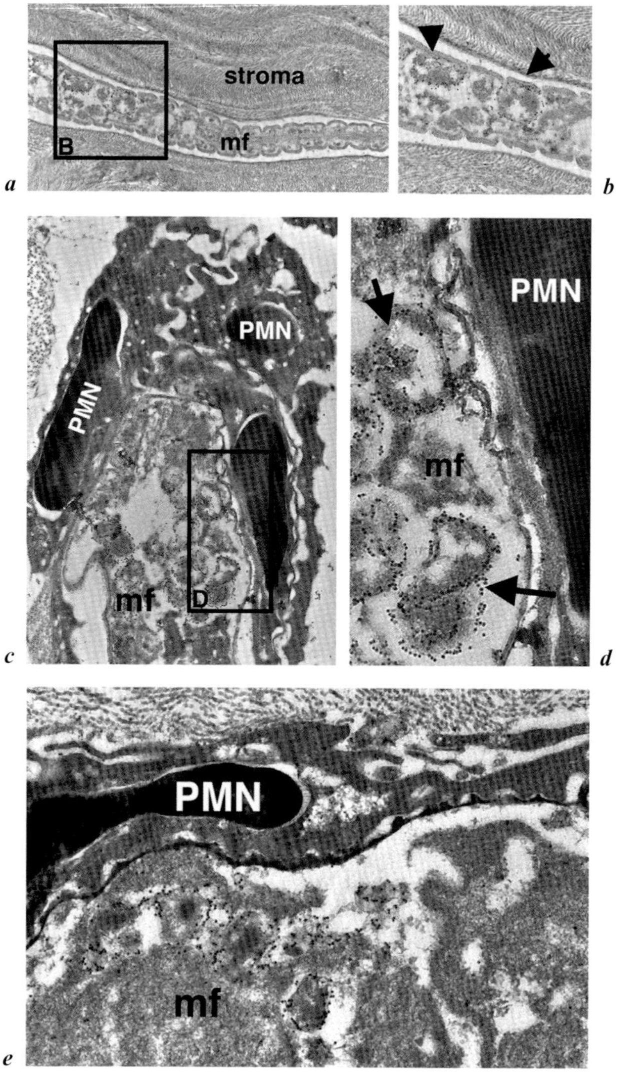

Fig. 2. Proximity of neutrophils to *Wolbachia* in the nematode hypodermis. C57BL/6 mice were injected with microfilariae into the corneal stroma, corneas were removed after 4 or 18 h, and thin sections were immunostained with anti-WSP and visualized with IgG conjugated to 15-nm gold particles. Sections were counterstained with uranyl acetate and lead citrate, and examined by electron microscopy. ***a***, ***b*** 4 h after injection, WSP was clearly detected inside microfilariae in the corneal stroma (arrows). mf = Microfilariae. ***c–e*** 18 h after injection, microfilariae containing *Wolbachia* were surrounded by neutrophils (PMN). WSP-labeled with gold particles (arrows) are present in the microfilariae adjacent to the neutrophils in either unimmunized (***c***) or immunized (***e***) mice. ***a*** ×4,800. ***b*** ×8,400. ***c*** ×5,300. ***d*** ×16,000. ***e*** ×14,57500 (reprinted with permission [36]).

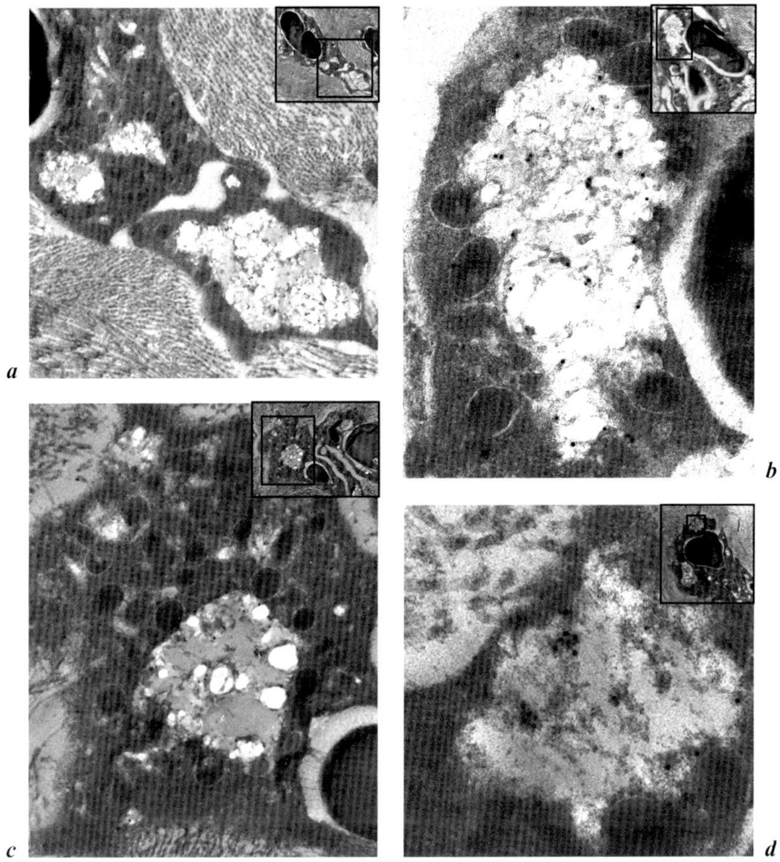

Fig. 3. *Wolbachia* in neutrophil vacuoles: immunoelectron microscopy of neutrophils 18 h after injection of microfilariae. Immunogold particles specific for WSP were prominent in neutrophil vacuoles of both immunized (***a***, ***b***) and unimmunized (***c***, ***d***) mice. ***a*** ×11,400. ***b*** ×45,000. ***c*** ×24,000. ***d*** ×67,500 (reprinted with permission [36]).

role for TLR2, TLR4 and MyD88 is therefore ingestion of *Wolbachia* and activation of neutrophils at this site. As neutrophils express functional TLR2, TLR4 and TLR9 [46], they can produce TNF-α MIP-2 and KC in response to *Wolbachia* [36], which stimulate further neutrophil infiltration, degranulation and secretion of cytotoxic products such as nitric oxide and myeloperoxidase and oxygen radicals. A cytotoxic effect on keratocytes and corneal endothelial cells will lead to loss of corneal clarity.

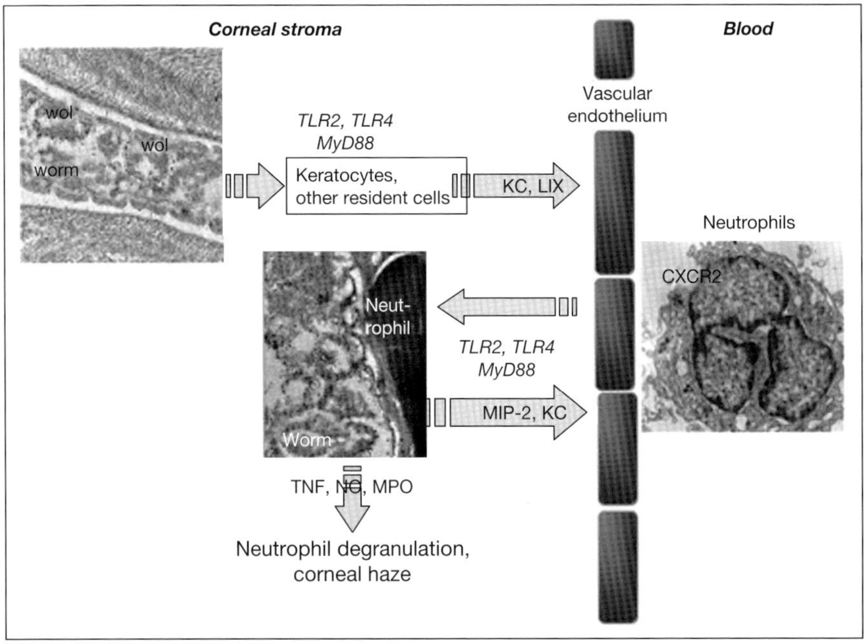

Fig. 4. Proposed sequence of events in innate immune responses underlying *Onchocerca* keratitis. MPO = Myeloperoxidase; NO = nitric oxide.

In chronically infected, untreated individuals, there is also an ongoing adaptive immune response, repeated invasion of microfilariae into the corneal stroma, and consistent worm degeneration and release of *Wolbachia*. The sustained inflammatory response in the presence of antibody and infiltration of eosinophils and macrophages combine to cause corneal opacification, loss of vision and blindness.

Conclusion

Studies using animal models of river blindness have helped our understanding of the pathogenesis of this disease. Most prominently, they have shown the essential role for endosymbiotic Wolbachia bacteria and the innate immune response in development of keratitis. Future studies will examine the role of TLRs in development of adaptive immunity in this important disease, and may identify targets for immune intervention.

Acknowledgments

This work was supported by NIH grants EY10320, EY11373, and by the Research to Prevent Blindness Foundation and the Ohio Lions Eye Research Foundation. E.P. is also a recepient of an RPB Senior Investigator Award.

References

1 Pearlman E, Toe L, Boatin BA, Gilles AA, Higgins AW, Unnasch TR: Eotaxin expression in *Onchocerca volvulus*-induced dermatitis after topical application of diethylcarbamazine. J Infect Dis 1999;180:1394–1397.
2 Maizels RM, Balic A, Gomez-Escobar N, Nair M, Taylor MD, Allen JE: Helminth parasites – masters of regulation. Immunol Rev 2004;201:89–116.
3 Goodridge HS, Wilson EH, Harnett W, Campbell CC, Harnett MM, Liew FY: Modulation of macrophage cytokine production by ES-62, a secreted product of the filarial nematode *Acanthocheilonema viteae*. J Immunol 2001;167:940–945.
4 Ottesen EA, Weller PF, Heck L: Specific cellular immune unresponsiveness in human filariasis. Immunology 1977;33:413–421.
5 Brattig NW: Pathogenesis and host responses in human onchocerciasis: impact of Onchocerca filariae and Wolbachia endobacteria. Microbes Infect 2004;6:113–128.
6 Steel C, Nutman TB: CTLA-4 in filarial infections: implications for a role in diminished T cell reactivity. J Immunol 2003;170:1930–1938.
7 Doetze A, Satoguina J, Burchard G, Rau T, Loliger C, Fleischer B, Hoerauf A: Antigen-specific cellular hyporesponsiveness in a chronic human helminth infection is mediated by T_h3/T_r1-type cytokines IL-10 and transforming growth factor-β but not by a T_h1 to T_h2 shift. Int Immunol 2000;12:623–630.
8 Hoerauf A, Satoguina J, Saeftel M, Specht S: Immunomodulation by filarial nematodes. Parasite Immunol 2005;27:417–429.
9 Taylor MD, LeGoff L, Harris A, Malone E, Allen JE, Maizels RM: Removal of regulatory T cell activity reverses hyporesponsiveness and leads to filarial parasite clearance in vivo. J Immunol 2005;174:4924–4933.
10 Kozek WJ, Marroquin HF: Intracytoplasmic bacteria in *Onchocerca volvulus*. Am J Trop Med Hyg 1977;26:663–678.
11 Taylor MJ, Hoerauf A: A new approach to the treatment of filariasis (comment). Curr Opin Infect Dis 2001;14:727–731.
12 Taylor MJ, Bilo K, Cross HF, Archer JP, Underwood AP: 16S rDNA phylogeny and ultrastructural characterization of *Wolbachia* intracellular bacteria of the filarial nematodes *Brugia malayi*, *B. pahangi*, and *Wuchereria bancrofti*. Exp Parasitol 1999;91:356–361.
13 McGarry HF, Egerton GL, Taylor MJ: Population dynamics of Wolbachia bacterial endosymbionts in *Brugia malayi*. Mol Biochem Parasitol 2004;135:57–67.
14 Taylor M: One in the eye for river blindness. Trends Parasitol 2001;17:358.
15 Hoerauf A, Mand S, Adjei O, Fleischer B, Buttner DW: Depletion of wolbachia endobacteria in *Onchocerca volvulus* by doxycycline and microfilaridermia after ivermectin treatment. Lancet 2001;357:1415–1416.
16 Hoerauf A, Mand S, Volkmann L, Buttner M, Marfo-Debrekyei Y, Taylor M, Adjei O, Buttner DW: Doxycycline in the treatment of human onchocerciasis: kinetics of Wolbachia endobacteria reduction and of inhibition of embryogenesis in female Onchocerca worms. Microbes Infect 2003;5: 261–273.
17 Taylor MJ, Makunde WH, McGarry HF, Turner JD, Mand S, Hoerauf A: Macrofilaricidal activity after doxycycline treatment of *Wuchereria bancrofti*: a double-blind, randomised placebo-controlled trial. Lancet 2005;365:2116–2121.

18 Cross HF, Haarbrink M, Egerton G, Yazdanbakhsh M, Taylor MJ: Severe reactions to filarial chemotherapy and release of Wolbachia endosymbionts into blood (comment). Lancet 2001;358: 1873–1875.
19 Keiser PB, Reynolds SM, Awadzi K, Ottesen EA, Taylor MJ, Nutman TB: Bacterial endosymbionts of *Onchocerca volvulus* in the pathogenesis of posttreatment reactions. J Infect Dis 2002;185:805–811.
20 Brattig NW, Buttner DW, Hoerauf A: Neutrophil accumulation around Onchocerca worms and chemotaxis of neutrophils are dependent on Wolbachia endobacteria. Microbes Infect 2001;3: 439–446.
21 Taylor MJ, Cross HF, Bilo K: Inflammatory responses induced by the filarial nematode *Brugia malayi* are mediated by lipopolysaccharide-like activity from endosymbiotic Wolbachia bacteria. J Exp Med 2000;191:1429–1436.
22 Pearlman E: Experimental onchocercal keratitis. Parasitol Today 1996;12:261–267.
23 Hoerauf A, Buttner DW, Adjei O, Pearlman E: Onchocerciasis. BMJ 2003;326:207–210.
24 Chakravarti B, Herring TA, Lass JH, Parker JS, Bucy RP, Diaconu E, Tseng J, Whitfield DR, Greene BM, Chakravarti DN: Infiltration of CD4+ T cells into cornea during development of *Onchocerca volvulus*-induced experimental sclerosing keratitis in mice. Cell Immunol 1994;159: 306–314.
25 Chakravarti B, Lass JH, Bardenstein DS, Diaconu E, Roy CE, Herring TA, Chakravarti DN, Greene BM: Immune-mediated *Onchocerca volvulus* sclerosing keratitis in the mouse. Exp Eye Res 1993;57:21–27.
26 Chakravarti B, Lagoo-Deenadayalan S, Parker JS, Whitfield DR, Lagoo A, Chakravarti DN: In vivo molecular analysis of cytokines in a murine model of ocular onchocerciasis. I. Up-regulation of IL-4 and IL-5 mRNAs and not IL-2 and IFN gamma mRNAs in the cornea due to experimental interstitial keratitis. Immunol Lett 1996;54:59–64.
27 Hall LR, Pearlman E: Pathogenesis of onchocercal keratitis (river blindness). Clin Microbiol Rev 1999;12:445–453.
28 Pearlman E, Lass JH, Bardenstein DS, Kopf M, Hazlett FE Jr, Diaconu E, Kazura JW: Interleukin 4 and T helper type 2 cells are required for development of experimental onchocercal keratitis (river blindness). J Exp Med 1995;182:931–940.
29 Hall LR, Diaconu E, Pearlman E: A dominant role for Fc gamma receptors in antibody-dependent corneal inflammation. J Immunol 2001;167:919–925.
30 Hall LR, Lass JH, Diaconu E, Strine ER, Pearlman E: An essential role for antibody in neutrophil and eosinophil recruitment to the cornea: B cell-deficient (μMT) mice fail to develop Th2-dependent, helminth-mediated keratitis. J Immunol 1999;163:4970–4975.
31 Hall LR, Diaconu E, Patel R, Pearlman E: CXC chemokine receptor 2 but not C-C chemokine receptor 1 expression is essential for neutrophil recruitment to the cornea in helminth-mediated keratitis (river blindness). J Immunol 2001;166:4035–4041.
32 Kaifi JT, Diaconu E, Pearlman E: Distinct roles for PECAM-1, ICAM-1, and VCAM-1 in recruitment of neutrophils and eosinophils to the cornea in ocular onchocerciasis (river blindness). J Immunol 2001;166:6795–6801.
33 Kaifi JT, Hall LR, Diaz C, Sypek J, Diaconu E, Lass JH, Pearlman E: Impaired eosinophil recruitment to the cornea in P-selectin-deficient mice in *Onchocerca volvulus* keratitis (river blindness). Invest Ophthalmol Vis Sci 2000;41:3856–3861.
34 Rothenberg ME, MacLean JA, Pearlman E, Luster AD, Leder P: Targeted disruption of the chemokine eotaxin partially reduces antigen-induced tissue eosinophilia. J Exp Med 1997;185:785–790.
35 Saint Andre A, Blackwell NM, Hall LR, Hoerauf A, Brattig NW, Volkmann L, Taylor MJ, Ford L, Hise AG, Lass JH, Diaconu E, Pearlman E: The role of endosymbiotic Wolbachia bacteria in the pathogenesis of river blindness. Science 2002;295:1892–1895.
36 Gillette-Ferguson I, Hise AG, McGarry HF, Turner J, Esposito A, Sun Y, Diaconu E, Taylor MJ, Pearlman E: Wolbachia-induced neutrophil activation in a mouse model of ocular onchocerciasis (river blindness). Infect Immun 2004;72:5687–5692.
37 Takeda K, Akira S: Toll receptors and pathogen resistance. Cell Microbiol 2003;5:143–153.
38 Takeda K, Kaisho T, Akira S: Toll-like receptors. Annu Rev Immunol 2003;21:335–376.

39 Brattig NW, Bazzocchi C, Kirschning CJ, Reiling N, Buttner DW, Ceciliani F, Geisinger F, Hochrein H, Ernst M, Wagner H, Bandi C, Hoerauf A: The major surface protein of Wolbachia endosymbionts in filarial nematodes elicits immune responses through TLR2 and TLR4. J Immunol 2004;173:437–445.
40 Blaxter M, Daub J, Guiliano D, Parkinson J, Whitton C: The *Brugia malayi* genome project: expressed sequence tags and gene discovery. Trans R Soc Trop Med Hyg 2002;96:7–17.
41 Gillette-Ferguson I, Hise AG, Sun Y, Diaconu E, McGarry HF, Taylor MJ, Pearlman E: *Wolbachia* and *Onchocerca volvulus*-induced keratitis (river blindness) is dependent on myeloid differentiation factor 88 (MyD88). Infect Immun 2006;74:2442–2445.
42 Johnson AC, Heinzel FP, Diaconu E, Sun Y, Hise AG, Golenbock D, Lass JH, Pearlman E: Activation of Toll-like receptor (TLR)2, TLR4, and TLR9 in the mammalian cornea induces MyD88-dependent corneal inflammation. Invest Ophthalmol Vis Sci 2005;46:589–595.
43 Song PI, Abraham TA, Park Y, Zivony AS, Harten B, Edelhauser HF, Ward SL, Armstrong CA, Ansel JC: The expression of functional LPS receptor proteins CD14 and Toll-like receptor 4 in human corneal cells. Invest Ophthalmol Vis Sci 2001;42:2867–2877.
44 Zhang J, Xu K, Ambati B, Yu FS: Toll-like receptor 5-mediated corneal epithelial inflammatory responses to *Pseudomonas aeruginosa* flagellin. Invest Ophthalmol Vis Sci 2003;44:4247–4254.
45 Cubitt CL, Tang Q, Monteiro CA, Lausch RN, Oakes JE: IL-8 gene expression in cultures of human corneal epithelial cells and keratocytes. Invest Ophthalmol Vis Sci 1993;34:3199–3206.
46 Hayashi F, Means TK, Luster AD: Toll-like receptors stimulate human neutrophil function. Blood 2003;102:2660–2669.

Note Added in Proof

Further studies have demonstrated that TLR2 rather than TLR4 is the predominant receptor for *Wolbachia* [1].

1 Hise AG, Daehnel K, Gillette-Ferguson I, Cho E, McGarry HF, Taylor MJ, Golenbock DT, Fitzgerald KA, Kazura JW, Pearlman E: Innate immune responses to endosymbiotic *Wolbachia* bacteria in *Brugia malayi* and *Onchocerca volvulus* are dependent on TLR2, TLR6, MyD88 and Mal, but not TLR4, TRIF or TRAM. J Immunol 2006, in press.

Dr. Eric Pearlman
Department of Ophthalmology, Case Western Reserve University
10900 Euclid Avenue
Cleveland, OH 44106–7286 (USA)
Tel. +1 216 368 1856, Fax +1 216 368 4825, E-Mail Eric.Pearlman@case.edu

Niederkorn JY, Kaplan HJ (eds): Immune Response and the Eye.
Chem Immunol Allergy. Basel, Karger, 2007, vol 92, pp 266–275

Role of Bacterial and Host Factors in Infectious Endophthalmitis

Meredith Gregory[a], *Michael S. Gilmore*[a], *Michelle C. Callegan*[b]

[a]Schepens Eye Research Institute, Harvard Medical School, Boston, Mass.,
[b]Dean A. McGee Eye Institute, University of Oklahoma Health Sciences Center, Oklahoma City, Okla., USA

Abstract

Endophthalmitis is a frequent blinding complication of globe-penetrating injury and ocular surgery. The outcome of this intraocular infection depends both on the organism involved and management of the ensuing inflammation. The role of various toxins and bacterial factors in the pathogenesis of this infection is beginning to be delineated, but appears to be organism specific. Because of the immune-privileged environment of the eye, principles important in the resolution of infection at extraocular sites cannot be extrapolated to understanding the host-parasite dynamics in eye infection. Moreover, some factors that suppress the intraocular immune environment appear to have unexpected roles in activating phagocytic cells of the innate immune system in response to the presence of bacteria. Therefore, considerable additional information characterizing the precise role of bacterial and host factors in the pathogenesis of endophthalmitis will be required in order to develop new therapies to improve the outcome of this often blinding infection.

Epidemiology and Etiology of Endophthalmitis

Endophthalmitis results from the seeding of microorganisms into the posterior segment of the eye. It is most commonly a complication of intraocular surgery (postoperative) or penetrating injury of the globe (posttraumatic), but may result from migration of microorganisms into the eye from a distant site of infection (endogenous), especially in immune-compromised individuals. Bacteria usually associated with endophthalmitis range from relatively avirulent normal flora to pathogens. Infection outcomes range from complete recovery of vision to blindness and occasionally loss of the eye itself despite early and aggressive antibiotic, anti-inflammatory, and surgical treatment.

The majority of reported endophthalmitis cases follow intraocular surgery. The incidence of postoperative endophthalmitis (POE) following ocular surgery is low, at approximately 0.01–0.05% [1], but recent reports indicate that the incidence after cataract surgery is increasing [2], with many isolates becoming resistant to prophylactic antibiotics [3]. The most common organisms associated with POE are those capable of colonizing the eyelid margin and the tear film. Coagulase-negative staphylococci, commonly found as normal flora of the ocular environment, cause the majority of acute endophthalmitis following cataract surgery. Other organisms frequently encountered include *Staphylococcus aureus*, viridans streptococci, other Gram-positive bacteria, and Gram-negative bacteria. Clinical outcomes of POE caused by non-coagulase-negative staphylococci are generally worse than those caused by coagulase-negative staphylococci [3, 4]. Late-onset POE may occur weeks to several months following surgery, and is often indolent and recurs despite treatment. These infections may be due to either the sequestration of avirulent organisms introduced during surgery, or from delayed inoculation of organisms through incision defects, sutures, vitreous wicks or filtering blebs. The organisms most commonly found in late-onset POE are relatively avirulent [4].

Posttraumatic endophthalmitis (PTE) is common (3–17% of globe-penetrating injuries) and often associated with a poor visual outcome. Important factors associated with the development of endophthalmitis following open globe injury include cleanliness of the wound, retained intraocular foreign body, lens capsule rupture and significantly delayed primary repair [4, 5]. PTE is caused by a wide variety of bacteria, including those that originate from the environment and exist on contaminated globe-penetrating objects. Gram-negative endophthalmitis occurs at a higher rate following traumatic injury (5–25%) than following intraocular surgery. The predominant pathogens involved in PTE include coagulase-negative staphylococci, non-coagulase-negative staphylococci, and *Bacillus* species [4, 5].

Endogenous endophthalmitis (EE) is relatively infrequent, and results from seeding of the eye with organisms as a complication of bacteremia or septicemia. Populations at greatest risk for EE included immunocompromised patients, those with prolonged use of indwelling devices, and intravenous drug users. Since patients with EE commonly have systemic infection, the associated mortality is relatively high. *Bacillus* species, *Candida* and *Aspergillus* are the most frequent causes of EE [6].

Bacterial Virulence Influences Outcome

Bacillus cereus *Endophthalmitis*

In *Bacillus* PTE, poor outcomes are common, despite prompt therapeutic and surgical intervention. More than two thirds of infected eyes lose all useful vision, including approximately half that must be eviscerated or enucleated. *B. cereus* is often introduced into the eye on contaminated foreign objects following a penetrating injury or following septicemia. Bacilli replicate and migrate rapidly within the eye, and an explosive intraocular inflammatory response parallels deteriorating retinal structure and function. The infection may also spread into periocular tissues leading to panophthalmitis [7].

B. cereus produces a number of toxins and proteases that may contribute to severity. A group of toxins under the direct control of *plcR*, a quorum-sensing regulator of toxin transcription, has been found to contribute to virulence during experimental *Bacillus* endophthalmitis [8]. However, membrane-damaging toxins, when tested individually, have been found to contribute modestly to the overall pathogenesis of disease [9]. These results suggest that the toxins involved in the virulence of *Bacillus* endophthalmitis may do so in a coordinated manner or that as yet uncharacterized toxins play a central role in pathogenesis. *B. cereus* is also motile and migrates rapidly throughout the eye during endophthalmitis. *Bacillus* strains deficient in motility do not migrate throughout the eye, do not grow as well in the vitreous, and are significantly less virulent than wild-type motile bacilli [8]. These results highlight quorum-sensing systems and bacterial motility as potential therapeutic targets for *B. cereus* endophthalmitis.

S. aureus *Endophthalmitis*

S. aureus causes significant visual loss in more than half of endophthalmitis cases. This organism produces a panoply of virulence factors that are controlled by the quorum-sensing systems *sar* (staphylococcal accessory regulator) and *agr* (accessory gene regulator). In experimental models, eyes infected with wild-type *S. aureus* were significantly more virulent than *S. aureus* with mutations in *agr*, *sar* or both quorum-sensing systems. Mutants deficient in α- or β-toxin expression were also less virulent than wild-type *S. aureus*, but not to the extent seen with the *agr*/*sar* quorum-sensing mutant [10].

Recent studies examined the value of intravitreal immunoglobulin against sterile toxin-induced endophthalmitis. Pooled human immunoglobulin was reported to attenuate the toxic effects of culture supernatants containing *S. aureus* exotoxins [11]. Lysostaphin, an enzyme that lyses staphylococci, was also effective against antibiotic-resistant *S. aureus* in experimental endophthalmitis [12]. In the future, these types of therapeutics may be useful against staphylococci that have developed resistance to most currently used antibiotics.

Enterococcus faecalis *Endophthalmitis*

E. faecalis is frequently isolated from infected filtering blebs following glaucoma surgery, and is the cause of 4–8% of POE. Visual outcomes of

E. faecalis endophthalmitis are frequently poor, with as many as 80% of cases resulting in a final visual acuity of 20/200 or worse [13].

Approximately half of *E. faecalis* ocular isolates produce a cytolysin that disrupts cell membranes. In an experimental rabbit endophthalmitis model, infection with cytolysin-producing *E. faecalis* was more virulent than noncytolytic *E. faecalis*, and completely refractory to intravitreal antibiotic and anti-inflammatory treatment despite the susceptibility of both strains to the antibiotics used [14]. *E. faecalis* also expresses two proteases that are under the control of the quorum-sensing system *fsr*. A deletion mutant of *fsrB* had significantly reduced virulence in a rabbit model of experimental endophthalmitis, which was greater than the level of attenuation observed for mutants in the proteases alone [15], suggesting that *fsrB* may have pleiotropic effects on the cell beyond regulating expression of these two proteases.

Propionibacterium acnes *Endophthalmitis*

The Gram-positive anaerobe *P. acnes* is a common cause of chronic and recurrent endophthalmitis following intraocular surgery or trauma [4]. Despite therapeutic and surgical intervention, late-onset treatment failures and persistent infections are common with *P. acnes* intraocular infection. Recurrence is thought to result from a failure of the host and antibiotics to clear *P. acnes* sequestered in bacterial plaques within the posterior segment, intraocular lenses or other prosthetic implants [4, 16]. The roles of virulence factors in *P. acnes* endophthalmitis have not been analyzed. However, *P. acnes* produces proteases and a fibronectin-binding protein that may contribute to tissue damage and adhesion to intraocular lenses or structures, respectively, during infection.

Gram-Negative Causes of Endophthalmitis

Gram-negative bacteria cause a small percentage of endophthalmitis cases, and are isolated more frequently from cases of PTE or EE. The visual outcome of Gram-negative cases of PTE and EE are generally poor. *Klebsiella pneumoniae*, a common Gram-negative EE pathogen, has been associated with a specific site of infection and underlying immunocompromise, and highly associated with EE following metastatic spread from hepatobiliary infections, especially in diabetics [17]. For *K. pneumoniae*, the link between specific *K. pneumoniae* virulence factors and endophthalmitis virulence has not been made. However, *K. pneumoniae* EE strains have been shown to be genetically related, and most have virulence factors associated with tissue invasion [18].

Host Response in Endophthalmitis

Significant progress has been made over the last several decades in elucidating the mechanisms involved in maintaining ocular immune privilege. However, the studies have, until recently, largely focused on immune privilege as it pertains to adaptive immunity and T cell-mediated inflammation. Immune privilege also affects innate immunity. The aqueous humor contains multiple factors that directly inhibit innate immunity including: (i) TGF-β, soluble Fas ligand (FasL), and α-melanocyte-stimulating hormone (which inhibit neutrophil activation), (ii) calcitonin gene-related peptide (which inhibits nitric oxide release from activated macrophages), and (iii) CD46, CD55, and CD59 (which inhibit complement activation) [reviewed in ref. 19]. While these mechanisms evolved to limit local tissue destruction and preserve the clarity of the visual axis, they also leave the eye more vulnerable to infection.

Despite immune privilege, ocular inflammation in response to an invading bacterial pathogen occurs and can be either acute or chronic. Acute inflammation is most commonly associated with more virulent bacteria (*B. cereus*, *E. faecalis*, and *S. aureus*) and a poor visual outcome [10]. As early as 48 h after infection, both anterior and posterior segments are involved resulting in corneal edema, cellular infiltration within the cornea and aqueous humor, vitritis, and retinal periphlebitis [4]. In contrast, chronic inflammation is associated with less virulent bacteria (*P. acnes* and *Staphylococcus epidermidis*), and a better visual outcome [4]. The onset of chronic inflammation is commonly delayed and clinically much milder.

Chronic Inflammation

In cases of chronic inflammation induced by *P. acnes*, inflammation can run a protracted course of 3–4 months. Initially, the inflammation responds to corticosteroid therapy but with time the inflammation becomes persistent and refractory to corticosteroid therapy [4, 16]. *P. acnes* is resistant to killing by macrophages and neutrophils, and, thus, can persist within the eye [20]. Clinical examination reveals the presence of white plaques inside the posterior capsule that have been shown to contain live bacterial organisms [4]. The removal of the lens capsule that contains these plaques often eliminates the nidus of infection, with the result that the inflammation subsides and vision is retained [16]. Early diagnosis and eradication of residual bacteria appear to be keys for successful treatment of bacterially induced chronic inflammation.

Acute Inflammation

Possible Role of Adaptive Immunity

Acute inflammation involves primarily components of the innate immune system. Although a role for T cell-mediated adaptive immunity has yet to be established for bacterial endophthalmitis, there appears to be a role for adaptive immunity in bacterial keratitis. CD4+ T cells were observed to contribute to the pathogenesis of *P. aeruginosa* keratitis in C57BL/6 mice [21]. It was also observed that T cell infiltration into the cornea during bacterial keratitis is central to the persistence of inflammation, although tissue damage was largely attributed to neutrophils. While these data raise the possibility that T cells may also play an important role in the course of endophthalmitis, studies directly testing this possibility have yet to be performed. Evidence has also emerged suggesting a possible role for B cell-mediated adaptive immunity in *S. aureus* endophthalmitis [22]. In a rabbit model, significant levels of IgG antibody specific for ribitol teichoic acid, a component of the *S. aureus* cell wall, were detected 3 days after inoculation [22]. Because the production of IgG antibodies is dependent upon the help of antigen-specific T cells, these data also suggest that T cells are at least responsive to events in acute endophthalmitis, if not contributing to the course and severity.

Innate Immunity

The first line of defense against invading pathogens consists of physical, anatomic, and chemical barriers. Several studies demonstrate that bacteria often enter the anterior chamber during cataract extraction, with contamination rates ranging from 29 to 43% [4]. However, the rate of endophthalmitis following cataract extraction is between 0.01 and 0.05% [1]. As early as 1955, it was shown that injection of bacteria into the vitreous of rabbits resulted in endophthalmitis, while the injection of the same inoculum into the anterior chamber was rapidly cleared [23]. Defensins are antimicrobial peptides which have recently been identified within the aqueous and vitreous of the eye [24]. β-Defensin 2 is inducible by inflammatory cytokines such as IL-1β, and, therefore, may be produced in response to inflammatory cytokine signals during infection and contribute to the clearance of the organisms [24].

In addition to the antimicrobial effects of aqueous humor, studies have demonstrated the significance of the posterior capsule as a physical and/or anatomic barrier against the development of bacterial endophthalmitis. *S. aureus* injected into the anterior chamber of primates failed to induce endophthalmitis in monkeys with an intact posterior capsule [25]. In contrast, 60% of the monkeys developed endophthalmitis when the posterior capsule was breeched following a posterior capsulectomy. These data demonstrate that invading bacterial organisms are more readily cleared from the aqueous as compared to the vitreous. While these studies have indicated a critical role for aqueous humor in the early clearance of bacterial infections, much work still remains in fully elucidating the mechanisms by which the bacteria are cleared from the anterior chamber, and the antibacterial components of aqueous humor remain to be identified.

Toll-like receptors (TLRs) are a family of pattern recognition receptors that recognize specific bacterial motifs and are expressed on cells of the innate system such as neutrophils, monocytes, macrophages, dendritic cells, and mast cells [26]. TLRs have emerged as key components of the innate immune system. The activation of cells via TLRs triggers a cascade of events: (i) the release of multiple pro-inflammatory cytokines that activate inflammation, (ii) enhancement of the phagocytosis of invading bacterial pathogens, and (iii) the release of cytokines, such as IFN-γ, that are critical in the development of adaptive immunity [26]. Recently, it was demonstrated that TLRs are expressed on human retinal pigment epithelial cells, where they may serve as an important defense against invading bacterial pathogens in the posterior segment [27]. However, a specific role for TLRs has not been established in bacterial endophthalmitis.

The complement system is also a component of innate immunity. Complement activation provides a very effective host defense mechanism against invading organisms by generating anaphylatoxins that: (i) trigger inflammation; (ii) chemotactically attract phagocytes to the site of infection; (iii) promote the opsonization and lysis of invading bacteria, and (iv) cause vasodilation and increased vascular permeability [28]. While each of these functions promotes clearance of bacteria, the same mechanisms, under uncontrolled circumstances, can also lead to extensive damage of host tissue. Thus, in an immune-privileged site such as the eye, where inflammation is detrimental to vision, the inflammatory response is tightly regulated. Using a mouse that lacks the central component of the complement system (C3−/−), it was shown that the absence of complement was inconsequential to the outcome of *S. aureus* endophthalmitis [29]. This study indicates that while complement may contribute to the early inflammatory response in the eye, it does not play a significant role in the clearance of the organism or the outcome of endophthalmitis in the murine model tested.

The primary function of the innate immune system is to detect invading pathogens and clear them. To achieve this, the innate system must: (i) trigger an immediate response; (ii) amplify the response; (iii) clear the pathogens, and (iv) activate the adaptive system in case the pathogen cannot be cleared quickly. Within 6 h after intravitreal inoculation with *S. aureus*, TNF-α, IL-1β, and cytokine-induced neutrophil chemoattractant (the rat homologue of IL-8) were detected within the vitreous [30]. The adhesion molecules ICAM-1 and E-selectin are also upregulated early in iris, ciliary body, and retinal vessels, serving to enhance the infiltration of leukocytes to the site of infection [31]. IFN-γ is not detected until 24 h after infection and correlates with increased infiltration of macrophages/monocytes and lymphocytes [30]. These studies did not determine whether induction of these molecules played a cause or effect role in the clinical outcome of endophthalmitis.

It was recently found that FasL plays an important role in the clearance of bacteria from the posterior segment, suggesting a direct role in recruiting or activating neutrophils [29]. FasL is constitutively expressed within the normal eye and has been shown to play a critical role in maintaining the immune-privileged environment by inducing apoptosis in infiltrating inflammatory cells [32]. It was found that while normal mice readily cleared an infection with 500 colony-forming units of *S. aureus*, mice deficient in FasL were unable to clear the same size inoculum [29]. In the absence of FasL, bacteria grew more rapidly, and fewer neutrophils were recruited to the site of infection. These findings suggest additional functions for FasL consistent with emerging data that FasL plays a critical role in the activation of the early innate immune response within the eye [33]. Membrane-bound FasL appears to activate innate immunity, whereas soluble FasL appears to inhibit inflammation. Therefore, the different forms of FasL may play a critical role in regulating host inflammation triggered by invading bacterial pathogens.

Anti-Inflammatory Reagents

Dexamethasone is frequently used as adjunctive therapy in the management of endophthalmitis [4] but remains the subject of debate. An inflammatory response is required to rapidly eradicate the infection, but the magnitude and persistence of such a response may be important determinants of bystander tissue damage. Corticosteroids are effective in blocking inflammation-mediated tissue damage and inhibiting production of pro-inflammatory cytokines. Nevertheless, the efficacy of corticosteroid treatment in clinical cases of endophthalmitis remains controversial [34].

Using a rabbit model of endophthalmitis, it was observed that intravitreal administration of dexamethasone, in conjunction with antibiotics, was effective in preserving vision in eyes infected with a non-cytolytic strain of *E. faecalis*. In contrast, corticosteroids had no effect on eyes infected with a cytolytic strain of *E. faecalis* [14]. These data reveal a main problem in ascertaining the value of anti-inflammatory drugs as adjunctive treatments in endophthalmitis – outcome depends strongly on the toxigenic status of the offending organism. Further, this therapy may be reserved in practice for the most severe cases which are caused by toxigenic microorganisms – ironically, cases where it may be least effective. A review of clinical data indicates that the use of intravitreal steroids may be detrimental and may lead to increased loss of vision following endophthalmitis [35], but this may be attributable to the latter bias in practice. Few studies have examined whether these agents improve outcome when cases are stratified by microbe. It remains to be determined whether observations made in one well-controlled model of endophthalmitis are generalizable to disease caused by other bacteria or to human cases.

Conclusion

Understanding of the host and microbe factors that influence the outcome of endophthalmitis is in its infancy. It is becoming clear that certain factors, such as whether a toxin plays an important role in pathogenesis, may be pathogen specific. It is also clear that successful resolution of endophthalmitis caused by virulent organisms will require careful management of the host response. A more detailed understanding of these interrelationships will be required before this knowledge can be translated into clinical practice.

References

1 Miller JJ, Scott IU, Flynn HW, Smiddy WE, Newton J, Miller D: Acute-onset endophthalmitis after cataract surgery (2000–2004): incidence, clinical settings, and visual acuity outcomes after treatment. Am J Ophthalmol 2005;139:983–987.

2 Taban M, Behrens A, Newcomb RL, Nobe MY, Saedi G, Sweet PM, McDonnell PJ: Acute endophthalmitis following cataract surgery: a systematic review of the literature. Arch Ophthalmol 2005;123:613–620.

3 Recchia FM, Busbee BG, Pearlman RB, Carvalho-Recchia CA, Ho AC: Changing trends in the microbiologic aspects of postcataract endophthalmitis. Arch Ophthalmol 2005;123:341–346.

4 Mandelbaum S, Foster RK: Exogenous endophthalmitis; in Pepose JS, Holland GN, Wilhelms KR (eds): Ocular Infection and Immunity. St. Louis, Mosby, 1996, pp 1298–1320.

5 Essex RW, Yi Q, Charles PG, Allen PJ: Post-traumatic endophthalmitis. Ophthalmology 2004;111: 2015–2022.

6 Schiedler V, Scott IU, Flynn HW Jr, Davis JL, Benz MS, Miller D: Culture-proven endogenous endophthalmitis: clinical features and visual acuity outcomes. Am J Ophthalmol 2004;137: 725–731.

7 Callegan MC, Kane ST, Cochran DC, Gilmore MS: Molecular mechanisms of Bacillus endophthalmitis pathogenesis. DNA Cell Biol 2002;21367–21373.

8 Callegan MC, Kane ST, Cochran C, Novosad B, Gilmore MS, Gominet M, Lereclus D: Bacillus endophthalmitis: roles of bacterial toxins and motility during infection. Invest Ophthalmol Vis Sci 2005;46:3233–3238.

9 Callegan MC, Cochran DC, Kane ST, Gilmore MS, Gominet M, Lereclus D: Contribution of membrane-damaging toxins to Bacillus endophthalmitis pathogenesis. Infect Immun 2002;70: 5381–5389.

10 Callegan MC, Engelbert M, Parke DW 2nd, Jett BD, Gilmore MS: Bacterial endophthalmitis: epidemiology, therapeutics, and bacterium-host interactions. Clin Microbiol Rev 2002;15:111–124.

11 Perkins SL, Han DP, Burke JM, Schlievert PM, Wirostko WJ, Tarasewicz DG, Skumatz CM: Intravitreally injected human immunoglobulin attenuates the effects of *Staphylococcus aureus* culture supernatant in a rabbit model of toxin-mediated endophthalmitis. Arch Ophthalmol 2004;122: 1499–1506.

12 Dajcs JJ, Thibodeaux BA, Girgis DO, Shaffer MD, Delvisco SM, O'Callaghan RJ: Immunity to lysostaphin and its therapeutic value for ocular MRSA infections in the rabbit. Invest Ophthalmol Vis Sci 2002;43:3712–3716.

13 Scott IU, Loo RH, Flynn HW Jr, Miller D: Endophthalmitis caused by *Enterococcus faecalis*: antibiotic selection and treatment outcomes. Ophthalmology 2003;110:1573–1577.

14 Jett BD, Jensen JG, Atkuri RV, Gilmore MS: Evaluation of therapeutic measures for treating endophthalmitis caused by isogenic toxin-producing and toxin-nonproducing *Enterococcus faecalis* strains. Invest Ophthalmol Vis Sci 1995;36:9–15.

15 Engelbert M, Mylonakis E, Ausubel FM, Calderwood SB, Gilmore MS: Contribution of gelatinase, serine protease, and fsr to the pathogenesis of *Enterococcus faecalis* endophthalmitis. Infect Immun 2004;72:3628–3633.
16 Aldave AJ, Stein JD, Deramo VA, Shah GK, Fischer DH, Maguire JI: Treatment strategies for postoperative *Propionibacterium acnes* endophthalmitis. Ophthalmology 1999;106:2395–2401.
17 Chen YJ, Kuo HK, Wu PC, Kuo ML, Tsai HH, Liu CC, Chen CH: A 10-year comparison of endogenous endophthalmitis outcomes: an east Asian experience with *Klebsiella pneumoniae* infection. Retina 2004;24:383–390.
18 Ma LC, Fang CT, Lee CZ, Shun CT, Wang JT: Genomic heterogeneity in *Klebsiella pneumoniae* strains is associated with primary pyogenic liver abscess and metastatic infection. J Infect Dis 2005;192:117–128.
19 Streilein JW: Ocular immune privilege: therapeutic opportunities from an experiment of nature. Nat Rev Immunol 2003;3:879–889.
20 Webster G, Leyden JJ, Musson RA, Douglas SD: Susceptibility of *Propionibacterium acnes* to killing and degradation by human neutrophils and monocytes in vitro. Infect Immun 1985;49: 116–121.
21 Kwon B, Hazlett LD: Association of CD4+ T cell-dependent keratitis with genetic susceptibility to *Pseudomonas aeruginosa* ocular infection. J Immunol 1997;159:6283–6290.
22 Engstrom RE, Modino BJ, Glasgow BJ, Pitchekian-Halabi H, Adamu SA: Immune response to *Staphylococcus aureus* endophthalmitis in a rabbit model. Invest Ophthalmol Vis Sci 1991;32: 1523–1533.
23 Maylath FR, Leopold JH: Study of experimental ocular infection. Am J Ophthalmol 1955;40:86–101.
24 Haynes RJ, McElveen JE, Dua HS, Tighe PJ, Liversidge J: Expression of human beta-defensins in intraocular tissues. Invest Ophthalmol Vis Sci 2000;41:3026–3031.
25 Beyer TL, Vogler G, Sharma D, O'Donnell FE Jr: Protective barrier effect of the posterior lens capsule in exogenous bacterial endophthalmitis: an experimental primate study. Invest Ophthalmol Vis Sci 1984;25:108–112.
26 Takeda K, Akira S: Toll-like receptors in innate immunity. Int Immunol 2005;17:1–14.
27 Kumr V, Nagineni CN, Chin MS, Hooks JJ, Detrick B: Innate immunity in the retina: Toll-like receptor (TLR) signaling in human retinal pigment epithelial cells. J Neuroimmunol 2004;153:7–15.
28 Tosi MF: Innate immune responses to infection. J Allergy Clin Immunol 2005;116:241–249.
29 Engelbert M, Gilmore MS: Fas ligand but not complement is critical for control of experimental *Staphylococcus aureus* endophthalmitis. Invest Ophthalmol Vis Sci 2005;46:2479–2486.
30 Giese MJ, Sumner HL, Berliner JA, Mondino BJ: Cytokine expression in a rat model of *Staphylococcus aureus* endophthalmitis. Invest Ophthalmol Vis Sci 1998;39:2785–2790.
31 Giese MJ, Shum DC, Rayner SA, Mondino BJ, Berliner JA: Adhesion molecule expression in a rat model of *Staphylococcus aureus* endophthalmitis. Invest Ophthalmol Vis Sci 2000;41:145–153.
32 Griffith T, Brunner T, Fletcher SM, Green DR, Ferguson TA: Fas ligand-induced apoptosis as a mechanism of immune privilege. Science 1995;270:1189–1192.
33 Gregory MS, Repp AC, Hohlbaum AM, Saff RR, Marshak-Rothstein A, Ksander BR: Membrane Fas ligand activates innate immunity and terminates ocular immune privilege. J Immunol 2002;169:2727–2735.
34 Meredith TA, Aguilar HE, Drews C, Sawant A, Gardner S, Wilson LA, Grossniklaus HE: Intraocular dexamethasone produces a harmful effect on treatment of experimental *Staphylococcus aureus* endophthalmitis. Trans Am Ophthalmol Soc 1996;94:241–257.
35 Shah GK, Stein JD, Sharma S, Sivalingam A, Benson WE, Regillo CD, Brown GC, Tasman W: Visual outcomes following the use of intravitreal steroids in the treatment of postoperative endophthalmitis. Am Acad Ophthalmol 2000;107:486–489.

Dr. M. Gilmore
Schepens Eye Research Institute
20 Staniford Street
Boston, MA 02114 (USA)
Tel. +1 617 912 7448, Fax +1 617 912 0115, E-Mail mgilmore@vision.eri.harvard.edu

Niederkorn JY, Kaplan HJ (eds): Immune Response and the Eye.
Chem Immunol Allergy. Basel, Karger, 2007, vol 92, pp 276–289

Influence of Immune Surveillance and Immune Privilege on Formation of Intraocular Tumors

Peter W. Chen[a], *Bruce R. Ksander*[b]

[a]Department of Ophthalmology, University of Texas Southwestern Medical Center at Dallas, Dallas, Tex., [b]Schepens Eye Research Institute, Harvard Medical School, Boston, Mass., USA

Abstract

The immune surveillance theory proposed almost half a century ago stated that the immune system was responsible for preventing the formation of spontaneous tumors by identifying and eliminating neoplastic cells early in their development. Recent studies demonstrating that innate and adaptive immune effector cells participate in preventing tumor growth and are effective in reducing the frequency of tumors have revived interest in immune surveillance. Paradoxically, other recent studies demonstrate that the immune system can also promote tumor progression by altering the immunogenic phenotype of developing tumors in a process called immunoediting. These data raise new questions regarding whether immune surveillance and immunoediting occur within the immune-privileged ocular environment where the innate and adaptive immune effector cells are inhibited and/or participate in the development of regulatory T cells.

Immune surveillance is an 'old' theory first proposed almost 50 years ago that hypothesized that one function of the immune system was to monitor cells throughout the host for changes that signified the start of malignant transformation. Recognition and elimination of these early premalignant cells would protect the host from the formation of spontaneous tumors. Although this theory was intellectually appealing to immunologists, the experimental evidence that accumulated in the 1970s failed to support the hypothesis and immunologists abandoned the idea of immune surveillance. However, recent data have emerged that clearly and convincingly support the immune surveillance theory in mouse models of spontaneous and induced tumors. In addition, new data demonstrate the existence of immune surveillance in human spontaneous tumors. In these more recent studies, a second important mechanism was discovered that is intimately associated with immune surveillance. This mechanism was termed 'immunoediting' and describes the effect of immune surveillance on tumor progression in circumstances when immune surveillance fails to prevent the formation of tumors. Immunoediting results in a reduction in the frequency of tumor rejection and the expression of a less immunogenic antigen repertoire by the tumor. In other words, immune surveillance had the effect of 'editing' out some of the antigens normally expressed by tumor cells in the absence of immune surveillance. These two concepts, immune surveillance and immunoediting, are likely to become the cornerstones by which immunologists view the development of tumors and will be critical in developing successful strategies for cancer immunotherapy.

The revival of immune surveillance and the emergence of immunoediting pose new questions in the development of ocular tumors and the study of immune privilege, starting with: Does immune surveillance and immunoediting occur within the eye during the development of intraocular tumors? If the answer is yes, then how does it occur since the eye is an immune-privileged site in which innate and adaptive immunity is downregulated? If the answer is no, then how does this impact on the pathogenesis and treatment of ocular tumors and their metastases? The first half of this study will review the new data that support immune surveillance and immunoediting. The second half will address if, and how, the development of ocular tumors within an immune-privileged site is linked to immune surveillance and immunoediting.

Beginnings of the Immune Surveillance Theory

In the early 1900s, Ehrlich [1] proposed that a critical function of the immune system was to detect and eliminate carcinomas from the host. Thomas [2] and Burnet [3] developed the theory of immune surveillance proposing that tumor cells developed frequently and expressed tumor antigens that triggered the host to generate an immune-mediated response that eliminated the tumor. Studies by Old and Boyse [4] and Klein [5] in the 1960s confirmed the existence of tumor antigens on chemically or virally transformed murine tumors, and observed that tumors expressing these antigens were rapidly eliminated in syngeneic hosts. If the theory of immune surveillance was correct, then there would be an increase in spontaneous tumor incidence in immunocompromised hosts compared to tumor incidence in immunocompetent hosts. However, tumor studies in nude mice that lack functional T and B cells demonstrated no changes in the incidence of spontaneous tumor development compared to immunocompetent hosts [6]. Supporters of the immune surveillance theory argued that nude mice were not completely immunodeficient, since nude mice, while defective in T cell immunity, still possessed an intact innate immune response that may be critical in immune surveillance [7]. Even though this argument proved much later to be correct, at the time, there were no experimental models that could rigorously test the role of innate immunity in immune surveillance, and in the absence of data, the theory quickly lost favor among immunologists.

The Revival of Immune Surveillance

Experimental support of immune surveillance began to emerge in the middle 1990s with the development and testing of a variety of mutant mice that were deficient in one or more components of innate or adaptive immune systems. The first evidence came from a series of experimental models that eliminated interferon (IFN)-γ, an important cytokine produced mainly by T cells, natural killer (NK) cells, and NKT cells. Mice treated with neutralizing antibodies for IFN-γ and then given transplanted fibrosarcoma tumors exhibited a significant incidence of tumor growth [8]. Kaplan et al. [9] demonstrated that at least one effect of IFN-γ was to directly inhibit tumor growth. They expressed dominant-negative IFN-γ receptors in fibrosarcomas that were then transplanted into recipient mice. Tumors that could not respond to IFN-γ grew significantly faster than tumors with functional IFN-γ receptors. The most convincing evidence for an important role of IFN-γ in protecting the host from developing tumors came from experiments using either IFN-γ gene knockout, or IFN-γ receptor gene knockout mice [9, 10]. Exposure of these knockout mice to the chemical carcinogen methylcholanthrene (MCA) resulted in a 10- to 20-fold increase in tumor formation. In addition, tumors formed more rapidly and grew faster in these knockout mice than in mice with an intact response to IFN-γ. Together, the data indicated that: (i) IFN-γ production protected the mice from the induction of chemically induced tumors, and (ii) protection was partly due to a direct inhibitory effect of IFN-γ on tumor growth. Evidence that cytolytic immune effector cells participate in preventing tumor growth was demonstrated in experiments which used perforin gene knockout mice [11]. Perforin is a pore-forming protein released by cytotoxic T cells and NK cells that is essential in lysing the target cell. If perforin knockout mice were treated with MCA, there was a significant increase in tumor incidence compared to tumor incidence in the normal counterparts.

Further evidence that T cells, NKT cells, and B cells protected mice from tumor development was provided by experiments in RAG-1 or RAG-2 gene knockout mice. The RAG gene encodes an enzyme that repairs breaks in double-stranded DNA. Mice that lack the RAG gene are unable to rearrange lymphocyte antigen receptors and therefore, completely lack T cells, NKT cells, and B cells. MCA treatment of these mice also resulted in an increased incidence of tumors [12]. Finally, a role for innate immune effectors was provided by targeted mutations that specifically eliminated either: NKT cells, NK cells, or γδ T cells [13, 14]. These mutant mice all displayed increased sensitivity to MCA-induced tumors.

One of the previous criticisms of the immune surveillance theory was that data supporting a role for immune protection were largely obtained by the induction of tumors with chemical carcinogens, such as MCA. To address this criticism, mice that possess p53 mutations were crossed with the mutant mice described above. Mice with p53 mutations develop a variety of spontaneous tumors [9]. However, if the p53 mutant mice were crossed with either RAG-1, or IFN-γ knockout mice, there was a significant increase in the incidence of spontaneous tumors [15, 16]. These data strongly support a protective role of innate and adaptive immune effector cells in preventing the development of tumors.

Involvement of Innate and Adaptive Immunity in Immune Surveillance

Innate immunity provides effective first-line immune responses against invading pathogens and consists of NK cells, dendritic cells (DCs), mast cells, macrophages, and natural IgM antibody-producing B cells [17]. Cells involved in innate immunity recognize conserved glycolipid or glycoprotein patterns rather than individual specific cell surface determinants to distinguish between self and non-self. Recent studies have demonstrated that the innate immune system has the capacity to discriminate between malignant cells and normal cells suggesting that innate immunity mediates tumor immune surveillance. Abnormal glycolipids and glycoproteins are frequently synthesized and expressed on the tumor cell surface, and many of these structures elicit strong IgM production by CD5+ B cells of the innate immune system. Tumor-reactive IgM antibodies that recognize abnormal carbohydrates expressed by mutated epithelial cells have been identified and isolated in patients with gastric cancer [18]. These antibodies can directly elicit tumor cell elimination by mediating apoptosis of malignant epithelial cells, or indirectly by inducing complement activation, or antibody-mediated cellular cytotoxicity. Interestingly, IgM antibodies isolated from healthy donors also recognized transformed epithelial cells from cancer patients suggesting that healthy individuals already possess naturally occurring

IgM antibodies capable of recognizing mutated glycolipid or glycoprotein patterns.

Studies in mice using models deficient in adaptive immune responses (SCID, nude and RAG knockout models) have demonstrated that NK cells play an important role in tumor recognition. NK cells recognize and kill tumor cells deficient in major histocompatibility complex (MHC) class I molecule expression. The activation and function of NK cells are regulated by a balance of inhibitory and activating signals through a number of receptors. Mice depleted of NK cells using either anti-NK1.1 or anti-asialo GM1 demonstrated increased susceptibility to spontaneous MCA-induced tumors [19]. Recently, human MHC class I chain-related proteins A and B (MICA/B) have been identified and characterized, and represent polymorphic nonclassical MHC class I type molecules that are stress-induced proteins [20]. Constitutive MICA/B expression has been found on tumors of the breast, lung, colon, kidney, liver, and skin melanoma but is not expressed by normal tissues with the exception of the epithelial lining of the gastrointestinal tract [20, 21]. MICA/B on tumor cells bind to their NK cell ligand NKG2D, a constitutively expressed disulfide-linked homodimer comprised of two NKG2D subunits associated with the transmembrane adaptor protein DAP10, which together serve as an NK cell activation molecule [22]. It is interesting to note that tumors from advanced stages of disease are capable of shedding MICA/B from the cell surface, and binding of soluble MICA/B downregulates expression of NKG2D on NK cells [23]. These results suggest that tumor cells have compensatory mechanisms that enable them to escape immune recognition.

NKT cells are a recently characterized subpopulation of T cells that express both NK markers and an invariant T cell receptor that may play a role in immunoregulation and in tumor immune surveillance. Human NKT cells express the NKR-P1A NK marker and the invariant T cell α chain Vα24-JαQ, whereas mice express NK1.1, a NK cell marker and the invariant T cell α chain Vα14-Jα281 [24]. Both human and mouse NKT cells are restricted by the MHC class I-like molecule CD1 which recognizes glycolipid antigens. Initial evidence that NKT cells play a role in tumor immune surveillance was demonstrated by two studies. First, mice treated with the NKT cell-activating compound α-galactosylceramide demonstrated a lower incidence of spontaneous chemically induced tumors [25]. Second, Jα281 knockout mice which lack Vα14-Jα281-expressing NKT cells developed a higher incidence of MCA-induced tumors than their wild-type counterparts [26]. Upon activation, NKT cells differentially produce cytokines that are dependent on activation via specific receptors; activation through the T cell receptor elicits interleukin-4 production while activation through the NK receptor elicits production of IFN-γ [24]. The production of these cytokines by NKT cells may play an important role not only in NKT cell activation and development, but also in the activation and maturation of macrophages and DCs involved in innate and adaptive immune responses against tumors.

In summary, there is ample evidence that the innate immune system participates in tumor immune surveillance and functions as a first responder by delaying tumor growth. However, in most cases, innate immune responses against tumors are insufficient to completely eliminate tumors. Therefore, innate immune responses triggered by tumors must also play an important role by providing support in activating immune responses mediated by the adaptive immune system.

The Immunoediting Hypothesis

Dunn et al. [27] recently proposed the immunoediting hypothesis which they considered an extension of the immune surveillance theory that explained situations in which immune surveillance failed to protect the host from malignant transformation. It is obvious that, even in an immune-competent host, spontaneous tumors still develop. This means that although immune surveillance is fully functional, some tumors still escape immune detection and grow progressively. Thus, immune surveillance appeared to be an 'all or none' effect in which it either prevented or failed to prevent tumor formation. The immunoediting hypothesis proved that this concept was wrong and demonstrated that tumor formation in the presence of immune surveillance has a profound effect on the tumor phenotype.

The immunoediting hypothesis was developed when Kaplan et al. [9] examined the immunogenicity of tumors that formed within either immunocompetent or immunodeficient mice. These experiments are diagramed in figure 1. As discussed earlier, there is a significant increase in the incidence of tumors that form in RAG-2 knockout mice exposed to MCA compared with normal mice exposed to the same carcinogen. A series of tumors were recovered from either normal or RAG-2 knockout mice and then injected into a second group of naïve immunocompetent mice. When the tumors recovered from normal mice were injected into the naïve recipients, 100% of the tumors grew progressively. By contrast, when the tumors recovered from RAG-2 knockout mice were injected into the naïve recipients, only 40% of the tumors grew progressively [12]. Therefore, tumors that formed in the presence of immune surveillance were *less immunogenic*, and tumors that formed in the absence of immune surveillance were *more immunogenic*. In light of their results, they proposed that immunoediting was responsible for editing or removing tumor antigens that were recognized by immune effector cells.

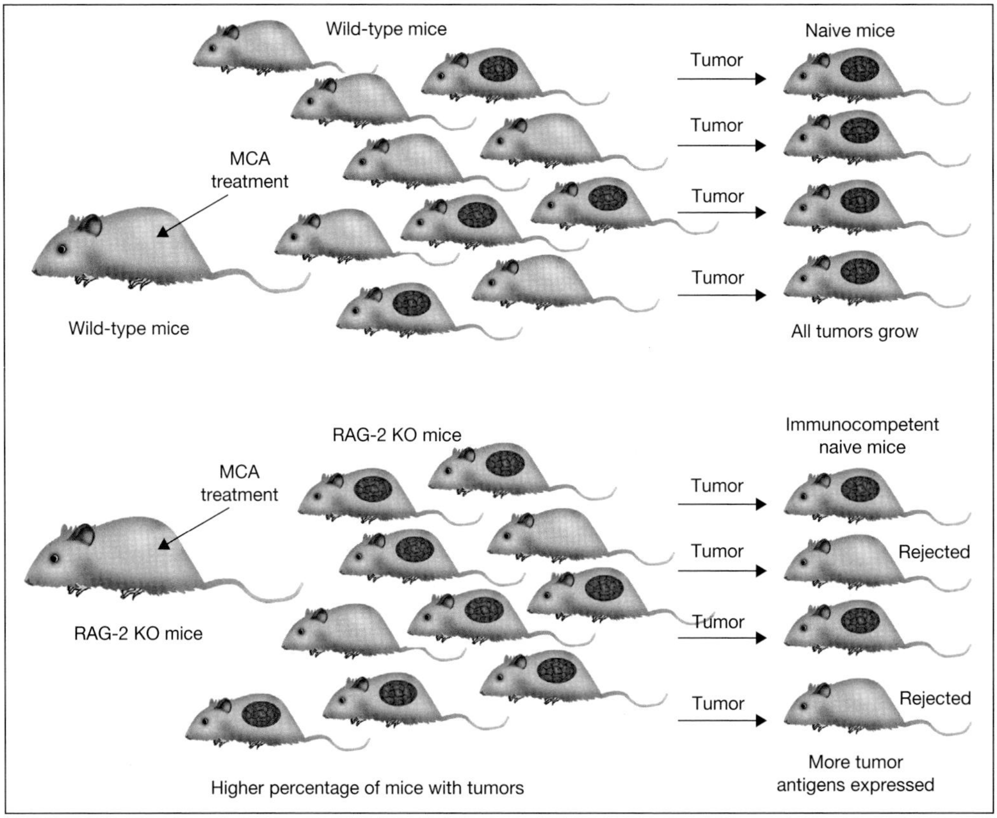

Fig. 1. Immunoediting of tumors that form within immunocompetent mice. Tumors are induced in immunocompetent wild-type, or RAG-2 knockout (KO) mice by treatment with the MCA carcinogen. Tumors are recovered from the mice and injected into a second group of immunocompetent naïve mice. Tumors derived from immunocompromised mice express more tumor antigens, resulting in some tumor rejection. By contrast, tumors derived from immunocompetent mice undergo immunoediting and express fewer tumor antigens, resulting in a higher frequency of progressively growing tumors.

The immunoediting hypothesis expanded the immune surveillance concept to be more than an 'all or none' effect on tumor growth. If tumors formed in the presence of immune surveillance, they expressed fewer tumor antigens than the same tumor formed in the absence of immune surveillance. This also revealed the paradox of immune surveillance; it is *protective* when it prevents tumor growth, but it can also *promote* tumor growth by making tumors less visible to the immune system. These two contradictory effects are possible because the immune effectors involved in surveillance have two functions: (i) eliminating antigen-positive tumors, and (ii) editing antigens from tumors that grow. The latter function is accomplished through the mechanism of selective pressure that is applied by the immune system on the tumor cells and leads to the formation of tumor escape mutants.

Selective Pressure and Tumor Escape

There is a wide variety of mechanisms that lead to the formation of tumor escape mutants [28]. The simplest form of tumor escape is via the loss of a tumor antigen expressed on a tumor cell. How the immune system applies selective pressure that leads to the formation of antigen-loss escape mutants is easily demonstrated in vitro. If cytotoxic T lymphocytes in cell cultures containing specific T cells plus tumor cells eliminate some, but not all of the tumor cells, then the tumor cells will undergo selective depletion. If the surviving tumor cells are allowed to proliferate and are re-exposed to another round of selection by T cells, and this process is repeated many times over a long period of time, the cell cultures will eventually develop escape mutant tumor cells that are completely resistant to elimination by the specific T cells [29]. The experiments of Dunn et al. [30] revealed that immune surveillance that fails to completely eliminate tumors provides this selective pressure for the development of escape mutations. It is believed that the inherent genetic instability of tumor cells induces random mutations in the proliferating tumor cells, and that specific T cells provide selective pressure for the survival of specific mutations that lead to immune escape. This selective T cell pressure is therefore an example of Darwinian natural selection at the cellular level. This mechanism of tumor escape has also been shown to occur in vivo in patients immunized against specific tumor antigens [31].

Does Immune Surveillance Occur within the Immune-Privileged Eye?

While this question may seem obvious, the critical experiments required to answer it have not been performed. There are several approaches to address this question. In one series of experiments, either normal or immunocompromised mice would receive an intraocular dose of a chemical carcinogen such as MCA. If immune surveillance occurs within the eye, then the incidence of tumors will increase in the immune-compromised mice. If immune surveillance does not occur within the eye, then the incidence of tumors will not change in the absence of an intact immune response. It will be important to examine a variety of innate and adaptive immunodeficient mice in order to determine if immune surveillance occurs within the eye.

A second type of experiment would utilize the recently developed transgenic models that spontaneously develop either retinoblastoma, or uveal melanoma [32, 33]. These transgenic mice would be crossed with immunodeficient mice, and the speed and size of tumor development would be monitored. If immune surveillance occurs in the eye, then the spontaneous tumors will appear sooner and grow more rapidly. If immune surveillance does not occur, then the appearance of the spontaneous tumors will remain unchanged. These experiments would conclusively prove whether immune surveillance occurs within the immune-privileged eye.

A third type of experiment would conclusively prove a close association between immune privilege and immune surveillance. In these experiments, MCA would be used to induce tumors in the eyes of immunocompetent mice in which immune privilege is terminated. If the frequency of tumors decreases in the absence of immune privilege in immunocompetent mice, then this will demonstrate that immune privilege blocks immune surveillance in the eye. The technical problem with conducting this type of experiment is that immune privilege would have to be terminated for many months in order to induce tumors with MCA. Currently, there is no method of terminating immune privilege in the eye for extended periods of time. However, the recent discovery of defects in immune privilege and anterior chamber-associated immune deviation in DBA/2J mice may provide the opportunity to conduct this type of experiment [34].

Regulation of Immune Surveillance Effectors within the Eye

Although there are no conclusive data on the role of immune surveillance in the eye, there are substantial data on the immune response against tumors transplanted or injected into the anterior chamber, and these data are useful in making predictions about whether or not immune surveillance occurs. The argument that immune surveillance does not occur in the eye is supported by data indicating that both innate and adaptive immune effector cells responsible for mediating surveillance are all negatively regulated within the eye. The effect of the ocular environment on each of these effector cell subpopulations is summarized below.

NK Cells

Apte et al. [35] discovered that macrophage migration inhibitory factor is present within aqueous humor and inhibits the cytolytic activity of NK cells.

DCs/Macrophages

A number of researchers have reported the inhibitory effects of the ocular environment on DCs/macrophages that prevent the development of both innate and adaptive immunity. For example, α-melanocyte-stimulating hormone inhibits the ability of DCs/macrophages to release nitric oxide, an important pro-inflammatory cytokine in innate immunity [36]. Transforming growth factor-β_2 alters the ability of DCs/macrophages to effectively stimulate CD4 and CD8 T cells, resulting in the activation of T regulatory (T_{reg}) cells that inhibit effectors of delayed hypersensitivity [37].

NKT Cells

Faunce and Stein-Streilein [38] discovered that NKT cells are critical in the activation of antigen-specific T_{reg} cells following injection of antigen into the anterior chamber of the eye. While the data that NKT cells participate in blocking the development of protective immunity are very convincing, other laboratories have reported a protective role for NKT cells in tumor formation and spread [25]. Further studies are required to understand the functions of this important effector cell population.

γδ T Cells

When antigen is injected into the anterior chamber of the eye, γδ T cells participate in the induction of T_{reg} cells through the induction of anterior chamber-associated immune deviation [39]. This was demonstrated in experiments using γδ T cell knockout mice, in which the injection of soluble antigen into the anterior chamber did not result in the activation of T_{reg} cells, resulting in the activation of primed T cells that mediate delayed hypersensitivity.

CD4+ and CD8+ T Cells

Investigators from different laboratories demonstrated that injection of antigen into the anterior chamber results in downregulation of delayed hypersensitivity via the induction of T_{reg} cells. CD4 T_{reg} cells inhibit the afferent phase, while CD8 T_{reg} cells inhibit the efferent phase of adaptive immunity [40, 41].

Together, these data argue against the idea that immune surveillance can occur within an immune-privileged site, since all of the effector cells that participate in immune surveillance are either inhibited or involved in the activation of T_{reg} cells. However, it is important to remember that immune privilege is not absolute and does not completely exclude the activation of immune effector cells within the eye. The extent of immune privilege that is experienced by tumors that are injected into the anterior chamber varies dramatically. Some tumors escape immune elimination completely and grow progressively, while others are rejected with the same speed and vigor as tumors that are placed

Table 1. Influence of ocular immune privilege on intraocular tumor rejection

Tumor	Strain of origin	Recipient strain	Antigens	Immunogenicity	Immune privilege	Tumor growth
P815	DBA/2	DBA/2	tumor Ags	weak	yes	progression
P815	DBA/2	BALB/c	minor	weak	yes	progression
B16F10	C57BL/6	LP/J	tumor Ags	weak	yes	progression
D5.164	C57BL/6	C57BL/6	tumor Ags	weak	yes	progression
P815	DBA/2	A/J	MHC	strong	transient	rejection
P815	DBA/2	C57BL/6	MHC + minor H	strong	transient	rejection
P91	DBA/2	DBA/2	mutated tumor Ag	strong	transient	rejection
UV-5C25	BALB/c	BALB/c	UV induced	strong	transient	rejection
SV40 FVN	FVB/n	FVB/n	SV40 T Ag	strong	no	rejection
Ad5E1	C56BL/6	C37BL/6	adenovirus	strong	no	rejection

within non-immune-privileged sites (table 1). An important question in the study of immune privilege within the eye that remains unanswered is: what mechanisms control if, or when, immune privilege is terminated? Data in the literature support the concept that the ocular environment is critical in establishing immune privilege and it is the presence of immunosuppressive factors within aqueous humor that inhibits the induction of innate and adaptive immunity. So, why does this environment establish immune privilege for some tumors, but fails to establish immune privilege for other tumors?

One possible answer to this question is provided by data indicating that there is an inverse relationship between immune privilege and the immunogenicity of the tumors. In other words, tumors that express highly immunogenic tumor antigens experience weak immune privilege, while tumors that express weak tumor antigens experience robust immune privilege (table 1). Clearly, immune privilege is most effective in protecting weakly immunogenic tumors, while privilege is least effective in protecting strongly immunogenic tumors. It is unclear at this time exactly how strong immunogenic tumors are able to overcome the inhibitory mechanisms within the eye. Together, these data indicate that immune privilege inhibits the immune effector cells responsible for maintaining immune surveillance.

We propose that there is an inverse relationship between immune privilege and immune surveillance. This relationship is illustrated in figure 2. At the two extremes are: (i) high levels of immunogenic tumor antigens coincide with effective immune surveillance, and (ii) no antigens, or low levels of weak tumor antigens, coincide with the absence of immune surveillance. However, the more

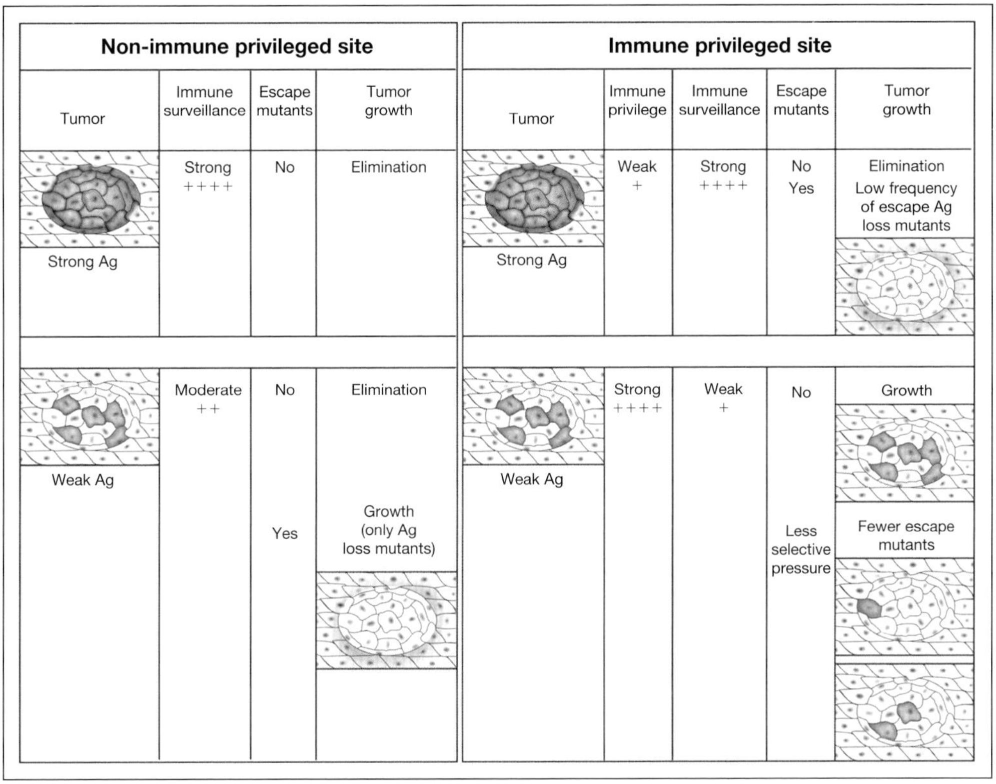

Fig. 2. The effect of immune privilege on immune surveillance, tumor antigens, and tumor growth. The predicted effects of immune privilege on tumors that express either strong tumor antigens (dark cells), or weak tumor antigens (shaded cells). Tumor antigen (Ag) escape mutants are displayed as white cells.

likely scenario is that ocular tumors display a range of tumor antigens. This mixture of antigens could be displayed sequentially or sporadically during malignant transformation. If this situation is compared between a tumor that develops within an immune-privileged site versus the same tumor that develops within a non-privileged site, then we predict that the effect of immune surveillance would be significantly delayed in the eye. This would result in tumors that form more frequently in the eye and express more tumor antigens.

In addition to immune privilege and immune surveillance, there are many other factors that affect malignant transformation in the eye that we have not discussed. For example, choroidal melanocytes have a very low rate of turnover and may be inherently more resistant to malignant transformation than melanocytes within the skin. Therefore, it will be important to determine not only whether immune surveillance is present within the eye, but also whether immune surveillance has a significant impact on tumor development and progression in human ocular tumors.

References

1 Ehrlich P: Ueber den jetzigen Stand der Karzinomforschung. Ned Tijdschr Geneeskd 1909;5: 273–290.
2 Thomas L: Reactions to homologous tissue antigens in relation to hypersensitivity; in Lawrence HS (ed): Cellular and Humoral Aspects of the Hypersensitive States. New York, Hoeber-Harper, 1959, pp 529–532.
3 Burnet FM: Immunological factors in the process of carcinogenesis. Br Med Bull 1964;20:154–158.
4 Old LJ, Boyse EA: Specific antigens of tumors and leukemias of experimental animals. Med Clin North Am 1966;50:901–912.
5 Klein G: Tumor antigens. Annu Rev Microbiol 1966;20:223–252.
6 Stutman O: Tumor development after 3-methylcholanthrene in immunologically deficient athymic-nude mice. Science 1974;183:534–536.
7 Herberman RB, Holden HT: Natural cell-mediated immunity. Adv Cancer Res 1978;27:305–377.
8 Dighe AS, Richards E, Old LJ, Schreiber RD: Enhanced in vivo growth resistance to rejection of tumor cells expressing dominant negative IFNγ receptors. Immunity 1994;1:447–456.
9 Kaplan DH, Shankaran V, Dighe AS, Stockert E, Aguet M, Old LJ, Schreiber RD: Demonstration of an interferon γ-dependent tumor surveillance system in immunocompetent mice. Proc Natl Acad Sci USA 1998;95:7556–7561.
10 Street SE, Trapani JA, MacGregor D, Smyth MJ: Suppression of lymphoma and epithelial malignancies effected by interferon γ. J Exp Med 1998;196:129–134.
11 van den Broek MF, Kagi D, Ossendorp F, Toes R, Vamvakas S, Lutza WK, Melief CJM, Zinkernagel RM, Hengartner H: Decreased tumor surveillance in perforin-deficient mice. J Exp Med 1996;184:1781–1790.
12 Shankaran V, Ikeda H, Bruce AT, White JM, Swanson PE, Old LJ, Schreiber RD: IFNγ and lymphocytes prevent primary tumour development and shape tumour immunogenicity. Nature 2001;410: 1107–1111.
13 Smyth MJ, Crowe NY, Godfrey DI: NK cells and NKT cells collaborate in host protection from methylcholanthrene-induced fibrosarcoma. Int Immunol 2001;13:459–463.
14 Girardi M, Oppenheim DE, Steele CR, Lewis JM, Glusac E, Filler R, Hobby P, Sutton B, Tigelaar RE, Hayday AC: Regulation of cutaneous malignancy by γδ T cells. Science 2001;294:605–609.
15 Nacht M, Jacks T: V(D)J recombination is not required for the development of lymphoma in p53-deficient mice. Cell Growth Differ 1998;9:131–138.
16 Liao MJ, Zhang XX, Hill R, Gao J, Qumsiyeh MB, Nichols W, Van Dyke T: No requirement for V(D)J recombination in p53-deficient thymic lymphoma. Mol Cell Biol 1998;18:3495–3501.
17 Diefenbach A, Raulet DH: Innate immune recognition by stimulatory immunoreceptors. Curr Opin Immunol 2003;15:37–44.
18 Brandlein S, Pohle T, Ruoff N, Wozniak E, Muller-Hermelink HK, Vollmers HP: Natural IgM antibodies and immunosurveillance mechanisms against epithelial cancer cells in humans. Cancer Res 2003;63:7995–8005.
19 Algarra I, Ohlen C, Perez M, Ljunggren HG, Klein G, Garrido F, Karre K: NK sensitivity and lung clearance of MHC-class-I-deficient cells within a heterogeneous fibrosarcoma. Int J Cancer 1989;44:675–680.
20 Vetter CS, Groh V, thorStraten P, Spies T, Brocker EB, Becker JC: Expression of stress-induced MHC class I related chain molecules on human melanoma. J Invest Dermatol 2002;118:600–605.
21 Groh V, Rhinehart R, Secrist H, Bauer S, Grabstein KH, Spies T: Broad tumor-associated expression and recognition by tumor-derived γδ T cells of MICA and MICB. Proc Natl Acad Sci USA 1999;96:6879–6884.

22 Gilfillan S, Ho EL, Cella M, Yokoyama WM, Colonna M: NKG2D recruits two distinct adapters to trigger NK cell activation and costimulation. Nat Immunol 2002;3:1150–1155.
23 Salih HR, Rammensee HG, Steinle A: Cutting edge: down-regulation of MICA on human tumors by proteolytic shedding. J Immunol 2002;169:4098–4102.
24 Taniguchi M, Seino K, Nakayama T: The NKT cell system: bridging innate and acquired immunity. Nat Immunol 2003;4:1164–1165.
25 Smyth MJ, Thia KY, Street SE, Cretney E, Trapani JA, Taniguchi M, Kawano T, Pelikan SB, Crowe NY, Godfrey DI: Differential tumor surveillance by natural killer (NK) and NKT cells. J Exp Med 2000;191:661–668.
26 Crowe NY, Coquet JM, Berzins SP, Kyparissoudis K, Keating R, Pellicci DG, Hayakawa Y, Godfrey DI, Smyth MJ: Differential antitumor immunity mediated by NKT cell subsets in vivo. J Exp Med 2005;202:1279–1288.
27 Dunn GP, Bruce AT, Ikeda H, Old LJ, Schreiber RD: Cancer immunoediting: from immunosurveillance to tumor escape. Nat Immunol 2002;3:991–998.
28 Schreiber H, Wu TH, Nachman J, Kast WM: Immunodominance and tumor escape. Semin Cancer Biol 2002;12:25–31.
29 Matsui S, Ahlers JD, Vortmeyer AO, Terabe M, Tsukui T, Carbone DP, Liotta LA, Berzofsky JA: A model for CD8+ CTL tumor immunosurveillance and regulation of tumor escape by CD4 T cells through an effect on quality of CTL. J Immunol 1999;163:184–193.
30 Dunn GP, Old LJ, Schreiber RD: The immunobiology of cancer immunosurveillance and immunoediting. Immunity 2004;21:137–148.
31 Khong HT, Restifo NP: Natural selection of tumor variants in the generation of 'tumor escape' phenotypes. Nat Immunol 2002;3:999–1005.
32 O'Brien JM, Marcus DM, Bernards R, Carpenter JL, Windle JJ, Mellon PL, Albert DM: A transgenic mouse model for trilateral retinoblastoma. Arch Ophthalmol 1990;108:1145–1151.
33 Morilla-Grasa A: Animal models in uveal melanoma: establishment and research. Can J Ophthalmol 2004;39:433–440.
34 Mo JS, Anderson MG, Gregory M, Smith RS, Savinova OV, Serreze DV, Ksander BR, Streilein JW, John SWM: By altering ocular immune privilege, bone marrow-derived cells pathogenically contribute to DBA/2J pigmentary glaucoma. J Exp Med 2003;197:1335–1344.
35 Apte RS, Sinha D, Mayhew E, Wistow GJ, Niederkorn JY: Cutting edge: role of macrophage migration inhibitory factor in inhibiting NK cell activity and preserving immune privilege. J Immunol 1998;160:5693–5696.
36 Taylor AW: The immunomodulating neuropeptide alpha-melanocyte-stimulating hormone (α-MSH) suppresses LPS-stimulated TLR4 with IRAK-M in macrophages. J Neuroimmunol 2005;162: 43–50.
37 Kezuka T, Streilein JW: Analysis of in vivo regulatory properties of T cells activated in vitro by $TGF\beta_2$-treated antigen presenting cells. Invest Ophthalmol Vis Sci 2000;41:1410–1421.
38 Faunce DE, Stein-Streilein J: NKT cell-derived RANTES recruits APCs and CD8+ T cells to the spleen during the generation of regulatory T cells in tolerance. J Immunol 2002;169:31–38.
39 Skelsey ME, Mellon J, Niederkorn JY: γδ T cells are needed for ocular immune privilege and corneal graft survival. J Immunol 2001;166:4327–4333.
40 Skelsey ME, Mayhew E, Niederkorn JY: CD25+, interleukin-10-producing CD4+ T cells are required for suppressor cell production and immune privilege in the anterior chamber of the eye. Immunology 2003;110:18–29.
41 Kezuka T, Streilein JW: In vitro generation of regulatory CD8+ T cells similar to those found in mice with anterior chamber-associated immune deviation. Invest Ophthalmol Vis Sci 2000;41:1803–1811.

Dr. Peter W. Chen
Department of Ophthalmology, UT Southwestern Medical Center at Dallas
5323 Harry Hines Boulevard
Dallas, TX 75390–9057 (USA)
Tel. +1 214 648 3677, Fax +1 214 648 9061, E-Mail Peter.Chen@UTSouthwestern.edu

Niederkorn JY, Kaplan HJ (eds): Immune Response and the Eye.
Chem Immunol Allergy. Basel, Karger, 2007, vol 92, pp 290–299

Immunogenicity and Immune Privilege of Corneal Allografts

Junko Hori[a], *Jerry Y. Niederkorn*[b]

Departments of Ophthalmology, [a]Nippon Medical School, Tokyo, Japan, [b]University of Texas Southwestern Medical Center, Dallas, Tex., USA

Abstract

Corneal allografts enjoy a remarkable success rate when compared to all other forms of organ transplants. In routine keratoplasties, HLA matching and systemic immunosuppressive drugs are not employed, yet 90% of the uncomplicated transplants survive. The success of corneal allografts was recognized over half a century ago and led to the term 'immune privilege'. The original explanation for the immune privilege of corneal allografts attributed the escape of immune rejection to the avascular and alymphatic nature of the corneal graft bed, which sequestered the corneal allograft from the immune apparatus. In the past 20 years, the widespread use of animal models of keratoplasty has shed light on the mechanisms of corneal immune privilege and has revealed that the success of corneal allografts is due to a combination of properties of the corneal graft bed and the cornea itself.

Keratoplasty is the oldest, most common, and arguably, the most successful form of solid tissue transplantation [1]. First time, uncomplicated, corneal transplants in human subjects can expect a 90% success rate, even in the absence of tissue typing and use of systemic immunosuppressive drugs [2]. This year marks the 100th anniversary of the first documented successful keratoplasty in a human and, thus, is a timely occasion to reconsider the basis for the remarkable immune privilege of corneal transplants [3]. Clinicians sometimes protest that corneal transplants do not express immune privilege, as keratoplasties can fail and immune rejection remains the leading cause of such failures. In this regard, it is useful to define immune privilege and provide specific examples. Studies using rodents help to define the immune privilege of corneal allografts and demonstrate that immune privilege is not an 'all or none' phenomenon. In many donor-host combinations, corneal allografts that are mismatched with the host at

Table 1. Survival of corneal and skin allografts across different histocompatibility barriers

Donor/host mismatch	Incidence of immune rejection, %	
	skin allograft	corneal allograft
MHC + minors	100	50–55
MHC class I only	100	35
MHC class II only	100	0–10

References found in a previously published review [4].

the entire major histocompatibility complex (MHC) plus multiple minor histocompatibility (H) loci are permanently accepted in over 50% of the hosts [4]. By contrast, skin allografts transplanted across the same barriers are invariably rejected [5]. Immune privilege is even more evident when the histocompatibility disparities are reduced (table 1). Two fundamental observations demonstrate the immune privilege of corneal allografts: (1) histocompatibility matching and systemic immunosuppressive drugs are not normally needed in routine keratoplasty, and (2) corneal allografts enjoy a profoundly greater success rate when compared to all other forms of solid tissue transplantation. Two factors contribute to the immune privilege of corneal allografts: (1) the reduced immunogenicity of the corneal graft itself, and (2) the unique properties of the eye and graft bed into which the corneal transplant is placed.

The Immunogenicity of Corneal Allografts: Heterotopic Corneal Transplantation in Animal Models

The normal corneal allograft possesses immunologic privilege. Even corneas grafted into eyes of pre-immunized recipients (mice) often fail to succumb to immune rejection [6]. Interpretation of results of this type is complicated by the fact that the graft bed itself is regarded as an immune-privileged site. Each layer of the cornea has the potential of contributing to the immunogenicity of this tissue as a graft. However, when full-thickness corneal allografts are placed orthotopically in eyes of experimental animals, it is difficult to discern the immunogenic potential of the various layers because the graft is placed in an immune-privileged site [1, 4, 7, 8]. Any analysis of immune responses to alloantigens expressed on orthotopic corneal grafts is complicated by the immunoregulatory properties of the avascular corneal graft bed and the underlying anterior chamber (AC) [4, 8–10].

Skin and Subcutaneous Space

Although the site of engraftment is immune privileged, the cornea itself has also been considered to be an immune-privileged tissue. Early experiments by Barker and Billingham [11] and Medawar [12] showed that the cornea has the capacity to escape destruction by the alloimmune rejection process. To eliminate the contribution of the immune privilege of the site to graft outcome, allogeneic corneas have been grafted to the skin, or placed in subcutaneous pouches – sites known *not* to be immune privileged [13]. Whether conducted in rabbits, rats, or mice, experiments of this type have revealed that rejection of allogeneic corneal grafts usually takes place at these heterotopic sites. The only exception is when the alloantigens confronting the recipient are encoded solely by genes within the MHC class II region. Because the normal cornea does not constitutively express MHC class II antigen-bearing cells [14–16], disparate corneal grafts of class II alone are not rejected in the skin [17].

Subcapsular Space of Kidney

The skin is a particularly inhospitable site for solid tissue grafts. By contrast, the subcapsular sinus of the kidney is a heterotopic site that is regarded by transplantation immunologists as 'conventional', i.e. not privileged. The subcapsular space of the kidney resembles the skin in its possession of lymphatics that drain via a superficial capsular system and a deeper hilar system to the para-aortic nodes [18]. The capsular microcapillary network is supplied by interlobular arteries of the kidney [19]. The kidney capsule contains antigen-presenting cells such as macrophages. Numerous reports indicate that allografts of the kidney, liver, skin, and islets of Langerhans are acutely rejected when placed beneath the kidney capsule [20–22]. In fact, it was the acceptance of allogeneic testis grafts beneath the kidney capsule that led Bellgrau et al. [23] to conclude that testicular tissue is indeed immune privileged, and that immune privilege in this instance arises from constitutive expression of CD95 ligand (CD95L) on Sertoli cells within the grafts. To follow on this lead, Hori et al. [24, 25] showed that the cornea's potential to display immune privilege is manifest at this site, and this property is largely derived from the endothelium.

Immunogenic Potential and Immune Privilege of Each Layer of the Corneal Allograft

The different layers of the normal cornea display either immunogenicity or immune privilege. Moreover, the properties of one layer can influence the properties and fate of another layer. Khodadoust and Silverstein [26] conducted a series of experiments in which individual layers of the cornea from outbred rabbits were placed for 4 weeks at orthotopic sites in eyes of allodisparate rabbit hosts. The allogeneic corneal tissue was then removed and grafted back into the fellow eye of the original donor. All of the grafts were rejected, and the conclusion was drawn that all three layers (epithelium, stroma, and endothelium) were immunogenic. However, the authors were unaware at that time of the ability of bone marrow-derived cells (such as Langerhans cells, LCs) to infiltrate into the corneal epithelium when it resurfaces a wound, and to migrate into the stroma of a corneal graft. In light of recent information indicating that grafted corneal tissue acquires recipient bone marrow-derived cells (expressing MHC class II molecules) in both the epithelial and stromal layers, the grafts used by Khodadoust and Silverstein [26], which were parked for 4 weeks on the rabbit hosts, were most likely repopulated with bone marrow-derived cells from the second rabbit host. Thus, these results do not reveal unequivocally whether each layer of the normal cornea is immunogenic in the absence of recipient-derived antigen-presenting cells.

When each layer of the cornea is placed beneath the kidney capsule, the epithelium and the stroma independently display alloimmunogenic potential at this site [25]. Either layer of the cornea is capable of inducing donor-specific delayed-type hypersensitivity responses to the donor alloantigens and succumbing to immune destruction. Only the corneal endothelium appears to lack these properties. In fact, the corneal endothelium not only lacks inherent immunogenicity, but it also prevents allosensitization by allogeneic corneal stroma that has been grafted into naive mice. The endothelium is even able to resist its own elimination when grafted into mice pre-sensitized to donor alloantigens. Thus, at least in this heterotopic grafting model, the immune privilege of the cornea resides solely with the endothelium. The capacity of the corneal endothelium to promote immune privilege is, however, overwhelmed if the corneal epithelium is included in the graft placed beneath the kidney capsule [25]. In this situation, the overwhelming immunogenicity of the epithelium prevents corneal allografts from surviving at the heterotopic site. Since full-thickness corneal allografts often survive indefinitely when placed orthotopically, the potent immunogenicity of corneal epithelium revealed beneath the kidney capsule is at least partially eclipsed in the eye.

Constitutive expression of CD95L on corneal endothelium is critical to its immune-privileged status [27, 28]. CD95L renders corneal endothelium resistant to immune destruction as revealed by the persistence of endothelial cells in allografts at heterotopic sites of pre-sensitized mice, where the stroma is being destroyed [25]. Moreover, some evidence indicates an immunomodulatory role for CD95L in the induction of alloimmunity [25]. Stroma-endothelial allografts induced donor-specific delayed-type hypersensitivity and rejection only if the corneal grafts failed to express CD95L. Thus, CD95L interferes with allosensitization and perhaps promotes tolerance induction by mechanisms that have yet to be characterized.

Strategies to Eliminate the Immunogenicity of Orthotopic Corneal Allografts

Full-thickness (epithelium-containing) allogeneic corneal allografts induce donor-specific sensitization when: (a) grafted orthotopically [29–31]; (b) when implanted into the AC [32, 33], or (c) when placed beneath the kidney capsule [24, 25]. Corneal epithelium also expresses MHC class I antigens more strongly than do either keratocytes or corneal endothelial cells [15, 16, 34]. In fact, 90% of the MHC class I antigen expression is found in the corneal epithelium [35].

These findings have led to the proposal that the primary immunogenicity of the cornea as an allograft resides within the epithelium. The validity of this proposal is challenged, however, by the observation that corneal allografts from which the epithelial layer had been removed proved to be much more immunogenic and vulnerable to rejection than full-thickness allogeneic corneas [36]. Moreover, simply covering an epithelium-deprived allogeneic cornea graft (stroma plus endothelium) with an epithelium that was genetically identical to the graft recipient virtually eliminated the aforementioned high risk for rejection when transplanted into low-risk graft beds [36].

Reconstitution of Immune Privilege and Promoting Corneal Allograft Acceptance in High-Risk Eyes

Whereas a significant proportion of orthotopic corneal allografts survive indefinitely when transplanted into normal eyes of mice and rats [37, 38], corneal allografts are inevitably rejected when transplanted into prevascularized, 'high-risk' eyes [39]. Full-thickness allogeneic corneal allografts transplanted into graft beds that have been prevascularized by insertion of sutures, are typically rejected within 14 days by an intense inflammatory and destructive reaction [39]. A similarly poor outcome occurs when corneal transplants are performed in high-risk human eyes [40]. In fact, the failure rate of corneas transplanted into human high-risk eyes is at least as high as the failure rate of other solid tissue grafts in humans (kidney, heart, liver, or islets of Langerhans). Moreover, clinically available immunosuppressive therapy aimed at reversing corneal graft rejection in high-risk eyes is often inadequate [40–42].

The use of murine composite corneal allografts has led to important insights into the relative immunogenicity of individual layers of the corneal allograft. A composite corneal allograft consists of a corneal epithelium that is prepared from the recipient mouse strain and is placed over a stroma and endothelium from an unrelated, allogeneic donor mouse. Such composite corneal allografts experience high acceptance rates, even in high-risk eyes of mice [43]. Recipients of these grafts show no evidence of donor-specific sensitization, implying that graft acceptance might result from immunologic ignorance. The corneal epithelium appears to reduce the immunogenicity of the composite graft, but does not affect its antigenicity. That is, composite corneal grafts do not provoke alloimmune responses in naïve hosts, but are susceptible to immune attack if the hosts have been previously sensitized to the donor's alloantigens [43].

Immune Privilege of Corneal Allografts: Contributions of the Corneal Graft Bed and the Eye

The graft bed and eye contribute to the immune privilege of corneal allografts. Three fundamental factors contribute to the immune privilege of corneal allografts: (a) afferent blockade of the inductive stage of the immune response; (b) deviation of the systemic immune response, and (c) efferent blockade of the efferent arm of the immune response. This privilege has been likened to a three-legged stool in which each of these factors contributes equally to the success of the corneal allograft [4, 44]. Removal or disruption of any of the three components leads to rejection.

Afferent Blockade of the Immune Response

The avascular and alymphatic nature of the corneal graft bed is the time-honored explanation to account for the immune privilege of corneal allografts. Corneal grafts placed into vascularized graft beds are invariably rejected [39]. However, the absence of blood and lymph vessels alone cannot explain the immune privilege of corneal allografts, as some corneal allografts placed into avascular graft beds undergo immune rejection. This occurs when factors in addition to an avascular graft bed prompt immune responses. One such factor comes from the corneal allograft itself. Normally, the cornea has few if any MHC class II+ antigen-presenting cells, such as LCs. However, various stimuli can induce the appearance of MHC class II+ LCs in the corneal epithelium [1, 4, 44].

MHC class II+ LCs express co-stimulatory molecules such as CD80 and are potent inducers of alloimmune responses. In fact, as few as 10 LCs can induce skin allograft rejection [45]. Corneal allografts prepared so as to contain MHC class II+ donor-derived LCs experience a dramatic increase in the incidence and tempo of rejection [46, 47], and depletion of these 'passenger cells' with UV irradiation or hyperbaric oxygen restores immune privilege and results in a dramatic reduction in the incidence of rejection [47]. Thus, the absence of resident, MHC class II+ LCs and the alymphatic and avascular nature of the graft bed conspire to block the afferent arm of the immune response and, thus, prevent the induction of allodestructive immune responses.

Deviation of the Systemic Immune Response to Corneal Allografts

Orthotopic corneal allografts are in direct contact with the AC and the corneal endothelium lines a significant portion of the AC. The juxtaposition of the corneal allograft with the AC is important in determining the fate of the corneal allograft. Antigens introduced into the AC are known to induce a deviant immune response in which delayed-type hypersensitivity and complement-fixing antibody responses are actively suppressed. This phenomenon has been termed AC-associated immune deviation (ACAID) and is closely correlated with the long-term survival of corneal allografts [4]. Mice with long-term corneal allografts demonstrate key features of ACAID [48], and maneuvers that prevent the induction of ACAID result in steep increases in the incidence of corneal allograft rejection [49]. Moreover, AC injection of donor alloantigens prior to corneal transplantation results in a significant reduction in corneal allograft rejection [50, 51].

Efferent Blockade of Immune Response

As mentioned previously, the presence of Fas ligand (FasL) on cellular elements of the corneal allograft serves to shield the graft from immune attack. Activated T cells and neutrophils express Fas receptor and are vulnerable to Fas-induced apoptosis. Corneal allografts prepared from gld/gld mice, which fail to express functional FasL, undergo rejection in 89–100% of the hosts, even if the grafts are placed into avascular graft beds [27, 28]. By contrast, only 50% of the FasL-expressing corneal allografts are rejected in the same donor-host combinations.

The role of alloantibody in corneal graft rejection is unresolved. The weight of evidence points to CD4+ T cell-dependent, cell-mediated immunity as the primary mechanism responsible for corneal allograft rejection [52]. However, there is evidence that alloantibody might, under certain circumstances, contribute to corneal allograft rejection. Passive transfer of alloantibody to T cell-deficient, nude mice results in the development of transient opacity and edema of the orthotopic corneal allografts, but does not culminate in frank graft rejection [53]. In vitro studies have shown that alloantibody produces extensive complement-dependent lysis of allogeneic corneal endothelial cells, but has no deleterious effect on corneal epithelial cells from the same donor strain [53]. The disparity in the resistance of corneal cells to complement-mediated cytolysis is referable to the expression of complement-regulatory proteins, e.g. decay-accelerating factor, on the corneal epithelium and its absence on the corneal endothelium [54, 55]. However, in vivo, the corneal endothelium is bathed in aqueous humor, which contains complement-regulatory proteins and protects against complement-mediated lysis [54, 55]. Thus, the buffering effects of the aqueous humor and the presence to two membrane-associated molecules (FasL and decay-accelerating factor) shield the corneal allograft from the effector elements of the alloimmune response.

Summary and Conclusions

The success of keratoplasty is often attributed to the avascular nature of the graft bed and the putative isolation of the corneal graft from the immune apparatus. Although there is merit in this appealingly simplistic explanation, the fate of corneal allografts is affected by a constellation of factors that conspire to prevent the induction and expression of allodestructive immune responses. Gaining a better understanding of how to enhance and restore immune privilege could have enormous benefit for promoting corneal allograft survival in the high-risk host.

References

1 Niederkorn JY: Immunology and immunomodulation of corneal transplantation. Int Rev Immunol 2002;21:173–196.
2 Aiken-O'Neill P, Mannis MJ: Summary of corneal transplant activity Eye Bank Association of America. Cornea 2002;21:1–3.
3 Zirm E: Eine erfolgreiche totale Keratoplastik. Graefes Arch Ophthalmol 1906;64:580–593.
4 Niederkorn JY: The immune privilege of corneal grafts. J Leukoc Biol 2003;74:167–171.
5 Auchincloss H Jr, Mayer T, Ghobrial R, Winn HJ: T-cell subsets, bm mutants, and the mechanisms of allogeneic skin graft rejection. Immunol Res 1989;8:149–164.
6 Sonoda Y, Streilein JW: Orthotopic corneal transplantation in mice – evidence that the immunogenetic rules of rejection do not apply. Transplantation 1992;54:694–704.
7 Streilein JW: Immune regulation and the eye: a dangerous compromise. FASEB J 1987;1:199–208.
8 Streilein JW: Ocular immune privilege: therapeutic opportunities from an experiment of nature. Nat Rev Immunol 2003;3:879–889.
9 Niederkorn J: Immune privilege of the eye; in Chen LS (ed): Animal Models of Human Inflammatory Skin Diseases. New York, CRC Press, 2004, p 564.
10 Niederkorn JY: Immune privilege in the anterior chamber of the eye. Crit Rev Immunol 2002;22:13–46.
11 Barker CF, Billingham RE: Immunologically privileged sites. Adv Immunol 1977;25:1–54.
12 Medawar PB: Immunity to homologous grafted skin. III. The fate of skin homografts transplanted to the brain, to subcutaneous tissue, and to the anterior chamber of the eye. Br J Exp Pathol 1948;29:58–69.
13 Streilein JW, McCulley J, Niederkorn JY: Heterotopic corneal grafting in mice: a new approach to the study of corneal alloimmunity. Invest Ophthalmol Vis Sci 1982;23:489–500.

14 Streilein JW, Toews GB, Bergstresser PR: Corneal allografts fail to express Ia antigens. Nature 1979;282:326–327.
15 Wang HM, Kaplan HJ, Chan WC, Johnson M: The distribution and ontogeny of MHC antigens in murine ocular tissue. Invest Ophthalmol Vis Sci 1987;28:1383–1389.
16 Whitsett CF, Stulting RD: The distribution of HLA antigens on human corneal tissue. Invest Ophthalmol Vis Sci 1984;25:519–524.
17 Rubsamen PE, McCulley J, Bergstresser PR, Streilein JW: On the Ia immunogenicity of mouse corneal allografts infiltrated with Langerhans cells. Invest Ophthalmol Vis Sci 1984;25:513–518.
18 Tisher CC, Madsen KM: Anatomy of the kidney. Lymphatics; in Brenner BM (ed): Brenner's and Rector's The Kidney. Philadelphia, Saunders, 1996.
19 Dworkin LD, Brenner BM: The renal circulations; in Brenner BM (ed): Brenner's and Rector's The Kidney. Philadelphia, Saunders, 1996.
20 Foglia RP, DiPreta J, Statter MB, Donahoe PK: Fetal allograft survival in immunocompetent recipients is age dependent and organ specific. Ann Surg 1986;204:402–410.
21 McCune JM, Namikawa R, Kaneshima H, Shultz LD, Lieberman M, Weissman IL: The SCID-hu mouse: murine model for the analysis of human hematolymphoid differentiation and function. Science 1988;241:1632–1639.
22 Reece-Smith H, Du Toit DF, McShane P, Morris PJ: Prolonged survival of pancreatic islet allografts transplanted beneath the renal capsule. Transplantation 1981;31:305–306.
23 Bellgrau D, Gold D, Selawry H, Moore J, Franzusoff A, Duke RC: A role for CD95 ligand in preventing graft rejection. Nature 1995;377:630–632.
24 Hori J, Joyce N, Streilein JW: Epithelium-deficient corneal allografts display immune privilege beneath the kidney capsule. Invest Ophthalmol Vis Sci 2000;41:443–452.
25 Hori J, Joyce NC, Streilein JW: Immune privilege and immunogenicity reside among different layers of the mouse cornea. Invest Ophthalmol Vis Sci 2000;41:3032–3042.
26 Khodadoust AA, Silverstein AM: Transplantation and rejection of individual cell layers of the cornea. Invest Ophthalmol 1969;8:180–195.
27 Stuart PM, Griffith TS, Usui N, Pepose J, Yu X, Ferguson TA: CD95 ligand (FasL)-induced apoptosis is necessary for corneal allograft survival. J Clin Invest 1997;99:396–402.
28 Yamagami S, Kawashima H, Tsuru T, Yamagami H, Kayagaki N, Yagita H, Okumura K, Gregerson DS: Role of Fas-Fas ligand interactions in the immunorejection of allogeneic mouse corneal transplants. Transplantation 1997;64:1107–1111.
29 Sano Y, Ksander BR, Streilein JW: Fate of orthotopic corneal allografts in eyes that cannot support anterior chamber-associated immune deviation induction. Invest Ophthalmol Vis Sci 1995;36: 2176–2185.
30 Sano Y, Okamoto S, Streilein JW: Induction of donor-specific ACAID can prolong orthotopic corneal allograft survival in 'high-risk' eyes. Curr Eye Res 1997;16:1171–1174.
31 Sonoda Y, Sano Y, Ksander B, Streilein JW: Characterization of cell-mediated immune responses elicited by orthotopic corneal allografts in mice. Invest Ophthalmol Vis Sci 1995;36:427–434.
32 Sonoda A, Sonoda Y, Muramatu R, Streilein JW, Usui M: ACAID induced by allogeneic corneal tissue promotes subsequent survival of orthotopic corneal grafts. Invest Ophthalmol Vis Sci 2000;41:790–798.
33 Yamada J, Streilein JW: Induction of anterior chamber-associated immune deviation by corneal allografts placed in the anterior chamber. Invest Ophthalmol Vis Sci 1997;38:2833–2843.
34 Treseler PA, Foulks GN, Sanfilippo F: The relative immunogenicity of corneal epithelium, stroma, and endothelium. The role of major histocompatibility complex antigens. Transplantation 1986;41: 229–234.
35 Tuberville AW, Foster CS, Wood TO: The effect of donor cornea epithelium removal on the incidence of allograft rejection reactions. Ophthalmology 1983;90:1351–1356.
36 Hori J, Streilein JW: Role of recipient epithelium in promoting survival of orthotopic corneal allografts in mice. Invest Ophthalmol Vis Sci 2001;42:720–726.
37 She SC, Steahly LP, Moticka EJ: A method for performing full-thickness, orthotopic, penetrating keratoplasty in the mouse. Ophthalmic Surg 1990;21:781–785.
38 Williams KA, Coster DJ: Penetrating corneal transplantation in the inbred rat: a new model. Invest Ophthalmol Vis Sci 1985;26:23–30.

39 Sano Y, Ksander BR, Streilein JW: Murine orthotopic corneal transplantation in high-risk eyes. Rejection is dictated primarily by weak rather than strong alloantigens. Invest Ophthalmol Vis Sci 1997;38:1130–1138.
40 Maguire MG, Stark WJ, Gottsch JD, Stulting RD, Sugar A, Fink NE, Schwartz A: Risk factors for corneal graft failure and rejection in the Collaborative Corneal Transplantation Studies. Collaborative Corneal Transplantation Studies Research Group. Ophthalmology 1994;101: 1536–1547.
41 The Collaborative Corneal Transplantation Studies Research Group: Effectiveness of histocompatibility matching in high-risk corneal transplantation. Arch Ophthalmol 1992;110:1392–1403.
42 Volker-Dieben HJ, Kok-van Alphen CC, Lansbergen Q, Persijn GG: Different influences on corneal graft survival in 539 transplants. Acta Ophthalmol (Copenh) 1982;60:190–202.
43 Hori J, Streilein JW: Survival in high-risk eyes of epithelium-deprived orthotopic corneal allografts reconstituted in vitro with syngeneic epithelium. Invest Ophthalmol Vis Sci 2003;44:658–664.
44 Niederkorn JY: The immune privilege of corneal allografts. Transplantation 1999;67:1503–1508.
45 McKinney EC, Streilein JW: On the extraordinary capacity of allogeneic epidermal Langerhans cells to prime cytotoxic T cells in vivo. J Immunol 1989;143:1560–1564.
46 Callanan D, Peeler J, Niederkorn JY: Characteristics of rejection of orthotopic corneal allografts in the rat. Transplantation 1988;45:437–443.
47 He YG, Niederkorn JY: Depletion of donor-derived Langerhans cells promotes corneal allograft survival. Cornea 1996;15:82–89.
48 Sonoda Y, Streilein JW: Impaired cell-mediated immunity in mice bearing healthy orthotopic corneal allografts. J Immunol 1993;150:1727–1734.
49 Skelsey ME, Mellon J, Niederkorn JY: $\gamma\delta$ T cells are needed for ocular immune privilege and corneal graft survival. J Immunol 2001;166:4327–4333.
50 Niederkorn JY, Mellon J: Anterior chamber-associated immune deviation promotes corneal allograft survival. Invest Ophthalmol Vis Sci 1996;37:2700–2707.
51 She SC, Steahly LP, Moticka EJ: Intracameral injection of allogeneic lymphocytes enhances corneal graft survival. Invest Ophthalmol Vis Sci 1990;31:1950–1956.
52 Niederkorn JY: The immunology of corneal transplantation. Dev Ophthalmol 1999;30:129–140.
53 Hegde S, Mellon JK, Hargrave SL, Niederkorn JY: Effect of alloantibodies on corneal allograft survival. Invest Ophthalmol Vis Sci 2002;43:1012–1018.
54 Bora NS, Gobleman CL, Atkinson JP, Pepose JS, Kaplan HJ: Differential expression of the complement regulatory proteins in the human eye. Invest Ophthalmol Vis Sci 1993;34:3579–3584.
55 Lass JH, Walter EI, Burris TE, Grossniklaus HE, Roat MI, Skelnik DL, Needham L, Singer M, Medof ME: Expression of two molecular forms of the complement decay-accelerating factor in the eye and lacrimal gland. Invest Ophthalmol Vis Sci 1990;31:1136–1148.

Dr. Junko Hori
Department of Ophthalmology
Nippon Medical School
1-5-1, Sendagi, Bunkyo, Tokyo, 113–8602 (Japan)
Tel. +81 3 3822 2131, Fax +81 3 5685 0988, E-Mail jhori-tky@umin.ac.jp

Niederkorn JY, Kaplan HJ (eds): Immune Response and the Eye.
Chem Immunol Allergy. Basel, Karger, 2007, vol 92, pp 300–316

Retinal Transplantation

Tat Fong Ng[a], Henry J. Klassen[a,b], Junko Hori[c], Michael J. Young[a]

Departments of Ophthalmology, [a]Schepens Eye Research Institute, Harvard Medical School, Boston, Mass., [b]University of California, Irvine, Calif., USA; [c]Nippon Medical School, Tokyo, Japan

Abstract

Degenerative diseases of the retina afflict millions of Americans, and very few effective treatments are available at present. Transplantation of solid tissue or stem cell grafts represents a promising, albeit challenging, approach to replace photoreceptor cells lost due to injury or disease. However, there remain a number of formidable obstacles to be overcome before these techniques can be applied in a clinical setting. Foremost of these challenges is immunological acceptance and survival of the graft. We will refer to studies performed in collaboration with J. Wayne Streilein over the past decade that address this issue. The immune-privileged status of the subretinal space, as well as the inherent immune privilege of retinal pigment epithelium, neuronal retina and neural stem cells will be described. The goal of these studies is to gain a better understanding of the immunological properties of both the donor tissues and recipient graft site in retinal transplantation. This information will allow for the development of strategies to improve graft outcome and lead to successful repair of the diseased eye.

There have been many attempts in the last 2 decades to graft neural tissues in an effort to treat central nervous system (CNS) diseases, including retinal degenerations. Relatively little success has been reported from these experiments, and poor graft survival has been a significant barrier to functional restoration of damaged CNS structures. This has prompted a reevaluation of two important questions: (1) does immune privilege actually exist within the brain and the retina, and (2) are brain and retinal tissues 'immune privileged'? Immunologic studies of the brain and the eye during the past 20 years have reaffirmed the existence of immune privilege within the brain [1], and within the posterior segment of the eye, including both the vitreous cavity [2] and the subretinal space [3]. However, the question of the immune-privileged status of brain and retinal tissue remained unanswered. Virtually all studies have placed these neuroectodermally derived tissues into immune-privileged sites. It is not possible to test the extent to which a particular cell or tissue is immune privileged if such grafts are placed into sites that are themselves immune privileged. Instead, assessment of graft immune privilege requires that the cells or tissue be transplanted to a non-privileged site where its vulnerability to immune rejection is not limited by the site.

Transplantation of Retinal Tissue and Retinal Pigment Epithelium to the Eye

In the early 90s, Jiang and Streilein [4–6] began work on the immunobiology of retinal and retinal pigment epithelium (RPE) transplants, and elucidated the importance of immune privilege in the success of these transplants. In this series of experiments, C57BL/6 (H-2K^b) donor tissue was grafted to BALB/c (H-2K^d) recipients. Implantation of either retinal fragments [4, 5] or RPE [6] in the subconjunctiva resulted in a strong immune response in the recipient mice. Delayed hypersensitivity (DTH) was assessed and the response was found to be directed against both alloantigens and retinal autoantigens. When neuronal retina was placed in the subretinal space, the graft thrived and survived for more than 12 days [2]. DTH to alloantigens was impaired in these recipients. Furthermore, this donor antigen-specific suppression could be adoptively transferred to naïve mice using spleen cells from the recipient mice.

These data demonstrated that the subretinal space is an immune-privileged site. However, the neuronal retina itself may possess inherent immune privilege. Wenkel and Streilein [7] transplanted P815 tumor cells (DBA/2 background) into the anterior chamber or subretinal space of BALB/c mice. Grafts placed in the subretinal space were rejected, but when placed into the anterior chamber these tumor cells grew progressively until day 14, and the recipients exhibited donor-specific immune deviation and concomitant immunity. These data demonstrated that the immune properties of the subretinal space are different from the anterior chamber.

Other studies have supported the notion that although the subretinal space is an immune-privileged site, its immune-privileged status is not absolute. Gregerson and Dou [8] used transgenic mice expressing β-galactosidase under control of the arrestin promoter to demonstrate that immune deviation to β-galactosidase occurred spontaneously in these mice. Microglia are one candidate cell type that might serve as antigen-presenting cells (APCs) responsible for this altered immune response. Ng and Streilein [9] demonstrated that exposure to high light levels caused microglial migration to the subretinal space.

Groups of albino BALB/c mice were exposed to different light levels for 2 weeks. Whole-mounted retinas or cryosections of the eye were immunostained with 5D4, a marker for resting microglia. Subretinal microglia in mice exposed to the highest light levels (500 lux) were round in shape with short processes (fig. 1a), but subretinal microglia in mice exposed to low light levels (100 lux) were ramified with long processes (fig. 1b). Electron-microscopic images demonstrated that mice exposed to bright light had subretinal microglia that contained photoreceptor outer segments in their cytoplasm (fig. 1c, d).

We wondered if the presence of a high density of subretinal microglia has a detrimental effect on the survival of allogeneic retinal grafts. Albino mice were again exposed to different light levels for 2 weeks, 'pre-conditioning' the subretinal space with 3 different densities of microglia [10]. Neonatal neuronal retina (NNR) from C57BL/6 mice served as the source of donor tissue. Recipients were kept in the same light conditions and were sacrificed on days 14, 35 and 56. The retinal grafts were examined, and their condition was scored and compared (table 1). The survival of the retinal allografts was best in dim light conditions, with 100% of the grafts surviving at least 56 days. Most of the retinal allografts in bright light conditions had a disorganized structure and were rejected by day 35. DTH specific to donor alloantigens was positive in recipients in bright light but not dim light conditions.

Previous work [11] showed that microglia derived from the brain could serve as potent APCs that prime naïve T cells. However, Gregerson and Yang [12] collected fresh, adult retinal microglia and demonstrated that the retinal microglia were neither efficient in priming naïve T cells, nor responsive to treatment with interferon (IFN)-γ, anti-CD40 and lipopolysaccharides. This suggests that retinal microglia possess different immune properties from brain microglia. Although we demonstrated that some subretinal microglia migrated from the inner retinal layers [9], we could not exclude the possibility that some cells identified as subretinal microglia were actually perivascular, or infiltrating macrophages. The greater rejection rate for retinal allografts in the subretinal space in the presence of a high density of microglia suggested that subretinal microglia are different from resident retinal microglia. Nevertheless, these results demonstrated that the presence of microglia could influence the survival of retinal allografts.

Immune-Privileged Status of Potential Donor Tissues

In addition to the phenomenon of site-specific immune privilege, as seen with transplantation to the eye, brain and testis [13–15], there is another form of immune privilege that pertains specifically to transplanted cells or tissues.

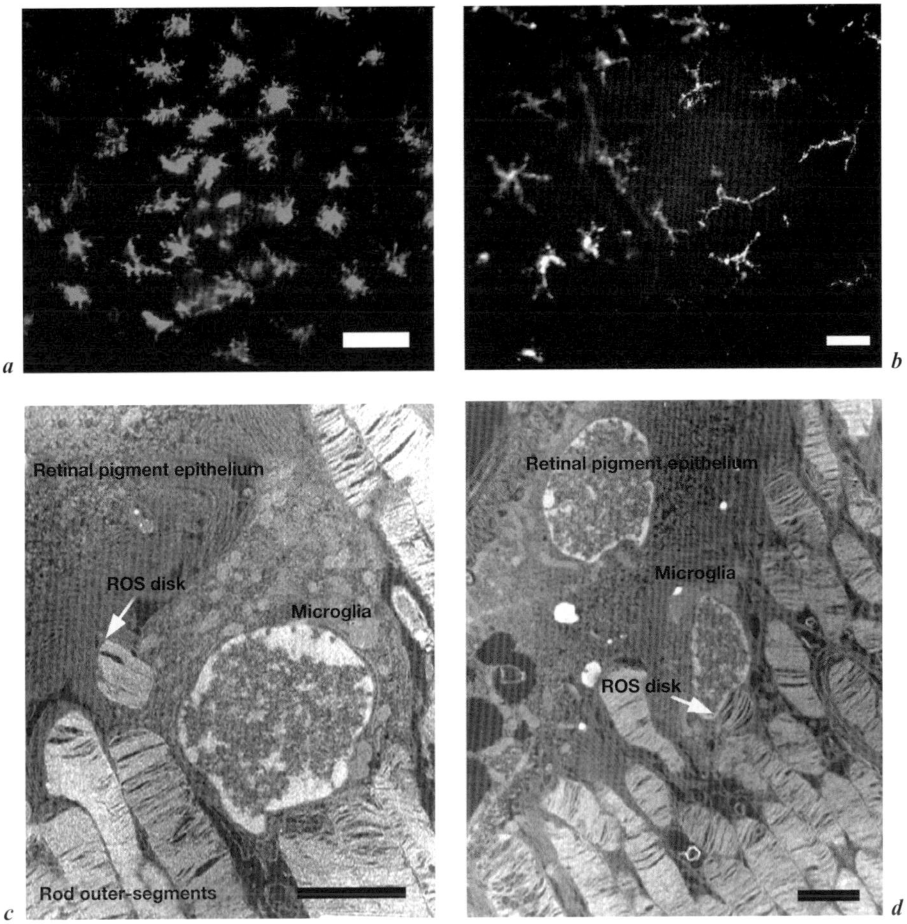

Fig. 1. Evidence that subretinal 5D4-positive cells are phagocytic. Eyes were enucleated from adult BALB/c mice that had been exposed to bright light (500 lux, continuous) for 2 weeks. ***a*** Light-microscopic image of 5D4-positive cells in the subretinal space: the cells have large, round cell bodies and short, stubby dendrites. ***b*** Light-microscopic image of 5D4-positive cells in the subretinal space of a BALB/c mouse placed in complete darkness for 2 weeks following a 2-week exposure to *bright* light: 5D4-positive cells have slender cell bodies and extensively ramified dendrites. ***c*** Electron-micrographic image of outer RPE layers: a microglia is present between photoreceptor cells and its cytoplasm contains phagocytized rod outer-segment (ROS) disks. ***d*** Electron-micrographic image of microglia with extensive profile of phagocytized rod outer-segment (ROS) disks: the cell is adjacent to an RPE cell. Scale bars: ***a***, ***b*** 3 μm. ***c***, ***d*** 20 μm. Reprinted in modified form with permission from Ng and Streilein [9].

Table 1. Influence of light conditions on graft survival

Conditions	Graft type	Score	Survival, %
Bright light	allogeneic B6	1+	33
Conventional light	allogeneic B6	4+	83
Dim light	allogeneic B6	5+	100
Bright light	syngeneic BALB/c	5+	100

Arbitrary scoring system reflecting the portion of the graft occupied by rosettes (0%: no graft identifiable): 5+ = >85%; 4+ = 70–85%; 1+ = <25%.

This cell- or tissue-specific immune privilege allows donor material to survive transplantation to an allogeneic host, even if the graft site does not exhibit characteristics of immune privilege. Therefore, in situations where donor cells survive transplantation to an allogeneic host either type of immune privilege, or both, could be involved. Survival of allogeneic cells in an immune-privileged site, as seen with brain-derived stem cells transplanted into the retina [16, 17], can be explained by the immunological properties of the recipient site alone, and therefore, does not address the question of whether the cells exhibit cell-specific immune privilege themselves.

Retinal Pigment Epithelium

RPE cells have an important role in maintaining immune privilege in the eye. The RPE has been shown to produce CD95 ligand, a gene product that can induce T cell apoptosis [18]. Furthermore, RPE secrete transforming growth factor-β, an important factor for the induction of tolerance, as well as its activator, thrombospondin. Finally, the RPE has been shown to suppress T cell proliferation induced by phytohemagglutinin [19], inhibit intraphotoreceptor retinoid binding protein-specific T cell activation [20], and even phagocytose T cells [21].

Wenkel and Streilein [22] investigated whether RPE is an immune-privileged tissue using transplantation to the kidney capsule. Neonatal RPE sheets from wild-type (C57BL/6) and gld/gld (CD95 ligand-deficient) mice were compared. Both were transplanted to the subcapsular space of the kidney and examined 1, 2 and 12 weeks after grafting. gld/gld RPE sheets did not survive and were rejected at 2 weeks. Interestingly, wild-type RPE sheets sensitized the recipients with a positive DTH, but the RPE grafts remained intact throughout the time course. This result is very different from previous data by Jiang and Streilein [4–6] who injected RPE suspensions into the subconjunctival space

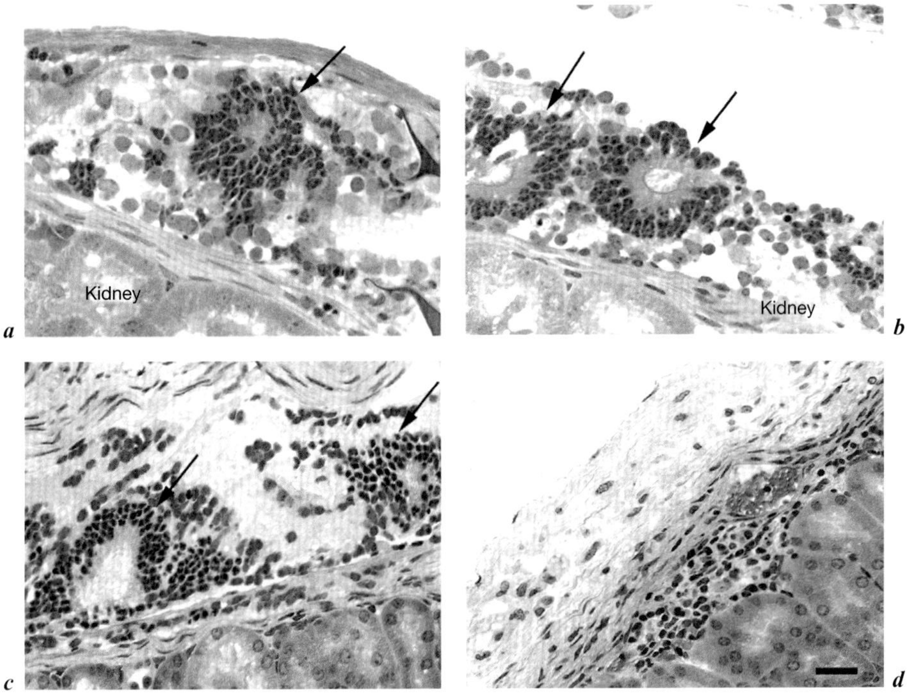

Fig. 2. Histologic appearance of BALB/c and C57BL/6 NNR grafts in the kidney subcapsular space. Syngeneic BALB/c (***a***, ***c***) and allogeneic C57BL/6 (***b***, ***d***) NNR grafts 12 (***a***, ***b***) and 20 days (***c***, ***d***) after implantation. Arrows: rosettes. Scale bar: 25 μm. Reprinted with permission from Ng et al. [23].

where the RPE suspension did not survive. This suggests that the tight junctions present in the RPE sheet are important for maintaining their immune privilege.

Neuronal Retina

To study the immune-privileged status of the neuronal retina, this tissue was transplanted to the kidney capsule [23]. The laminar integrity of both syngeneic and allogeneic adult neuronal retina was lost within 24 h, with the graft slowly degenerating thereafter even in the absence of an obvious immune response. However, neonatal neuronal retina (NNR) survived under the kidney capsule and differentiated into a structure resembling native retina. In the case of syngeneic NNRs, well-formed rosettes formed by photoreceptors were first observed on day 7, and these structure remained intact until day 20 (fig. 2a, c).

Allogeneic NNRs also survived and rosettes were found in the grafts up to day 14, but the graft became disorganized by day 20 (fig. 2b, d).

Microglia were found in the central lumen as previously reported [24]. Interestingly, DTH was impaired on day 14. Adoptive transfer of the lymphoid cells to naïve mice suppressed donor-specific DTH. However, DTH to alloantigens emerged on day 20. We concluded that NNRs do not possess absolute immune privilege as seen with neonatal RPE, but do display partial immune privilege.

The Immunological Properties of CNS Stem Cells

In the past decade a new cell type, known as a 'neural stem cell' or 'neural progenitor cell' has been isolated from various regions of the adult and embryonic CNS of mice, rats and humans, among other species [25]. These cells are multipotent, i.e. they can give rise to the three cell lineages of the CNS: neurons, astrocytes, and oligodendrocytes. Moreover, neural stem cells are self-renewing, i.e. they divide to give rise to at least one daughter cell that maintains 'stemness'. The plasticity of neural stem cells has generated interest as to whether these cells can be used to replace cells in the CNS. Studies in animal models have shown that neural stem cells can replace populations of diseased or damaged cells, in some cases leading to behavioral recovery [26]. The fact that these cells can be grown in large numbers ex vivo represents another advantage over conventional solid tissue grafts, especially in a clinical setting.

Neural stem cells derived from the rat hippocampus were able to integrate into degenerating retinas of both rd mice and Royal College of Surgeons rats [17]. No evidence of immune rejection was found in these experiments, raising questions concerning the immunogenicity of neural stem or progenitor cells. Might neural stem cells function as an immune-privileged tissue?

In order to illuminate this question we implanted syngeneic [transgenic green fluorescent protein (GFP)-negative C57BL/6 to C57BL/6] and allogeneic (transgenic GFP-negative C57BL/6 to BALB/c) neural stem cells beneath the kidney capsule of adult mice [14]. The implants were evaluated for survival by clinical inspection and immunohistochemical analysis. The ability of allogeneic neural stem cells to sensitize recipients when implanted beneath the kidney capsule was assessed. We also evaluated the vulnerability of implanted cells to rejection following specific sensitization of the recipient to transplantation antigens of the graft donor. Our results indicate that neural stem cells possess inherent immune privilege, suggesting that allografts have utility in the setting of CNS repair.

Survival of Neural Stem Cells Placed beneath the Kidney Capsule

Grafts in allogeneic recipients were indistinguishable from those in syngeneic recipients at all observation points. I-A^b and H-2K^b were not expressed in vitro, nor in the grafted cells placed beneath either allogeneic or syngeneic kidney capsules. No evidence of rejection or necrosis of neural stem cell grafts was seen over the course of this study, in contrast to control grafts of freshly isolated neonatal cerebellum. Irrespective of whether CNS stem cells were placed beneath the kidney capsule of syngeneic or allogeneic recipients, no evidence of major histocompatibility complex (MHC) class I expression was detected over the course of this study. Control grafts of neonatal cerebellum, however, showed clear staining for H-2K^b-positive cells 14 days after grafting. Importantly, we found no evidence, by morphology or by CD45+ staining, for the presence of 'bone marrow-derived' cell lineages within stem cell grafts.

Donor-Specific Delayed Hypersensitivity

We then examined whether allogeneic neural stem cell grafts could sensitize recipients harboring these grafts beneath the kidney capsule by assaying for donor-specific DTH. The data of a representative experiment are presented in figure 3a. Allogeneic neural stem cells grafted beneath the kidney capsule failed to induce DTH, in marked contrast to allogeneic spleen cells.

To determine whether the failure of induction of allospecific DTH was due to active suppression of DTH or to a failure of allosensitization, we examined the left ear pinna of the same set of mice that had been subjected to the DTH assay by rechallenging with irradiated C57BL/6 spleen cells. The results presented in figure 3b indicate the induction of DTH in mice receiving neural stem cell allografts. Thus, allogeneic neural stem cell grafts placed beneath the kidney capsule neither sensitized their recipients for DTH, nor rendered these mice incapable of becoming sensitized to donor alloantigens.

Presentation of Alloantigens to Primed T Cells

We next determined whether neural stem cells are capable of expressing alloantigens. As revealed in figure 3c, mice presensitized to C57BL/6 alloantigens on neural stem cells developed significant ear swelling responses compared to negative controls. This indicates that neural stem cells display histocompatibility antigens in a manner that permits presensitized T cells to recognize and respond to the cells.

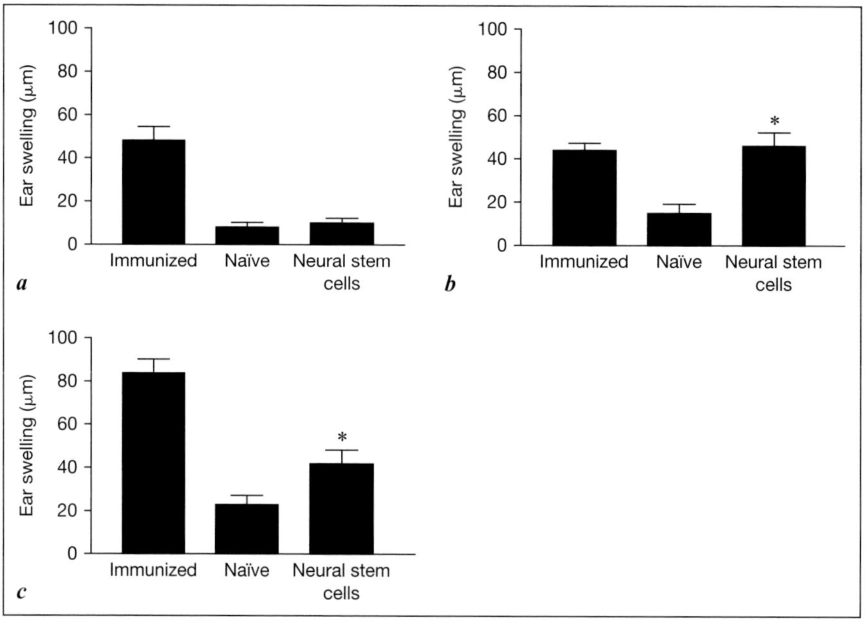

Fig. 3. Donor-specific DTH following CNS stem cell grafts. ***a*** Lack of induction of donor-specific DTH. We evaluated the induction of DTH following implantation of CNS stem cell allografts beneath the kidney capsule of BALB/c mice at 25 days. Positive immunization controls (Immunized) received subcutaneous injection of 10×10^6 donor spleen cells 1 week prior to assay. Right ear pinna received injection of irradiated C57BL/6 spleen cells (1×10^6) and ear swelling responses were assessed 24 and 48 h later. Negative control (naïve) received ear pinna challenge only. Mean 24-hour ear swelling responses are compared with negative controls. ***b*** Lack of active suppression of donor-specific DTH. Donor-specific DTH 24 h after initial ear challenge following implantation of neural stem cell allografts beneath the kidney capsule of allogeneic BALB/c mice. Left ear of the recipient mice received injection of irradiated C57BL/6 spleen cells (1×10^6), and ear swelling responses were assessed 24 and 48 h later. Positive (Immunized) and negative (Naïve) controls are similar to those described in the legend to ***a***. Mean ear swelling responses are compared with negative controls. $^*p < 0.001$ vs. negative control. ***c*** Neural stem cells present alloantigens to primed T cells. Elicitation of donor-specific DTH in BALB/c mice by injection of C57BL/6 neural stem cells following recipient presensitization with C57BL/6 spleen cells. Both test mice and positive controls first received subcutaneous immunization with 10×10^6 C57BL/6 spleen cells. One week later, positive (Immunized) and negative (Naïve) control mice received ear pinna challenge with 10 μl of irradiated C57BL/6 spleen cells (1×10^6), whereas test mice received ear pinna challenge with irradiated neural stem cells (10 μl of 1×10^6). Ear swelling responses were measured at 24 and 48 h. Mean ear swelling responses (+SEM) at 24 h are presented. $^*p < 0.01$ vs. negative control. Reprinted in modified form with permission from Hori et al. [35].

Survival of Neural Stem Cells before and after Sensitization in Mice

Finally, we determined whether neural stem cells could serve as a target of alloimmune rejection. The BALB/c mice with enhanced GFP (EGFP)-positive neural stem cells beneath the kidney capsule that had been challenged with C57BL/6 spleen cells were sacrificed, and the fate of the grafts observed by confocal microscopy. Results revealed that none of the recipient kidneys contained EGFP-positive cells. Instead, CD45+ cells accumulated at the graft site in all samples indicating that EGFP-positive neural stem cells had been eliminated after ear challenge with C57BL/6 spleen cells. To determine the capacity of neural stem cells to be a target of alloimmune rejection, allogeneic neural stem cells were placed beneath the kidney capsule of presensitized mice. Thirteen days after grafting, the kidneys were inspected clinically, then removed and examined by confocal microscopy. Both clinical inspection and confocal microscopy showed no EGFP-positive cells in any samples, but instead revealed an accumulation of CD45+ cells at the graft site. Thus, allogeneic neural stem cells, incapable of sensitizing recipients, are nonetheless vulnerable to rejection in specifically sensitized recipients regardless of whether sensitization preceded engraftment or took place after the graft had become established at its heterotopic site.

Stem cells harvested from the CNS of EGFP transgenic mice display the properties of immune-privileged tissues. When implanted at a non-immune privileged site, such as beneath the kidney capsule, both syngeneic and allogeneic CNS stem cells established residence and carried out a recognizable version of their development program by differentiating into cells with neural and glial phenotypes. Since allogeneic CNS stem cells formed stable grafts that continued to thrive for at least 4 weeks, and since allogeneic neonatal cerebellar grafts had been destroyed at this time, CNS stem cells displayed the properties of an immune-privileged tissue. Thus, allogeneic CNS stem cell grafts proved incapable of sensitizing their recipients, and therefore, lack the property of alloimmunogenicity but retain the property of alloantigenicity.

The finding that allogeneic CNS stem cells were unable to survive in recipients sensitized systemically to donor alloantigens deserves special comment. The terms 'immunogenic' and 'antigenic', when applied to tissue transplants, indicate (a) the ability of an allograft to sensitize its recipient and (b) the vulnerability of the graft to specific immune effectors of rejection, respectively. Allogeneic skin grafts placed beneath the kidney capsule display both immunogenicity and antigenicity. By contrast, our results indicate that similarly implanted allogeneic CNS stem cells lack immunogenicity but retain antigenicity.

In this study, we found no direct evidence for the expression of MHC antigens by the mouse neural stem cells, or their differentiated progeny, except when such expression was induced in vitro using IFN-γ. These data are consistent with our transplantation results showing grafted CNS stem cells to be non-immunogenic when transplanted to a conventional site. Alternatively, the rapid and complete rejection of CNS stem cells from beneath the kidney capsule following peripheral immunization with allogeneic spleen cells from identical donors indicates that the donor neural stem cells exhibited non-immunogenic antigenicity. The antigens initiating this rejection remain to be elucidated. One possibility is that MHC class I antigens were expressed at levels below the threshold of detection by either immunocytochemistry or flow cytometry [27]. Alternatively, minor transplantation antigens may be the target of the rejection response. Thus, the lack of immunogenicity we found in CNS stem cell allografts beneath the kidney capsule is no guarantee of universal acceptance of these grafts under any circumstance. Our evidence indicates that exposure to pro-inflammatory cytokines or the preexistence of donor-specific immunity within the recipient can render the graft vulnerable to rejection.

Together with the virtual absence of MHC alloantigens on CNS stem cells, the lack of immunogenicity of these grafts is understandable. It is relevant that allogeneic neonatal cerebellar grafts, which do contain passenger cells in the form of microglia, suffered a different fate from allogeneic CNS stem cell grafts. Previously, evidence has been presented that microglia within NNR grafts display properties similar to passenger leukocytes [24]. We suspect that microglia within the neonatal cerebellar grafts placed beneath the kidney capsule alerted the recipient's immune system to the graft, thereby initiating its eventual rejection.

Recent evidence that human embryonic stem [28] and germ [29] cells possess the intrinsic developmental capacity of pluripotent stem cells has generated considerable interest in the burgeoning field of regenerative medicine. Results from stem and progenitor cell transplantation experiments, in a variety of paradigms, suggest to us that it is worth revisiting the historical concepts of plasticity, fate commitment and lineage determination [30–32].

After more than a decade of human neural transplantation studies [33–35], our knowledge of the basic immunological properties of conventional embryonic and fetal donor tissue remains inadequate. In most cases, immunological concerns are not specifically addressed, with immunosuppressive drugs being applied to elderly patients suffering from neurodegenerative diseases, undergoing highly invasive neurosurgical procedures. The results we present here demonstrate that neuronal stem cells are a non-immunogenic immune-privileged tissue, and that they can be grafted into allogeneic recipients without the need to impose potentially toxic immunosuppressive regimens. These results are encouraging with respect to the ultimate immunological success of neural stem cell transplantation.

MHC and Fas Expression by Mammalian CNS Stem Cells

The mechanisms underlying the properties of cell-specific immune privilege exhibited by CNS stem cells have not been thoroughly examined and could, in principle, be quite complex. As an initial examination of this issue, we looked at the expression of immune-related surface molecules and immunomodulatory cytokines by these cells, both from the brain and the retina. In the course of these studies, we have examined CNS stem cells from a number of mammalian species, including mouse, rat, and human. These results are consistent with our previous work, both in vitro [36] and in vivo [37], and shed light on the molecular mechanisms by which brain- and retina-derived stem cells evade immune rejection, as we will now describe.

The molecules of the MHC represent surface antigens of particular interest in the setting of allogeneic transplantation. We used flow cytometry to evaluate the expression of MHC class I and class II molecules by CNS stem cells cultured from the brain and retina of various mammalian species. Results from these studies will be itemized by species and then summarized for potential significance between cell types and across species.

In the mouse (C57B6), CNS stem cells did not express any detectible MHC antigens under baseline culture conditions, including MHC class I (both heavy chain and β_2-microglobulin components) and MHC class II. This was the case for both brain-derived [38] and retina-derived (fig. 4) stem cells. In the rat, brain-derived stem cells (adult hippocampal) expressed low levels of MHC class I (including β_2-microglobulin), but did not express MHC class II molecules [36]. In the human, brain-derived stem cells strongly expressed MHC class I (including β_2-microglobulin), but did not express detectible MHC class II [38, 39]. Likewise, human retinal stem cells exhibited the same pattern as the brain-derived cells, with prominent expression of MHC class I but no class II expression that could be detected by flow cytometry [40].

Based on these data, we noted a number of trends worth pointing out since they can be used to generate testable hypotheses for future experiments. First of all, for a given species, both brain- and retina-derived stem cells appear to express a very similar MHC profile and certainly cannot be distinguished from each other on this basis. This was the case for both mouse and human cells, even though the results from these two species differed when compared directly to each other. It would be of interest to extend this result to additional mammalian species, including the rat, from which retinal stem cells have also been cultured [41, 42]. Interestingly, both sources for these cells, namely the brain and retina, exhibit evidence of being immune-privileged sites [1, 2].

Another trend evident across species was the absence of detectible MHC class II expression. This finding was consistent for mice, rats, and humans and

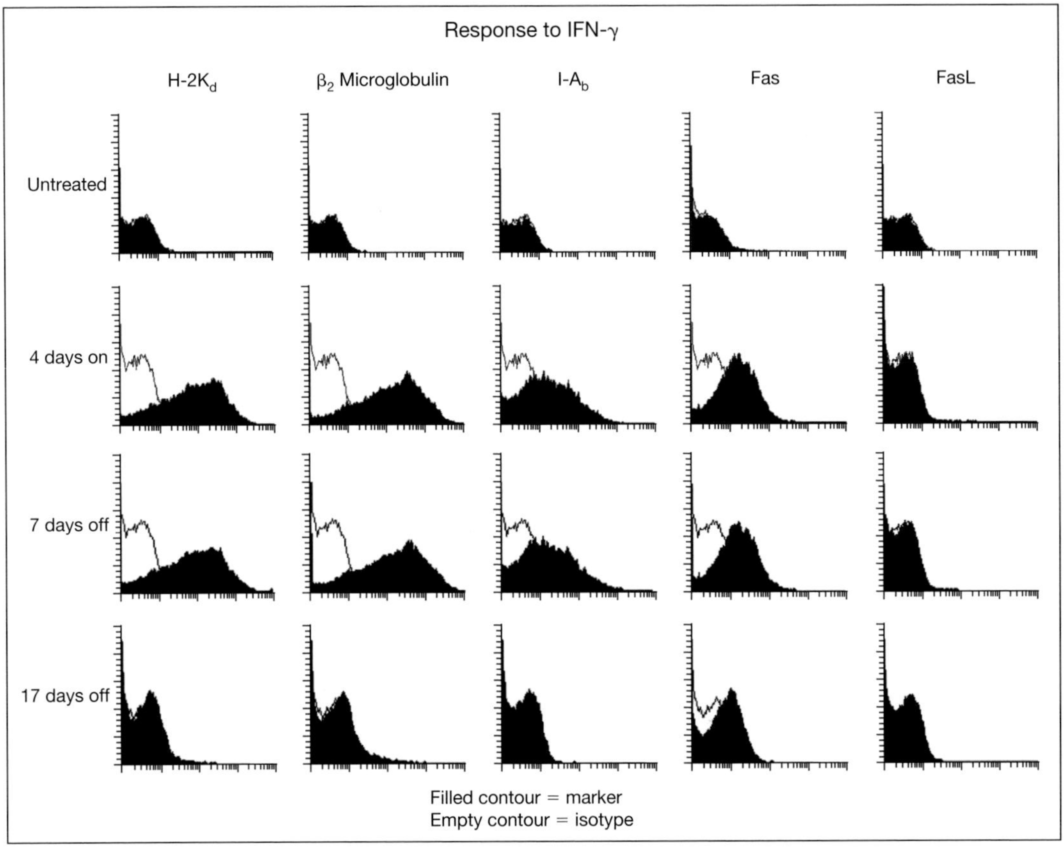

Fig. 4. Induction of MHC expression by treatment of retinal stem cells with IFN-γ. Under baseline culture conditions, retinal stem cells from GFP-negative transgenic mice do not express the MHC antigens H-2K^d (MHC class I heavy chain), β_2-microglobulin, or I-A^b (MHC class II), nor do they express Fas or Fas ligand (FasL) (top row). After 4 days of treatment with the pro-inflammatory cytokine IFN, class I and class II MHC antigens were induced, as was Fas, but not Fas ligand (second row). After termination of IFN-γ treatment, expression levels were sustained for 7 days (third row) but eventually returned to baseline (bottom row).

is of considerable importance in the setting of transplant immunology. Indeed, the classical rejection response involves the nonspecific recognition of foreign MHC class II molecules by CD4+ lymphocytes of the host. The absence of MHC class II molecules would therefore protect grafted stem cells from this important mechanism of graft rejection. Thus CNS stem cells differ from solid tissue grafts of either the brain or retina, which contain MHC class II-expressing cell types such as microglia, macrophages, and endothelium that increase the likelihood of classical immune rejection.

Finally, yet another trend we saw involved marked differences in MHC class I expression across species. Based on data from mice, rats, and humans, this trend appeared to show increasing expression of class I between species that was consistent with relative phylogenetic complexity. In this way, mouse CNS stem cells expressed the least class I (i.e. none), human stem cells the most, with rat stem cells intermediate. Again, it would be very useful to explore this trend across additional mammalian species. We have recently cultured CNS stem cells for the pig [43], and data from these cells, among others, would be helpful in looking for further evidence of a phylogenetic relationship for MHC class I expression by CNS stem cells. If confirmed as a general phenomenon, it would be of great interest to know whether this trend relates to increasing immunological complexity or, perhaps, reflects a role for traditional immunological molecules in neural development, as has been proposed by Huh et al. [27].

Interestingly, expression of Fas (CD95), a non-MHC molecule known to play a role in lymphocyte selection, showed a profile across species very similar to MHC class I. Fas was not expressed by the mouse CNS stem cells [38], lightly expressed by rat brain stem cells [36] and strongly expressed by human CNS stem cells [38, 40]. Fas is termed a 'death receptor' and is known to play a role in triggering apoptosis following binding of Fas ligand. Why Fas would be strongly expressed by human but not murine CNS stem cells from both the brain and retina remains unclear at this point, as is the reason for the apparent relationship of Fas and MHC I expression across species.

Changes in Immune Marker Expression in Response to IFN-γ

The baseline expression of MHC molecules by cultured mammalian CNS stem cells can be altered by stimulation with extrinsic cytokines. Consistent with results from other cell types, we have shown that these cells respond to species-specific IFN-γ by upregulating MHC. As described above, mouse brain-derived stem cells do not express detectable MHC expression under baseline conditions in culture. Three days after addition of murine recombinant IFN-γ, the cells expressed high levels of MHC class I, including β_2-microglobulin, as well as MHC class II. Cessation of IFN-γ exposure resulted in diminution of MHC expression, returning to undetectable levels (consistent with baseline) 11 days later.

We have obtained analogous results for retinal stem cells from the mouse (fig. 4). Again, MHC levels went from undetectable at baseline to strong expression of class I and moderate expression of class II within 4 days of IFN-γ treatment, together with induction of moderate expression of Fas. Cessation of IFN stimulation once again resulted in an eventual return to baseline for all of these markers by 17 days. In contrast, Fas ligand remained undetectable throughout.

Data from rat brain-derived stem cells also show dynamic upregulation of MHC class I in response to rat recombinant IFN-γ [38]. In addition, we obtained similar results with human brain-derived stem cells [Klassen et al., unpublished data]. Although class II levels are high at baseline in the human cells, levels increased even higher after 4-day exposure to human recombinant IFN-γ. MHC class II was also expressed at this time, as was the adhesion marker intercellular adhesion molecule (CD54), the latter result being consistent with the behavioral changes (increased flattening of cells and increased adhesion to substrate) seen in culture during this time.

These findings show that MHC gene expression by CNS stem cells is quite responsive to IFN-γ modulation, regardless of species, site of origin or baseline expression levels. While these cells appear to exhibit a high degree of immune privilege as a cell type, it must be borne in mind that this status could be altered by the microenvironment into which the cells are grafted. In the presence of an active inflammatory response, the immunological status of the stem cells could be altered. Induction of MHC class II by IFN-γ from the host could markedly increase the vulnerability of allogeneic stem cells to classical immune rejection.

Conclusion

The studies we have described lead to several conclusions. Firstly, the subretinal space possesses immune privilege, although the nature of this status differs somewhat from what has been described for the anterior chamber. It is also subject to modulation by the presence of microglial cells that migrate to this location following injury. Second, the cell types presently being employed for donor tissue in retinal transplantation all possess, to some degree, inherent immune privilege. This is true for RPE cells, neuronal retinal and stem cells derived from the CNS. There are a number of variables, such as graft organization or exposure to light damage or pro-inflammatory cytokines that can profoundly impact the immunogenicity of the graft. One must remain mindful of these conditions when designing experimental studies or when contemplating clinical translation of retinal transplantation.

References

1 Wenkel H, Streilein JW, Young MJ: Systemic immune deviation in the brain that does not depend on the integrity of the blood-brain barrier. J Immunol 2000;164:5125–5131.

2 Jiang LQ, Jorquera M, Streilein JW: Subretinal space and vitreous cavity as immunologically privileged sites for retinal allografts. Invest Ophthalmol Vis Sci 1993;34:3347–3354.

3 Wenkel H, Chen PW, Ksander BR, Streilein JW: Immune privilege is extended, then withdrawn, from allogeneic tumor cell grafts placed in the subretinal space. Invest Ophthalmol Vis Sci 1999;40:3202–3208.

4 Jiang LQ, Streilein JW: Immunity and immune privilege elicited by autoantigens expressed on syngeneic neonatal neural retina grafts. Curr Eye Res 1992;11:697–709.
5 Jiang LQ, Streilein JW: Immune responses elicited by transplantation and tissue-restricted antigens expressed on retinal tissues implanted subconjunctivally. Transplantation 1991;52:513–519.
6 Jiang LQ, Jorquera M, Streilein JW: Immunologic consequences of intraocular implantation of retinal pigment epithelial allografts. Exp Eye Res 1994;58:719–728.
7 Wenkel H, Streilein JW: Analysis of immune deviation elicited by antigens injected into the subretinal space. Invest Ophthalmol Vis Sci 1998;39:1823–1834.
8 Gregerson DS, Dou C: Spontaneous induction of immunoregulation by an endogenous retinal antigen. Invest Ophthalmol Vis Sci 2002;43:2984–2991.
9 Ng TF, Streilein JW: Light-induced migration of retinal microglia into the subretinal space. Invest Ophthalmol Vis Sci 2001;42:3301–3310.
10 Ng TF, Cho KS, Osawa H, Streilein JW: Bright light, by recruiting microglia to the subretinal space prejudices survival of neonatal neuronal retina allografts (abstract). Invest Ophthalmol Vis Sci 2002;43:2291.
11 Ma N, Streilein JW: T cell immunity induced by allogeneic microglia in relation to neuronal retina transplantation. J Immunol 1999;162:4482–4489.
12 Gregerson DS, Yang J: CD45-positive cells of the retina and their responsiveness to in vivo and in vitro treatment with IFN-gamma or anti-CD40. Invest Ophthalmol Vis Sci 2003;44:3083–3093.
13 Hori J, Joyce N, Streilein JW: Epithelium-deficient corneal allografts display immune privilege beneath the kidney capsule. Invest Ophthalmol Vis Sci 2000;41:443–452.
14 Reece-Smith H, Du Toit DF, McShane P, Morris PJ: Prolonged survival of pancreatic islet allografts transplanted beneath the renal capsule. Transplantation 1981;31:305–306.
15 Bellgrau D, Gold D, Selawry H, Moore J, Franzusoff A, Duke RC: A role for CD95 ligand in preventing graft rejection. Nature 1995;377:630–632.
16 Takahashi M, Palmer TD, Takahashi J, Gage FH: Widespread integration and survival of adult-derived neural progenitor cells in the developing optic retina. Mol Cell Neurosci 1998;12: 340–348.
17 Young MJ, Ray SJO, Whiteley SJO, Klassen HJ, Gage FH: Integration of transplanted neural progenitor cells into the retina of immature and mature dystrophic rats. Mol Cell Neurosci 2000;16: 197–205.
18 Farrokh-Siar L, Rezai KA, Semnani RT, Patel SC, Ernest JT, Peterson EJ, Koretzky GA, van Seventer GA: Human fetal retinal pigment epithelial cells induce apoptosis in the T-cell line Jurkat. Invest Ophthalmol Vis Sci 1999;40:1503–1511.
19 Kaestel CG, Lovato P, Odum N, Nissen MH, Ropke C: The immune privilege of the eye: human retinal pigment epithelial cells selectively modulate T-cell activation in vitro. Curr Eye Res 2005;30:375–383.
20 Sun D, Enzmann V, Lei S, Sun SL, Kaplan HJ, Shao H: Retinal pigment epithelial cells activate uveitogenic T cells when they express high levels of MHC class II molecules, but inhibit T cell activation when they express restricted levels. J Neuroimmunol 2003;144:1–8.
21 Willermain F, Caspers-Velu L, Nowak B, Stordeur P, Mosselmans R, Salmon I, Velu T, Bruyns C: Retinal pigment epithelial cells phagocytosis of T lymphocytes: possible implication in the immune privilege of the eye. Br J Ophthalmol 2002;86:1417–1421.
22 Wenkel H, Streilein JW: Evidence that retinal pigment epithelium functions as an immune-privileged tissue. Invest Ophthalmol Vis Sci 2000;41:3467–3473.
23 Ng TF, Osawa H, Hori J, Young MJ, Streilein JW: Allogeneic neonatal neuronal retina grafts display partial immune privilege in the subcapsular space of the kidney. J Immunol 2002;169: 5601–5606.
24 Ma N, Streilein JW: Contribution of microglia as passenger leukocytes to the fate of intraocular neuronal retinal grafts. Invest Ophthalmol Vis Sci 1998;39:2384–2393.
25 Gage FH, Ray J, Fisher LJ: Isolation, characterization, and use of stem cells from the CNS. Annu Rev Neurosci 1995;18:159–192.
26 Yandava BD, Billinghurst LL, Snyder EY: 'Global' cell replacement is feasible via neural stem cell transplantation: evidence from the dysmyelinated *shiverer* mouse brain. Proc Natl Acad Sci USA 1999;96:7029–7034.

27 Huh GS, Boulanger LM, Du H, Riquelme PA, Brotz TM, Shatz CJ: Functional requirement for class I MHC in CNS development and plasticity. Science 2000;290:2155–2159.
28 Thomson JA, Itskovitz-Eldor J, Shapiro SS, Waknitz MA, Swiergiel JJ, Marshall VS, Jones JM: Embryonic stem cell lines derived from human blastocysts. Science 1998;282:1145–1147.
29 Shamblott MJ, Axelman J, Wang S, Bugg EM, Littlefield JW, Donovan PJ, Blumenthal PD, Huggins GR, Gearhart JD: Derivation of pluripotent stem cells from cultured human primordial germ cells. Proc Natl Acad Sci USA 1998;95:13726–13731.
30 Bjornson CR, Rietze RL, Reynolds BA, Magli MC, Vescovi AL: Turning brain into blood: a hematopoietic fate adopted by adult neural stem cells in vivo. Science 1999;283:534–537.
31 Clarke DL, Johansson CB, Wilbertz J, Veress B, Nilsson E, Karlstrom H, Lendahl U, Frisen J: Generalized potential of adult neural stem cells. Science 2000;288:1660–1663.
32 Lagasse E, Connors H, Al-Dhalimy M, Reitsma M, Dohse M, Osborne L, Wang X, Finegold M, Weissman IL, Grompe M: Purified hematopoietic stem cells can differentiate into hepatocytes in vivo. Nat Med 2000;6:1229–1234.
33 Madrazo I, Leon V, Torres C, Aguilera MC, Varela G, Alvarez F, Fraga A, Drucker-Colin R, Ostrosky F, Skurovich M, Franco R: Transplantation of fetal substantia nigra and adrenal medulla to the caudate nucleus in two patients with Parkinson's disease. N Engl J Med 1988;318:51.
34 Freed CR, Greene PE, Breeze RE, Tsai WY, DuMouchel W, Kao R, Dillon S, Winfield H, Culver S, Trojanowski JQ, Eidelberg D, Fahn S: Transplantation of embryonic dopamine neurons for severe Parkinson's disease. N Engl J Med 2001;344:710–719.
35 Hagell P, Schrag A, Piccini P, Jahanshahi M, Brown R, Rehncrona S, Widner H, Brundin P, Rothwell JC, Odin P, Wenning GK, Morrish P, Gustavii B, Bjorklund A, Brooks DJ, Marsden CD, Quinn NP, Lindvall O: Sequential bilateral transplantation in Parkinson's disease: effects of the second graft. Brain 1999;122:1121–1132.
36 Klassen H, Imfeld KL, Ray J, Young MJ, Gage FH, Berman MA: The immunological properties of adult hippocampal progenitor cells. Vision Res 2003;43:947–956.
37 Hori J, Ng TF, Shatos M, Klassen H, Streilein JW, Young MJ: Neural progenitor cells lack immunogenicity and resist destruction as allografts. Stem Cells 2003;21:405–416.
38 Klassen H, Schwartz MR, Bailey AH, Young MJ: Surface markers expressed by multipotent human and mouse neural progenitor cells include tetraspanins and non-protein epitopes. Neurosci Lett 2001;312:180–182.
39 Schwartz PH, Bryant PJ, Fuja TJ, Su H, O'Dowd DK, Klassen H: Isolation and characterization of neural progenitor cells from post-mortem human cortex. J Neurosci Res 2003;74:838–851.
40 Klassen H, Ziaeian B, Kirov II, Young MJ, Schwartz PH: Isolation of retinal progenitor cells from post-mortem human tissue and comparison with autologous brain progenitors. J Neurosci Res 2004;77:334–343.
41 Ahmad I, Dooley CM, Thoreson WB, Rogers JA, Afiat S: In vitro analysis of a mammalian retinal progenitor that gives rise to neurons and glia. Brain Res 1999;831:1–10.
42 Yang P, Seiler MJ, Aramant RB, Whittemore SR: Differential lineage restriction of rat retinal progenitor cells in vitro and in vivo. J Neurosci Res 2002;69:466–476.
43 Schwartz PH, Nethercott H, Kirov II, Ziaeian B, Young MJ, Klassen H: Expression of neurodevelopmental markers by cultured porcine neural precursor cells. Stem Cells 2005;23:1286–1294.

Dr. Michael J. Young
Schepens Eye Research Institute
Harvard Medical School, 20 Staniford Street
Boston, MA 02114 (USA)
Tel. +1 617 912 7419, Fax +1 617 912 0101, E-Mail mikey@vision.eri.harvard.edu

Niederkorn JY, Kaplan HJ (eds): Immune Response and the Eye.
Chem Immunol Allergy. Basel, Karger, 2007, vol 92, pp 317–327

Therapies Based on Principles of Ocular Immune Privilege

Jie Zhang-Hoover, Joan Stein-Streilein

Schepens Eye Research Institute, and Pulmonary and Critical Care Division, Department of Medicine, Brigham and Women's Hospital, Harvard Medical School, Boston, Mass., USA

Abstract

Anterior chamber (AC)-associated immune deviation (ACAID) is a form of ocular-derived peripheral tolerance that helps to maintain the immune privilege of the eye by suppressing both the priming and elicitation of adaptive immune responses. ACAID is known to facilitate the survival of corneal grafts and suppression autoimmune uveitis in the eye. Intravenous inoculation of in vitro generated ACAID tolerance-inducing antigen presenting cells (APCs) treated with transforming growth factor-β_2 (tolerogenic APCs) generates the kind of T regulatory cells found in in vivo ACAID when antigen is inoculated into the AC of the eye. Here, we review the application of peripheral tolerance induction by ACAID with either AC inoculation or in vitro generated tolerogenic ACAID-APCs in suppressing ongoing Th1- and Th2-mediated immune pathogenesis in naïve and presensitized hosts. Transfer of tolerogenic APCs has suppressed antigen-specific immune inflammation in animal models of experimental autoimmune encephalomyelitis, hapten immune pulmonary interstitial fibrosis, and ovalbumin-induced allergic pulmonary inflammation. The possibility of immune therapy by in vitro generated ACAID-like tolerogenic APCs in humans is discussed.

Studies in cellular and molecular mechanisms of ocular immune privilege help us to understand how the eye and immune system collaborate to preserve visual function while fighting off infections and insults. From 1974 to 1985, research done by Streilein and Kaplan, and later by Niederkorn showed that ocular immune privilege is, in part, maintained by an active suppression process that involves both the eye and the spleen [1–8]. This model of immune privilege and peripheral tolerance through the eye is known as anterior chamber

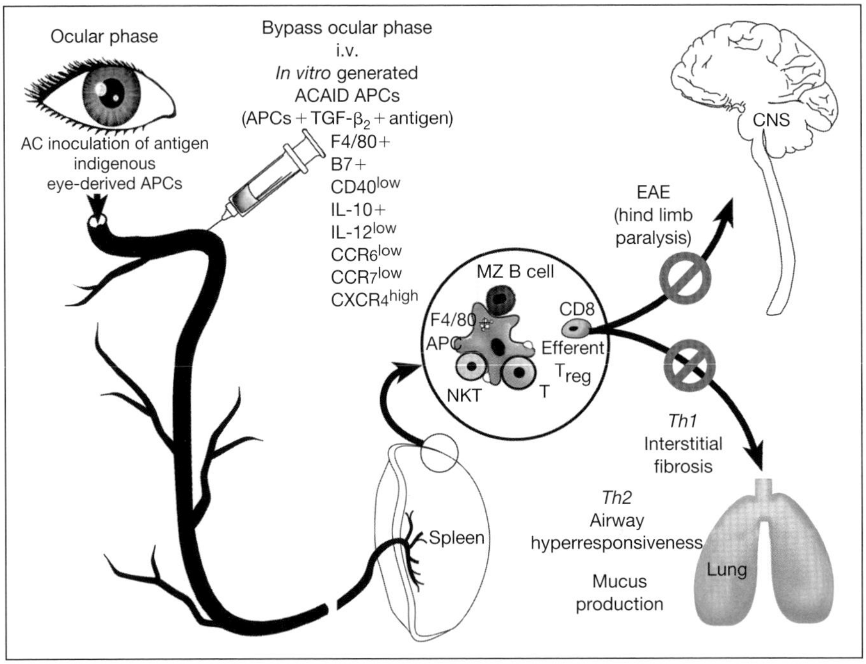

Fig. 1. Antigens introduced into the AC of the eye induce cellular and molecular processes that culminate in the development of T_{reg} cells that mitigate immune-mediated diseases in the eye, lung, and central nervous system (CNS). EAE = Experimental autoimmune encephalomyelitis.

(AC)-associated immune deviation (ACAID). ACAID prevents corneal graft rejection and autoimmune uveitis in the eye [9–16]. Indigenous eye-derived antigen presenting cells (APCs) that generate ACAID after intracameral inoculation of antigens can be reproduced in vitro by treating APCs with transforming growth factor (TGF)-β_2 and antigens [16–24]. Discoveries elucidating ACAID mechanisms generating peripheral tolerance and preventing inflammation in the eye allowed us to manipulate APCs in vitro to functionally mimic the eye-derived APCs. The fact that AC inoculation of antigens can be bypassed raised the possibility that induction of ACAID might be a cell-based therapy for regulating immune inflammation in general. In this review, we summarize the work that has been done recently to apply in vitro generated ACAID-like tolerogenic APCs as a therapy in various immune-mediated disease models outside of the eye (fig. 1).

F4/80+ Antigen-Presenting Cells: Messengers in the Camero-Splenic Axis during Anterior Chamber-Associated Immune Deviation

ACAID generates both CD4+ afferent and CD8+ efferent T regulatory (T_{reg}) cells in the spleen after AC inoculation of antigens [8, 25, 26]. The pathway that connects the eye and spleen and leads to the generation of T_{reg} cells in ACAID was dissected by Streilein and Niederkorn [8]. In the early 1990s, Wilbanks and Streilein [21–24, 27] identified eye-derived APCs as the link between the eye and the spleen during the generation of the T_{reg} cell and the induction of peripheral tolerance by ACAID. They showed that TGF-β_2 in aqueous humor transformed APCs (in this case, thioglycollate elicited peritoneal exudate cells, PECs) into tolerance-inducing APCs [21–24, 27]. Soon thereafter Niederkorn's group established ACAID in a dish (i.e. in vitro ACAID) and showed that TGF-β_2-treated antigen-pulsed PECs cultured with naïve spleen cells resulted in the development of the T_{reg} cell that could suppress delayed-type hypersensitivity in vivo [28].

Knowing that the eye-derived APCs interacted with cells in the spleen allowed our group to analyze the trafficking of F4/80+ APCs to the spleen. Faunce et al. [29] showed that F4/80+ APCs were located in the marginal zone (MZ) of the spleen during ACAID induction, and that they were physically in close contact with T cells and natural killer (NK) T cells. Others showed that ACAID F4/80+ APCs educated B cells and transformed them into APCs that induced tolerance through the Qa-1 molecule [28, 30–32]. Later Sonoda and Stein-Streilein [33] showed that it was MZ B cells and not follicular B cells that were required for ACAID induction. In summary, after AC inoculation of antigens specialized F4/80+ APCs from the iris and ciliary body take up antigens and migrate through the blood into the spleen MZ where they interact with cells, such as T cells, NKT cells, and MZ B cells, to induce tolerance. It is assumed that intravenous administration of in vitro generated ACAID-APCs induce the same cellular interactions to induce tolerance as does AC inoculation of antigens.

Mechanisms of Tolerance Induction by TGF-β_2-Treated, Antigen-Pulsed Antigen-Presenting Cells

APCs, particularly dendritic cells (DCs), are endowed with considerable plasticity in their ability to initiate an immune response. Maturation stage and external activation signals are some of the factors that determine the different functions of DCs [34, 35]. Plasmacytoid DCs and interleukin (IL)-10-producing DCs in the lung generate CD4+ T_{reg} cells and induce tolerance [36, 37]. Human monocyte-derived immature DCs that are grown in the presence of granulocyte-macrophage colony-stimulating factor and IL-4 induce the generation of antigen-specific IL-10-producing T cells when they are injected subcutaneously into human volunteers [38]. Tumor necrosis factor-α- or vitamin D_3 metabolite $1\alpha,25(OH)_2D_3$-treated in vitro monocyte-derived DCs induce the differentiation of IL-10-producing CD4+ T_{reg} cells [34, 39, 40]. In general, tolerogenic APCs have a semi-mature phenotype (MHC II^{high}, $B7^{high}$, $CD40^{low}$, $IL\text{-}12^{low}$, tumor necrosis factor-α^{low}, and $IL\text{-}6^{low}$), and functionally they are defined by their ability to suppress immune responses and induce the generation of T_{reg} cells [35].

ACAID-APCs have been generated in vitro with TGF-β_2 using PECs, macrophage hybridoma cells (No. 59) [21, 41, 42], and more recently, bone marrow (BM)-derived APCs [43]. In vitro generated ACAID-APCs are phenotypically similar to the so-called semi-mature DCs. ACAID-APCs have low or no expression of co-receptors like CD40 and IL-12 and an increased expression of IL-10 and TGF-β.

It is known that APCs treated with TGF-β_2 and antigen in vitro functionally mimic eye-derived APCs and generate CD4+ afferent and CD8+ efferent T_{reg} cells in both naïve and presensitized hosts. Transfer of in vitro generated ACAID-APCs suppresses both Th1- and Th2-mediated immunity [44, 45]. Little is known about the molecules and mechanisms used by ACAID CD8+ T_{reg} cells in efferent immune responses. Recent reports showed that Fas/Fas ligand [46] and CD103 pathways [47] may play a role in ACAID CD8+ T_{reg} suppression.

Therapeutic Application of Tolerance-Inducing Antigen-Presenting Cells in Disease Models

The effect of a variety of tolerogenic APCs has been tested in organ transplantation and autoimmune disease models. Intravenous injection of myeloid immature DCs generated in vitro with granulocyte-macrophage colony-stimulating factor prolonged the survival of pancreatic islet or heart allografts [35]. Splenic CD8+ DCs use both contact-dependent and -independent mechanisms to suppress Th2 responses and reverse Th2-mediated pathogenesis in a mouse model of asthma [48].

The feature of ACAID-APCs suppressing preexisting immune inflammation in an antigen-specific fashion is relatively unique and supports the idea that induction of ACAID tolerance by a cell-based therapy might be a successful approach for preexisting autoimmune and immune-inflammatory conditions. ACAID tolerance is known to be critical for the acceptance of a corneal graft and suppression of uveitis in experimental disease models in the eye [49, 50].

Studies using in vitro generated ACAID-APCs to reverse immune inflammation in the eye were first reported in 1992 when TGF-β_2-treated, interphotoreceptor retinol binding protein-pulsed PECs were intravenously transferred and blocked expression of experimental autoimmune uveitis in mice [16].

Experimental Autoimmune Encephalomyelitis

Since the induction of tolerance in the eye leads to both local and peripheral tolerance, it was reasoned that the transfer of ACAID-APCs might suppress ongoing inflammation in organs and tissues in addition to the eye. Faunce et al. [51] showed that ACAID-APCs generated tolerance that suppressed immune inflammation in myelin basic protein-induced experimental autoimmune encephalomyelitis. TGF-β_2-treated myelin basic protein-pulsed PECs inoculated 7 days after induction of the immune response delayed the onset of the symptoms and decreased both the severity and incidence of ongoing disease in mice [51]. Splenic T cells harvested from treated mice with experimental autoimmune encephalomyelitis, 30 days later, were able to transfer the suppression into another set of mice. The recipient mice were resistant to the development of experimental autoimmune encephalomyelitis by myelin basic protein plus adjuvant and the suppression was mediated by CD8+ T_{reg} cells that most likely suppressed the CD4+ T effector cells in the model. This study demonstrates that in vitro generated ACAID-APCs are able to generate T_{reg} cells during an ongoing robust Th1 inflammatory response and subsequently suppress the inflammation-mediated pathogenesis. Thus, ACAID-APCs are able to suppress immune responses in another example of an immune-privileged site, the central nervous system.

The Autoimmune Pulmonary Fibrosis Model

The ability of in vitro generated ACAID-APCs to induce antigen-specific tolerance suppressing immune-mediated pathogenesis in non-immune-privileged tissues was shown in an autoimmune pulmonary interstitial fibrosis model called adoptively transferred-hapten immune pulmonary interstitial fibrosis (ADT-HIPIF) [43]. The ADT-HIPIF model shares the characteristics of idiopathic pulmonary interstitial fibrosis, a devastating and recurring condition in humans that occurs in about 17/100,000 individuals yearly with unknown etiology and no effective treatment. Mice that received hapten 2,4,6-trinitrobenzene sulfonic acid-sensitized cells and challenged intratracheally in the lung with the immunizing hapten developed pulmonary interstitial fibrosis. However, intravenous transfer of TGF-β_2-treated 2,4,6-trinitrobenzene sulfonic acid-pulsed APCs to experimental mice even 1 day after pulmonary challenge reduced the collagen deposition and subsequent scarring in the interstitium of the lung. As in ACAID, ADT-HIPIF mice treated with tolerogenic APCs developed antigen-specific CD8+ T_{reg} cells that suppressed the efferent response by regulating the presensitized T effector cells.

There are several interesting points worth mentioning in this study. This is the first report to show that APCs derived from mouse BM cultures acquired ACAID-tolerogenic characteristics. The BM-derived ACAID-APCs were generated from mouse BM cells using L929 cell-conditioned medium in a dish in vitro and have a phenotype of F4/80+, CD11b+, CD11c^{dim}, CD40+, B7^{+} [43]. After TGF-β_2 treatment, BM-APCs reduced CD40 but maintained their surface expression of F4/80 and B7 [43]. In addition, gene analyses (gene array and RT-PCR) after TGF-β_2 treatment showed that chemokine receptor expression on BM-derived ACAID-APCs is modulated from CCR6^{high} CCR7^{low} CXCR4^{low} to CCR6^{low} CCR7^{low} CXCR4^{high} [45]. The expression pattern of chemokine receptors CCR6, CCR7, and CXCR4 on ACAID-APCs supports their unusual migration in the spleen [29]. Following AC inoculation, F4/80+ APCs that transport antigen to the spleen do not migrate to the T cell area (white pulp) of the spleen like inflammatory APCs (CCR6^{low} CCR7^{high}) would do in response to a chemokine (CCL19 and CCL21) gradient in the T cell area of secondary lymphoid organs. Instead they accumulate in the MZ of the spleen where they settle in close contact with T cells, MZ B cells, and NKT cells to generate T_{reg} cells [29]. Second, T_{reg} cells existed in both the spleen and the lung draining lymph nodes of experimental mice after ACAID-APC treatment [43]. However, it was not clear whether T_{reg} cells were generated by ACAID-APCs in the lung draining lymph nodes or they migrated to the lymph nodes from the spleen. Third, ADT-HIPIF shares etiological and pathological characteristics with a variety of human immune-inflammatory conditions of the lung that eventuate into interstitial fibrosis; these studies provide insight into potential therapies to alter the course of pulmonary fibrosis in humans.

The Th2-Mediated Asthma Model

Earlier in the study of ACAID, it was reasoned that mechanisms that mediated suppression of a Th1 response might in fact include a deviation toward a Th2 response. More recently, it has been clearly shown that at least the development of the CD8+ efferent T_{reg} cell is not dependent on a Th2 response [52]. Thus the question arose as to whether the efferent CD8+ T_{reg} cell might suppress Th2 responses, as well as Th1.

Historically, ACAID-APCs are shown to induce suppression of Th1-mediated immune responses. A recent publication by Katagiri et al. [44] showed that preemptive induction of ACAID could inhibit Th2 responses using a mouse model of ovalbumin (OVA)-induced, Th2-dependent pulmonary inflammation. Injecting OVA alone into the AC or injecting OVA-pulsed, TGF-β_2-treated PECs intravenously before sensitization blocked every aspect of Th2 inflammation that included OVA-specific IgE production, Th2 cytokine (IL-4, IL-5, and IL-13) production, and eosinophil and lymphocyte pulmonary infiltration.

Further study showed that ACAID-APCs given to Th2-presensitized mice suppressed most aspects of the Th2 response (i.e. reduced pulmonary inflammatory cell infiltration and Th2 cytokine production) as well as subsequent pathogenesis (i.e. airway hyperresponsiveness and mucus production) [45]. Furthermore, suppression of the presensitized Th2 response is also mediated by CD8+ T_{reg} cells in ACAID. However, there was no suppression of OVA-specific IgE in presensitized mice by ACAID-APC. Since IgE is produced by existing long-lived plasma cells in presensitized mice, the suppression of IgE may be a late phenomenon, one that occurs after the immune traits are recessed. The treatment with ACAID-APCs in both naïve and pre-sensitized mice did not alter interferon-γ production. Thus, ACAID-APC induced tolerance and not merely an induction of a Th1 response capable of suppressing Th2-mediated pathogenesis in a mouse model of human allergic asthma.

Early explanations of ACAID mechanisms suggested that Th1 responses were being modulated by generating a Th2 response. However, several pieces of evidence support ACAID not being a Th2 response. Kosiewicz and Streilein [53] reported that no Th2 cytokine-producing cells were found in spleen and lymph nodes of mice that only received intracameral inoculation of antigens. Instead, the splenic cells of these mice secreted only TGF-β when stimulated with OVA in vitro. Furthermore, mice deficient in IL-4/IL-13 and STAT6 genes that are critical for Th2 development readily acquired ACAID suppression after intracameral inoculation of antigens [52]. Finally, the ability of ACAID and ACAID-tolerogenic APCs to suppress Th2-mediated pathogenesis adds the additional evidence to put the notion that ACAID is similar to a Th2 response to rest.

Conclusions, Future Perspectives, and Possibilities in Humans

With the better understanding of cellular and molecular mechanisms of the phenomenon of the eye's ability to regulate immune responses, ACAID tolerance-inducing APCs were used to treat multiple immune-mediated disease models in various organs in mice. Several different kinds of APCs (PECs, macrophage hybridoma, and BM-grown APCs) were shown to induce ACAID tolerance after TGF-β_2 pretreatment. The success in modifying in vitro grown APCs (BM-derived APCs) to ACAID-inducing APCs in mice makes it possible to test whether human peripheral blood- or BM-derived APCs can be transformed into human ACAID-like tolerance-inducing APCs.

ACAID exists in rodents, rabbits, primates, and possibly in humans [54, 55]. It needs to be tested whether TGF-β_2 and antigen treatment modulates human APCs toward a tolerance-inducing phenotype. Once it is shown that human APCs are responsive to TGF-β treatment, it can be tested whether human TGF-β_2-treated, antigen-pulsed APCs are capable of suppressing inflammation in vitro using human peripheral blood mononuclear cells or inflammation-mediated pathogenesis in vivo using (human-SCID mouse) chimera disease models. The SCID mice are like test tubes that hold human immune cells because they lack T and B cells and cannot reject foreign tissues. In cases where disease pathogenesis is mediated by factors from human immune inflammatory cells, it may be possible to test the ACAID cell-based therapy. Furthermore, in the clinical setting, peripheral blood APCs from patients could be a source to be treated with TGF-β_2 and antigens (e.g. allergens and alloantigens) in vitro. After treatment, the modulated APCs may be monitored for tolerogenic characteristics and then administered intravenously back into the same patient.

Using ACAID-APCs in the treatment of immune-mediated pathogenesis in humans may become the therapy of choice since it is an adaptation of a natural immune-regulatory mechanism found in immune-privileged sites, a place where the regulation allows for protection but prevents damaging inflammation [54]. The unique features of tolerance mediated by ACAID and results from using in vitro generated ACAID-inducing APCs in disease models in mice raise the possibility that tolerance by ACAID-inducing APCs may be used to prevent and reduce immune-inflammatory disease with specificity, effectiveness and minimal side effects in a variety of tissues and organs in humans.

References

1 Kaplan HJ, Streilein JW: Do immunologically privileged sites require a functioning spleen? Nature 1974;251:553–554.

2 Kaplan HJ, Streilein JW, Stevens TR: Transplantation immunology of the anterior chamber of the eye. II. Immune response to allogeneic cells. J Immunol 1975;118:809–814.

3 Kaplan HJ, Streilein JW: Immune response to immunization via the anterior chamber of the eye. I. F1-lymphocyte-induced immune deviation. J Immunol 1977;118:809–814.

4 Kaplan HJ, Streilein JW: Immune response to immunization via the anterior chamber of the eye. II. An analysis of F1 lymphocyte-induced immune deviation. J Immunol 1978;120:689–693.

5 Niederkorn J, Streilein JW, Shadduck JA: Deviant immune responses to allogeneic tumors injected intracamerally and subcutaneously in mice. Invest Ophthalmol Vis Sci 1980;20:355–363.
6 Streilein JW, Niederkorn JY: Induction of anterior chamber-associated immune deviation requires an intact, functional spleen. J Exp Med 1981;153:1058–1067.
7 Niederkorn JY, Streilein JW: Alloantigens placed into the anterior chamber of the eye induce specific suppression of delayed type hypersensitivity but normal cytotoxic T lymphocyte responses. J Immunol 1983;131:2670–2674.
8 Streilein JW, Niederkorn JY: Characterization of the suppressor cell(s) responsible for anterior chamber-associated immune deviation (ACAID) induced in BALB/c mice by P815 cells. J Immunol 1985;134:1381–1387.
9 Niederkorn JY, Mellon J: Anterior chamber-associated immune deviation promotes corneal allograft survival. Invest Ophthalmol Vis Sci 1996;37:2700–2707.
10 Sonoda A, Sonoda Y, Muramatu R, Streilein JW, Usui M: ACAID induced by allogeneic corneal tissue promotes subsequent survival of orthotopic corneal grafts. Invest Ophthalmol Vis Sci 2000;41:790–798.
11 Sonoda Y, Streilein JW: Impaired cell-mediated immunity in mice bearing healthy orthotopic corneal allografts. Immunology 1993;150:1727–1734.
12 Sonoda Y, Sano Y, Ksander B, Streilein JW: Characterization of cell-mediated immune responses elicited by orthotopic corneal allografts in mice. Invest Ophthalmol Vis Sci 1995;36:427–434.
13 Streilein JW: Immunobiology and immunopathology of corneal transplantation; in Streilein JW (ed): Immune Response and the Eye. Chem Immunol. Basel, Karger, 1999, vol 73, pp 186–206.
14 Hara Y, Caspi RR, Wiggert B, Chan CC, Wilbanks GA, Streilein JW: Suppression of experimental autoimmune uveitis in mice by induction of anterior chamber-associated immune deviation with interphotoreceptor retinoid-binding protein. J Immunol 1992;148:1685–1692.
15 Mizuno K, Altman NF, Clark AF, Streilein JW: Histopathologic analysis of experimental autoimmune uveitis attenuated by intracameral injection of S-antigen. Curr Eye Res 1989;8:113–121.
16 Hara Y, Caspi RR, Wiggert B, Dorf M, Streilein JW: Analysis of an in vitro-generated signal that induces systemic immune deviation similar to that elicited by antigen injected into the anterior chamber of the eye. J Immunol 1992;149:1531–1538.
17 Cousins SW, McCabe MM, Danielpour D, Streilein JW: Identification of transforming growth factor-beta as an immunosuppressive factor in aqueous humor. Invest Ophthalmol Vis Sci 1991;32:2201–2211.
18 Hara Y, Okamoto S, Rouse B, Streilein JW: Evidence that peritoneal exudate cells cultured with eye-derived fluids are the proximate antigen-presenting cells in immune deviation of the ocular type. J Immunol 1993;151:5162–5171.
19 Kezuka T, Streilein JW: In vitro generation of regulatory $CD8^+$ T cells similar to those found in mice with anterior chamber associated immune deviation. Invest Ophthalmol Vis Sci 2000;41: 1803–1811.
20 Kezuka T, Streilein JW: Analysis of in vivo regulatory properties of T cells activated in vitro by TGFβ2-treated antigen presenting cells. Invest Ophthalmol Vis Sci 2000;41:1410–1421.
21 Wilbanks GA, Mammolenti M, Streilein JW: Studies on the induction of anterior chamber-associated immune deviation (ACAID). III. Induction of ACAID depends upon intraocular transforming growth factor-beta. Eur J Immunol 1992;22:165–173.
22 Wilbanks GA, Mammolenti M, Streilein JW: Studies on the induction of anterior chamber-associated immune deviation (ACAID). II. Eye-derived cells participate in generating blood-borne signals that induce ACAID. J Immunol 1991;146:3018–3024.
23 Wilbanks GA, Streilein JW: Studies on the induction of anterior chamber-associated immune deviation (ACAID). I. Evidence that an antigen-specific, ACAID-inducing, cell-associated signal exists in the peripheral blood. J Immunol 1991;146:2610–2617.
24 Wilbanks GA, Streilein JW: Fluids from immune privileged sites endow macrophages with the capacity to induce antigen-specific immune deviation via a mechanism involving transforming growth factor-beta. Eur J Immunol 1992;22:1031–1036.
25 Wilbanks GA, Streilein JW: Characterization of suppressor cells in anterior chamber-associated immune deviation (ACAID) induced by soluble antigen. Evidence of two functionally and phenotypically distinct T-suppressor cell populations. Immunology 1990;71:383–389.

26 Kosiewicz MM, Okamoto S, Miki S, Ksander BR, Shimizu T, Streilein JW: Imposing deviant immunity on the presensitized state. J Immunol 1994;153:2962–2973.
27 Wilbanks GA, Streilein JW: Macrophages capable of inducing anterior chamber associated immune deviation demonstrate spleen-seeking migratory properties. Reg Immunol 1992;4: 130–137.
28 Niederkorn JY, Mayhew E: Role of splenic B cells in the immune privilege of the anterior chamber of the eye. Eur J Immunol 1995;25:2783–2787.
29 Faunce DE, Sonoda KH, Stein-Streilein J: MIP-2 recruits NKT cells to the spleen during tolerance induction. J Immunol 2001;166:313–321.
30 D'Orazio TJ, Niederkorn JY: Splenic B cells are required for tolerogenic antigen presentation in the induction of anterior chamber-associated immune deviation (ACAID). Immunology 1998;95:47–55.
31 Skelsey ME, Mayhew E, Niederkorn JY: Splenic B cells act as antigen presenting cells for the induction of anterior chamber-associated immune deviation. Invest Ophthalmol Vis Sci 2003;44: 5242–5251.
32 D'Orazio TJ, Mayhew E, Niederkorn JY: Ocular immune privilege promoted by the presentation of peptide on tolerogenic B cells in the spleen. II. Evidence for presentation by Qa-1. J Immunol 2001;166:26–32.
33 Sonoda KH, Stein-Streilein J: CD1d on antigen-transporting APC and splenic marginal zone B cells promotes NKT cell-dependent tolerance. Eur J Immunol 2002;32:848–857.
34 Lutz MB, Schuler G: Immature, semi-mature and fully mature dendritic cells: which signals induce tolerance or immunity? Trends Immunol 2002;23:445–449.
35 Rutella S, Lemoli RM: Regulatory T cells and tolerogenic dendritic cells: from basic biology to clinical applications. Immunol Lett 2004;94:11–26.
36 Bilsborough J, George TC, Norment A, Viney JL: Mucosal CD8α+ DC, with a plasmacytoid phenotype, induce differentiation and support function of T cells with regulatory properties. Immunology 2003;108:481–492.
37 Akbari O, DeKruyff R, Umetsu D: Pulmonary dendritic cells producing IL-10 mediate tolerance induced by respiratory exposure to antigen. Nat Immunol 2001;2:725–731.
38 Dhodapkar M, Steinman R, Krasovsky J, Munz C, Bhardwaj N: Antigen-specific inhibition of effector T cell function in humans after injection of immature dendritic cells. J Exp Med 2001;193:233–238.
39 Groux H, Fournier N, Cottrez F: Role of dendritic cells in the generation of regulatory T cells. Semin Immunol 2004;16:99–106.
40 Adorini L, Giarratana N, Penna G: Pharmacological induction of tolerogenic dendritic cells and regulatory T cells. Semin Immunol 2004;16:127–134.
41 Kuchroo VK, Minami M, Diamond B, Dorf ME: Functional analysis of cloned macrophage hybridomas. VI. Differential ability to induce immunity or suppression. J Immunol 1988;141: 10–16.
42 Masli S, Turpie B, Hecker KH, Streilein JW: Expression of thrombospondin in TGFß-treated APCs and its relevance to their immune deviation-promoting properties. J Immunol 2002;168: 2264–2273.
43 Zhang-Hoover J, Stein-Streilein J: Tolerogenic APC generate CD8+ T regulatory cells that modulate pulmonary interstitial fibrosis. J Immunol 2004;172:178–185.
44 Katagiri K, Zhang-Hoover J, Mo JS, Stein-Streilein J, Streilein JW: Using tolerance induced via the anterior chamber of the eye to inhibit Th2-dependent pulmonary pathology. J Immunol 2002;169:84–89.
45 Zhang-Hoover J, Finn P, Stein-Streilein J: Modulation of ovalbumin-induced airway inflammation and hyperactivity by tolerogenic APC. J Immunol 2005;175:7117–7124.
46 Kosiewicz MM, Alard P, Liang S, Clark SL: Mechanisms of tolerance induced by transforming growth factor-beta-treated antigen-presenting cells: CD8 regulatory T cells inhibit the effector phase of the immune response in primed mice through a mechanism involving Fas ligand. Int Immunol 2004;16:697–706.
47 Keino H, Masli S, Sasaki S, Streilen JW, Stein-Streilein J: CD8+ T regulatory cells use a novel genetic program that includes CD103 to suppress Th1 immunity in eye-derived tolerance. Invest Ophthalmol Vis Sci 2006;47:1533–1542.

48 Gordon JR, Li F, Nayyar A, Xiang J, Zhang X: CD8α+, but not CD8α−, dendritic cells tolerize Th2 responses via contact-dependent and -independent mechanisms, and reverse airway hyperresponsiveness, Th2, and eosinophil responses in a mouse model of asthma. J Immunol 2005;175:1516–1522.
49 Okamoto S, Kosiewicz MM, Caspi RR, Streilein JW: ACAID as a potential therapy for established experimental autoimmune uveitis; in Nussenblatt RB, Whitcup SM, Caspi RR, Gery I (eds): Advances in Ocular Immunology Amsterdam, Elsevier, 1994, pp 195–198.
50 Streilein JW: Ocular immune privilege: the eye takes a dim but practical view of immunity and inflammation. J Leukoc Biol 2003;74:179–185.
51 Faunce DE, Terajewicz A, Stein-Streilein J: Cutting edge: in vitro-generated tolerogenic APC induce CD8+ T regulatory cells that can suppress ongoing experimental autoimmune encephalomyelitis. J Immunol 2004;172:1991–1995.
52 Nakamura T, Terajewicz A, Stein-Streilein J: Mechanisms of peripheral tolerance following intracameral inoculation are independent of IL-13 or STAT6. J Immunol 2005;175:2643–2646.
53 Kosiewicz MM, Streilein JW: Is deviant immunity induced by intraocular injection of antigen dependent on Th2 cells? Invest Ophthalmol Vis Sci 1996;37:S1136.
54 Streilein JW: Ocular immune privilege: therapeutic opportunities from an experiment of nature. Nat Rev Immunol 2003;3:878–889.
55 Kezuka T, Sakai JI, Usui N, Streilein JW, Usui M: Evidence for antigen-specific immune deviation in patients with acute retinal necrosis. Arch Ophthalmol 2001;119:1044–1049.

Dr. Jie Zhang-Hoover
Schepens Eye Research Institute
20 Staniford Street
Boston, MA 02114 (USA)
Tel. +1 617 912 7493, Fax +1 617 912 0105, E-Mail jzhoover@vision.eri.harvard.edu

Author Index

Subject Index